Dementia Care

Dementia Care
International Perspectives

Edited by

Alistair Burns
Professor of Old Age Psychiatry
University of Manchester, UK

Philippe Robert
Professor of Psychiatry
University Côte d'Azur, France

In collaboration with the International Dementia
Alliance (IDEAL)
Norman Sartorius, Switzerland (Chair)
Alistair Burns, UK
Antonio Lobo, Spain
Marcel Olde Rikkert, The Netherlands
Philippe Robert, France
Maya Semrau, UK (Secretary)
Gabriela Stoppe, Switzerland

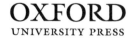

OXFORD
UNIVERSITY PRESS

OXFORD
UNIVERSITY PRESS

Great Clarendon Street, Oxford, OX2 6DP,
United Kingdom

Oxford University Press is a department of the University of Oxford.
It furthers the University's objective of excellence in research, scholarship,
and education by publishing worldwide. Oxford is a registered trade mark of
Oxford University Press in the UK and in certain other countries

© Oxford University Press 2019

The moral rights of the authors have been asserted

First Edition Published in 2019

Impression: 1

Published in the United States of America by Oxford University Press
198 Madison Avenue, New York, NY 10016, United States of America

British Library Cataloguing in Publication Data

Data available

Library of Congress Control Number: 2018966724

ISBN 978-0-19-879604-6

Printed and bound by
CPI Group (UK) Ltd, Croydon, CR0 4YY

Acknowledgements

We are most grateful to all the contributors for their time and excellent work, to Gillian Burns for administrative assistance, and to our publishers Peter Stevenson and Rachel Goldsworthy for their support.

Contents

Section 5 **North America**

Section 6 **South America**

Abbreviations

AB	amyloid beta protein	**BPSSD**	behavioural and psychological signs and symptoms of dementia
ABRAz	Brazilian Alzheimer's Association		
ACL	Administration for Community Living	**CAA**	Croatian Alzheimer Alliance
		CAS	Centre for Ageing Studies
Actifcare	ACcess to TImely Formal Care	**CCNA**	Canadian Consortium on Neurodegeneration in Aging
AD	Alzheimer's disease		
ADC	Alzheimer's Disease Chinese	**CDCD**	Centres for Cognitive Diseases and Dementia (*Centri per Disturbi Cognitivi e Demenze*)
ADI	Alzheimer's Disease International		
ADOK	Alzheimers and Dementia Organization Kenya		
		CDR	Clinical Dementia Rating
ADWG	Alzheimer's Disease Working Group	**CGA**	Comprehensive Geriatric Assessment
AE	Alzheimer Europe	**CHF**	Swiss franc
AHI	Allied Health Intervention	**CI**	confidence interval
AHP	allied health professionals	**CIEn**	*Centro Interdisciplinario de Envejecimiento*
AiBL	Australian Imaging Biomarkers and Lifestyle Study	**CIHI**	Croatian Institute for Health Insurance
AIC	Agency for Integrated Care		
AIDS	acquired immune deficiency syndrome	**CIHR**	Canadian Institutes for Health Research
		CIND	Cognitively Impaired Not Demented
AMHF	Africa Mental Health Foundation		
		CMES	Continuous Medical Education Sessions
AoA	Administration of Aging		
ARDSI	Alzheimer's and Related Disorders Society of India	**COPRAD**	*Corporación Profesional de Alzheimer y otras demencias*
ASHA	Accredited Social Health Activist	**C5R**	Consortium of Canadian Centers for Clinical Cognitive Research
AUDAS	*Asociación Uruguaya de Alzheimer y Similares*		
AUGE	*Acceso Universal con Garantías Explícitas*	**CREA**	State Reference Centre for the Care of Persons with Alzheimer's Disease and other Dementias
AWBZ	*Algemene Wet Bijzondere Ziektekosten*		
		CSF	cerebrospinal fluid
BDNF	brain-derived neurotrophic factor	**CT**	computerized tomography
		CZK	Czech koruna
BMI	body mass index	**DALY**	disability-adjusted life year
BPSD	behavioural and psychological symptoms of dementia	**DANE**	*Departamento Administrativo Nacional de Estadística*

DBMAS	Dementia Behaviour Management Advisory Service	**GP**	general practitioner
DFA	Dementia-Friendly America	**G-RACE**	Geriatric Psychiatry Out-Reach Assessment, Consultation and Enablement
DHB	district health board		
DNDI	Dementia and Neurodegeneration Ireland	**HABIT**	Healthy Actions to Benefit Independence and Thinking
DSIDC	Dementia Services Information and Development Centre	**HCP**	home care package
		HIQA	Health Information and Quality Authority
DSM-5	Diagnostic and Statistical Manual of Mental Disorders, fifth edition	**HIS**	Healthcare Improvement Scotland
		HR	hazard ratio
ECAQ	Elderly Cognitive Assessment Questionnaire	**HRB**	Health Research Board
		HRQol	health-related quality of life
ECHO	Extension for Community Healthcare Outcomes	**HRSA**	Health Resources Services Administration
EEG	electroencephalography		
ELSI	Ethical, Legal, and Social Impact (committee)	**HSC**	Health and Social Care
		HSE	Health Service Executive
EMPAM	*Examen Anual de Medicina Preventiva del Adulto Mayor*	**HVLTm**	modified Hopkins verbal learning test
EQ-5D	European Quality of Life-5 Dimension	**IAGMH**	Indian Association for Geriatric Mental Health
ERP	event-related potentials	**ICCS**	Integrated Community Care System
ERPI	residential structures for the elderly		
EU	European Union	**ICD-10**	International Classification of Diseases, tenth revision
EWT	Edhi Welfare Trust		
FAQ	Functional Activities Questionnaire	**ICMR**	Indian Council for Medical Research
FDG-PET	18-fluoro-deoxyglucose positron emission tomography	**ICT**	Information and Communication Technologies
FRSSD	Functional Rating Scale for Symptoms of Dementia	**IGA**	Integrated Geriatric Assessment
FUCAS	Functional Cognitive Assessment Scale	**I-IDRP**	Indianapolis-Ibadan Dementia Research Project
GAADRD	Greek Association of Alzheimer's Disease and Related Disorders	**ILO**	International Labour Organization
GCC	Grand Challenges Canada	**IMSS**	*Instituto Mexicano del Seguro Social*
GDP	gross domestic product		
GDS	Geriatric Depression Scale	**INEI**	National Institute of Statistics and Informatics
GHC	G-RACE Home Clinic	**INMAYORES**	*Instituto Nacional de las Personas Mayores*
GMS	Geriatric Mental State		

ISA	Ibadan Study of Aging	NAPA	National Alzheimer's Project Act
ISSSTE	*Instituto de Seguridad y Servicios Sociales de los Trabajadores del Estado*	NAPAD	National Action Plan on Alzheimer's Disease
JPND	Joint Programme–Neurodegenerative Disease Research	NCD	non-communicable disease
		NDSP	National Dementia Support Program
KMTC	Kenya Medical Training Institute College	NES	NHS Education for Scotland
KPA	Kenya Psychiatric Association	NGO	non-governmental organization
LEA	essential levels of care (*livelli essenziali di assistenza*)	NHIF	National Health Insurance Fund
		NHMRC	National Health and Medical Research Council
LMIC	low- and middle-income country	NHS	National Health Service
LTCI	Long-Term Care Insurance	NHSS	Nursing Homes Support Scheme
MBDC	Mindfulness-Based Dementia Care	NI	Northern Ireland
MBS	Medicare Benefits Schedule	NICE	National Institute for Health and Care Excellence
MCI	mild cognitive impairment	NIMHANS	National Institute of Mental Health and Neuro-Sciences
MD	medical doctor	NMDA	N-methyl-D-aspartate
mhGAP	Mental Health Gap Action Programme	NSDE	National Survey of Dependency in the Elderly
mhGAP-IG	WHO Mental Health Global Action Programme Intervention Guide	NSH	National Survey of Health
		NSSF	National Social Security Fund
MHLW	Ministry of Health, Labour, and Welfare	NUHS	National University Health System
MIDES	*Ministerio de Desarrolo Social*	NYUCI	New York University Caregiver Intervention (programme)
MMSE	Mini-Mental State Examination	NZ	New Zealand
MoCA	Montreal Cognitive Assessment	NZDC	New Zealand Dementia Cooperative
MOH	Ministry of Health	OECD	Organization for Economic Cooperation and Development
MOU	Memorandum of Understanding		
MRI	magnetic resonance imaging	OPAH	Older People in Acute Hospital
MSP	*Ministerio de Salud Pública*	PADL	personal activities of daily living
MWC	Mental Welfare Commission		
NADRC	National Alzheimer's and Dementia Resource Center	PADOMI	Home Care Programme (Peru)

PBS	Pharmaceutical Benefits Scheme	**SENAMA**	*Servicio Nacional del Adulto Mayor*
PCC	primary care centre	**SES**	socio-economic status
PET	positron emission tomography	**SNIC**	*Sistema Nacional Integrado de Cuidados*
PFADRD	Panhellenic Federation of Alzheimer's Disease and Related Disorders	**SNIS**	*Sistema Nacional Integrado de Salud*
PFAQ	Pfeffer Functional Activities Questionnaire	**SONEPSYN**	Chilean Society of Neurology, Psychiatry and Neurosurgery
PiB PET	Pittsburgh compound B positron emission tomography	**SPECT**	single-photon emission computerized tomography
P-Tau	phosphorylated Tau	**SSSC**	Scottish Social Services Council
QESDC	Quality and Excellence in Specialist Dementia Care	**SUS**	*Sistema Único de Saúde* (National Health System)
QoL	quality of life	**SveDem**	Swedish Dementia Registry
RCT	randomized controlled trial	**TAP**	Tailored Activity Program
RNCCI	National Network for Integrated Long-Term Care (*Rede Nacional de Cuidados Continuados Integrados*)	**TOP**	Teachers of Psychiatry
		T-Tau	total Tau
		UAE	United Arab Emirates
		UK	United Kingdom
ROI	Republic of Ireland	**UMI**	upper middle income
rTMS	repetitive transcranial magnetic stimulation	**UVA**	Alzheimer's Evaluation Units (*Unità di Valutazione per l'Alzheimer*)
SCIE	Social Care Institute for Excellence	**UVD**	Evaluation Units of Dementia
SCU	specific care unit		
SD	standard deviation	**WHO**	World Health Organization
SEK	Swedish krona		

Contributors

Amir IA Ahmed, Consultant Geriatrician and Clinical Pharmacologist, Department of Geriatric Medicine, Alzheimer's Center and the Department of Pharmacology and Toxicology, Radboud University Medical Center, The Netherlands

Abdullah Al Ali, Consultant Geriatric Medicine, Program Director of the Internal Medicine Residency Program, Zayed Military Hospital, United Arab Emirates

Salwa Alsuwaidi, Consultant Internal Medicine and Geriatrics, Dubai Health Authority, United Arab Emirates

Olatunde Olayinka Ayinde, World Health Organization Collaborating Centre for Research and Training in Mental Health, Neurosciences and Drug and Alcohol Abuse, Department of Psychiatry, College of Medicine, University of Ibadan, Nigeria

Conor Barton, Consultant Old Age Psychiatrist, Belfast Health and Social Care Trust, UK

Bastaman Basuki, Department of Community Medicine, University of Indonesia, Indonesia

Waldo Cárdenas Berrocal, Home care, Social Security Portal of Peru (ESSALUD), Peru

Jacqueline Arabia Buraye, Director of the Cali Alzheimer Foundation, Colombia

Alistair Burns, Professor of Old Age Psychiatry, University of Manchester, UK

Paulo R Canineu, Laboratory of Neuroscience, Department and Institute of Psychiatry, Faculty of Medicine, University of São Paulo, Brazil

Víctor Carcelén, Gerontology and Geriatrics Society of Peru, Scientific University of the South, Peru

Jane Casey, Mental Health Services for Older People, Auckland City Hospital, New Zealand

Santosh K Chaturvedi, Senior Professor, Department of Psychiatry, National Institute of Mental Health and Neurosciences, India

Gary Cheung, Department of Psychological Medicine, University of Auckland, New Zealand

Emma Louise Cunningham, Centre for Public Health, Queen's University, UK

Renaud David, Department of Gerontology, Memory Clinic, Nice University Hospital, France

Saïda Douki Dedieu, Emeritus Professor of Psychiatry, Medicine School of Tunis, Tunisia

Slavica Djukic-Dejanovic, Clinic for Mental Disorders 'Dr Laza Lazarevic', Serbia

Gorica Djokic, Clinic for Mental Disorders 'Dr Laza Lazarevic', Serbia

Catherine Dolan, Department of Psychiatry of Later Life, Sligo Leitrim Mental Health Service, Ireland

Hayriye Elbi, Division of Consultation Liaison Psychiatry, Department of Psychiatry, Ege University School of Medicine Hospital, Turkey

Knut Engedal, Department of Geriatrics, Oslo University Hospital and Norwegian Advisory Unit for Aging and Health, Vestfold County Hospital, Norway

Robert Pérez Fernández, Institute of Social Psychology, Faculty of Psychology, CIEN Interdisciplinary Center for Aging, University of the Republic, Uruguay

Rodolfo Ferrando, Nuclear Medicine and Molecular Imaging Center, Clinics Hospital, Faculty of Medicine, University of the Republic, Uruguay

Orestes V Forlenza, Department of Psychiatry, Faculty of Medicine, University of Sao Paulo Institute of Psychiatry, Hospital das Clinicas HCFMUSP, Brazil

Manuel A Franco-Martin, Head of Psychiatric Department, University Rio Hortega Hospital, Zamora Hospital, Spain

Jean Gajardo, Faculty of Health Sciences, Central University of Chile, Chile

Sundarnag Ganjekar, Associate Professor of Psychiatry, Department of Psychiatry, National Institute of Mental Health and Neurosciences, India

Serge Gauthier, Director, Alzheimer's Disease and Related Disorders Research Unit, McGill Center for Studies in Aging, Canada

Manuel Gonçalves-Pereira, CEDOC, Chronic Diseases Research Centre, Nova Medical School/Faculdade de Ciências Médicas, Universidade Nova de Lisboa, Portugal

Changsu Han, Korea University College of Medicine, South Korea

Iva Holmerová, Centre of Expertise in Longevity and Long-Term Care, Faculty of Humanities Charles University, Czech Republic

Akira Homma, Otafuku Clinic, Japan

Geanina Ilinoiu, Tees, Esk and Wear Valley NHS Foundation Trust, UK; University of Medicine and Pharmacy Tg Mures, Department M4 Psychiatry, Romania

Muhammad Iqbal Afridi, Dean, Jinnah Postgraduate Medical Centre and Chairman, Faculty of Psychiatry, Jinnah Sindh Medical University, Pakistan

Raden Irawati Ismail, Professor of Psychiatry, Faculty of Medicine Universitas Indonesia, Cipto Mangunkusumo General Hospital, Indonesia

Graham A Jackson, Alzheimer Scotland Centre for Policy and Practice, University of the West of Scotland, UK

Afzel Javed, Chairman of Pakistan Psychiatric Research Centre, Fountain House, Pakistan

Vesna Jelic, Memory Clinic, Karolinska University Hospital, Sweden

Rabaa Jomli, Department of Psychiatry A Hospital Razi, Tunisia

Marija Kušan Jukić, Department of Mental Health and Addiction Prevention, Andrija Štampar Teaching Institute of Public Health, Croatia

Lucy W Kamau, Africa Mental Health Foundation, Kenya

Muhammad Nasar Sayeed Khan, President of Pakistan Psychiatric Society, Pakistan

Özlem Kuman Tunçel, Department of Psychiatry, Ege University Faculty of Medicine, Turkey

Kua Ee Heok, Department of Psychological Medicine, Yong Loo Lin School of Medicine, National University of Singapore, Singapore

Brian Lawlor, Global Brain Health Institute, Trinity College Dublin, Ireland

António Leuschner, Magalhães Lemos Psychiatric Hospital, Portugal; University of Porto, Abel Salazar Biomedical Institute, Behavior Sciences Department, Portugal

John A Lucas, Department of Psychiatry and Psychology Mayo Clinic, USA

Angela M Lunde, Education Program Manager, Associate in Neurology, Mayo Clinic, USA

Valeria Manera, University of Nice Sophia Antipolis, France

Shanooha Mansoor, Department of Psychiatry, Indira Gandhi Memorial Hospital, Maldives

Raimundo Mateos, Department of Psychiatry and Psychogeriatric Unit, University of Santiago de Compostela, CHUS University Hospital, Spain

Seamus V McNulty, Elderly Mental Health NHS Ayrshire and Arran, Scotland

Adriana Mihai, University of Medicine and Pharmacy Tg Mures, Department M4 Psychiatry, IPPD Institute of Psychotherapy and Personal Development, Romania

Ninoslav Mimica, Department of Biological Psychiatry and Psychogeriatrics, University Psychiatric Hospital Vrapče, University of Zagreb School of Medicine, Croatia

Mamadou Bengaly Minthe, Department of Geriatrics, Our Lady of Grace Provincial Hospital, Spain

Fidiansjah Mursjid, Directorate of Prevention and Control of Mental Health Problem and Substance Abuse, Ministry of Health, Indonesia

Christine W Musyimi, Africa Mental Health Foundation, Kenya

Victoria N Mutiso, African Mental Health Foundation, Kenya

Fethi Nacef, Professor of Psychiatry, Psychiatry Service, Hospital Razi, Tunisia

Erick S Nandoya, Department of Research and Programs, Africa Mental Health Foundation, Kenya

David M Ndetei, University of Nairobi, Africa Mental Health Foundation, Kenya

Nikolay Neznanov, V M Bekhterev National Research Medical Center for Psychiatry and Neurology, Russia

Adefolakemi Temitope Ogundele, Old Age Unit, Neuropsychiatric Hospital, Aro, Abeokuta, Nigeria

Amador Ernesto Macias Osuna, Geriatric Medicine Coordinator, School of Medicine and Health Sciences, Monterrey Institute of Technology and Higher Education, Mexico

Uta Ouali, Department of Psychiatry A, Hospital Razi, Tunisia; Faculty of Medicine, University of Tunis El Manar, Tunisia

Fátima González Palau, Sanatorio Allende Hospital, CIATEC Foundation, Siglo 21 Business University, Argentina

Claudia Palumbo, Department of Psychiatry, ASST Papa Giovanni XXIII-Bergamo, Italy

Peter Passmore, Centre for Public Health, Queen's University, UK

Marta LGF Pereira, Laboratory of Neuroscience, Department and Institute of Psychiatry, Faculty of Medicine, University of São Paulo, Brazil

Ronald C Petersen, Department of Neurology Mayo Clinic, USA

Kanitpong Phabphal, Prince of Songkla University, Thailand

María Cristina Quijano Martínez, Department of Social Sciences, Pontificia University of Javeriana Cali, Colombia

Federico Ramos Ruiz, Psychiatry Research Coordinator, School of Medicine and Health Sciences, Monterrey Institute of Technology and Higher Education, Mexico

Ahmed Rasheed, Indira Gandhi Memorial Hospital, Ministry of Health, Maldives

Iris Rawtaer, Department of Psychological Medicine, National University Hospital, Singapore

Florian Riese, Division of Old Age Psychiatry, Psychiatric University Hospital Zurich, Switzerland

Marcel Olde Rikkert, Chair Dept Geriatrics/Radboudumc Alzheimer Centre, Donders Institute for Medical Neurosciences, Radboud University Medical Center, Nijmegen, The Netherlands

Philippe Robert, Professor of Psychiatry, CoBTeK Lab, Memory Centre, University Côte d'Azur, Association IA, France

Eric Salmon, Memory Clinic, Department of Neurology, University Hospital of Liege, Belgium

Per-Olof Sandman, Section for Clinical Geriatrics, NVS-Department Karolinska Institutet, Sweden

Martina Wiwie Setiawan Nasrun, Department of Psychiatry, Faculty of Medicine, Universitas Indonesia, Cipto Mangunkusumo General Hospital, Indonesia

Cheolmin Shin, Korea University College of Medicine, South Korea

Yumi Shindo, National Center for Geriatrics and Gerontology, Japan

Andrea Slachevsky, Gerosciences Center for Brain Health and Metabolism (GERO), University of Chile, Chile; Neuropsychiatry and Memory Disorders clinic (CMYN), Neurology Department, Hospital del Salvador and Faculty of Medicine, University of Chile, Chile

Assyatou Bobo Sow, Department of Geriatrics, Complejo Hospitalario de Segovia, Spain

Florindo Stella, Laboratory of Neuroscience, Department and Institute of Psychiatry, Faculty of Medicine, University of São Paulo, Brazil

Thitiporn Supasitthumrong, Department of Psychiatry, Faculty of Medicine, Chulalongkorn University, King Chulalongkorn Memorial Hospital, Thai Red Cross Society, Thailand

Sookjaroen Tangwongchai, Department of Psychiatry, Faculty of Medicine, Chulalongkorn University, Thailand

Jochen René Thyrian, German Center for Neurodegenerative Diseases (DZNE) Site Rostock/Greifswald, Germany

Stephen Todd, Care of the Elderly Medicine Western Health and Social Care Trust, Altnagelvin Hospital, UK

Maria-Silvia Trandafir, University of Medicine and Pharmacy Carol Davila Bucharest Department VI, Neurosciences - Department of Psychiatry, Psychiatric Hospital Prof. Dr. Alexandru Obregia, Bucharest, Romania

Magda Tsolaki, Chair of 1st Department of Neurology, Aristotle University of Thessaloniki, AHEPA University Hospital, Thessaloniki, Greece; Chair of Greek Federation of Alzheimer's Disease, Greece

Chavit Tunvirachaisakul, Department of Psychiatry, Faculty of Medicine, Chulalongkorn University, Thailand

Pichet Udomratn, Department of Psychiatry, Faculty of Medicine, Prince of Songkla University, Thailand

Umberto Volpe, Professor of Psychiatry, Department of Neuroscience, School of Medicine, Università Politecnica delle Marche, Italy

Lars-Olof Wahlund, Section for Clinical Geriatrics, NVS-Department Karolinska Institutet, Sweden

Huali Wang, Dementia Care and Research Center, Clinical Research Division, Peking University Institute of Mental Health, Peking University Sixth Hospital, China

Bob Woods, Dementia Services Development Centre Wales, Bangor University, UK

Hengge Xie, Department of Neurology, Chinese PLA General Hospital, China

Natalia Zalutskaya, Department of Geriatric Psychiatry, V M Bekhterev National Research Medical Center for Psychiatry and Neurology, Russia

Tatiana Castro Zamparella, National University of Córdoba, Argentina

Henry Zeimer, Aged Care Services, Austin Health, Australia

Yosra Zgueb, AHU in Psychiatry, Psychiatry Service, Hospital Razi, Tunisia

Stelios Zygouris, School of Medicine, Aristotle University of Thessaloniki, Greece; Network Aging Research, University of Heidelberg, Germany

Introduction

The primary aim of this book is to present arrangements for the care of people with dementia and their families in different parts of the world and to serve as a stimulus to develop new ideas for the provision of such care. In this way, the review builds on the previous efforts of our Committee [1].

According to estimates of the World Health Organization (WHO), the number of people living with dementia will double almost every 20 years for the foreseeable future. While, in 2010, there were 35.6 million people with dementia worldwide, this number is expected to increase to 65.7 million by 2030, and to 115.4 million by 2050 [2, 3]. Dementia has significant implications on the micro-, meso-, and macro-levels of society [4].

Dementia is not only a substantial burden for the person living with the illness; numerous studies have shown that family and carers of people with dementia are at a higher risk of stress, depression, anxiety, and other health complications, than carers of people with physical impairments and disability [5]. At the same time, dementia inflicts a significant burden on society and— already strained—health care systems. It is estimated that the total global costs of dementia in 2010 were US$604 billion (approximately €490 billion), which corresponds to 1.0% of the global gross domestic product (GDP) [3]. With the expected increase in prevalence, the cost of informal and formal professional care for dementia will grow even further in the near future.

The consequences of the increasing prevalence of dementia, and the need to describe the organization and coordination of dementia care within Europe, were recognized by the International Dementia Alliance (IDEAL) group [formerly European Dementia Consensus Network (EDCON)]. This group, formed in 2002, consists of leading European specialists from various disciplines with experience in research, diagnosis, and care of people with dementia, their families, and carers. The aim of IDEAL is to identify and build consensus statements about controversial issues concerning the recognition and care of people with dementia and to make recommendations about actions that would lead to an improvement of such care.

We have attempted to include, as far as we can, within the constraints of publishing a volume which is manageable and digestible for the reader, the descriptions of care for people with dementia in as many countries as we could, hoping that these descriptions will reflect the wide spread of countries, big and small, geographically diverse from all continents and encompassing the major language and culture groups. We apologize if, inadvertently, we have left anyone out and hope to include them in this type of review as well—we are looking forward already to our next edition.

While preparing this book, we asked the world's leading experts in the field of dementia five questions—having initially gathered information about these issues through an Internet search. The results of this enquiry are shown for 45 of the countries, and the summary is presented as follows.

Question 1: Is there a national dementia plan in that country?

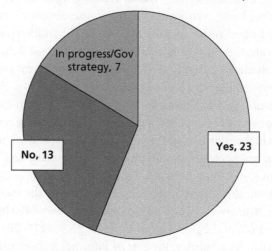

Question 2: Has there been an attempt to estimate the number of people with dementia in that country?

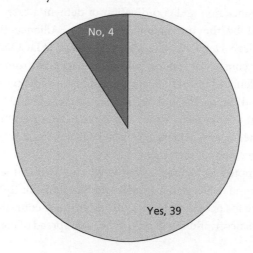

Question 3: Have anti-dementia drugs been licensed in that country?

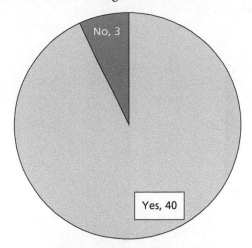

Question 4: Is there a national website for information on dementia?

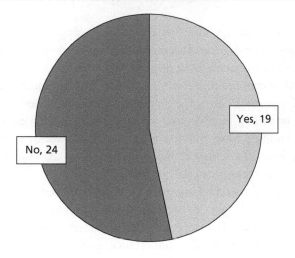

Question 5: Is there a National Alzheimer association that has a website giving independent advice?

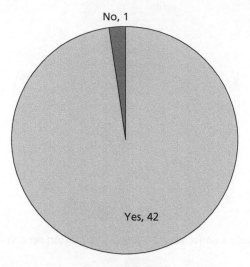

No, 1

Yes, 42

The answers to these questions were highly encouraging. More than half of the 43 countries have developed a national plan for the development of care for dementia, and in another quarter of them, the development of such a plan is in process. Most countries have websites which provide information about dementia, and more than half of the countries have created a non-governmental association providing independent advice for people with dementia, their carers, and families. Most countries have made an attempt to estimate the number of people with dementia, and drugs to treat dementia are widely available (although reimbursement policies differ).

It is interesting to reflect on how much progress has been made in dementia care around the world since our previous review summarized in our first book. There has been a huge increase in the general interest in dementia, prompted by an increasing awareness of its importance, and initiatives from organizations such as the WHO, the Global Dementia Observatory, and organizations like Alzheimer's Disease International (ADI). While everyone would appreciate that a cure is some way off, the interest and commitment to supporting people with dementia and looking at models of care have been gratifying, and as progress continues, in terms of awareness, post-diagnostic support, and a search for a cure, the future for dementia looks bright.

Country	Is there a national dementia plan?	Has there been an attempt to estimate the number of people with dementia in that country?	Have anti-dementia drugs been licensed in that country?	Is there a national website for information on dementia?	Is there a National Alzheimer charity that has a website that gives independent advice?
Argentina	Yes	Yes	Yes	No	Yes
Australia	Yes	Yes	Yes	Yes	Yes
Belgium	Yes	Yes	Yes	Yes	Yes
Brazil	No	Yes	Yes	Yes	Yes
Canada	No	Yes	Yes	Yes	Yes
Chile	Yes	Yes	Yes	No	Yes
China	No	Yes	Yes	Yes	Yes
Colombia	No	Yes	No	No	Yes
Croatia	No—non-gov strategy only	Yes	Yes	No	Yes
Czech Republic	Yes	Yes	Yes	No	Yes
France	Yes	Yes	Yes	Yes	Yes
Germany	No	Yes	Yes	Yes	Yes
Greece	Yes	Yes	Yes	No	Yes
India	No	Yes	Yes	Yes	Yes
Indonesia	Yes	Yes	Yes	No	Yes
Ireland	Yes	Yes	Yes	Yes	Yes
Italy	Yes	Yes	Yes	Yes	Yes
Japan	Yes	Yes	Yes	Yes	Yes
Kenya	No	No	No	No	Yes
Mali	No	No	No	No	Yes
Maldives	No	No	Yes	No	No
Mexico	Yes	Yes	Yes	No	Yes
Netherlands	Yes	Yes	Yes	Yes	Yes
New Zealand	Yes	Yes	Yes	Yes	Yes
Nigeria	No	No	Yes	No	Yes
Norway	Yes	Yes	Yes	Yes	Yes
Pakistan	No	Yes	Yes	No	Yes
Peru	No	Yes	Yes	No	Yes
Portugal	No—strategy only	Yes	Yes	No	Yes

Country	Is there a national dementia plan?	Has there been an attempt to estimate the number of people with dementia in that country?	Have anti-dementia drugs been licensed in that country?	Is there a national website for information on dementia?	Is there a National Alzheimer charity that has a website that gives independent advice?
Romania	No—non-gov strategy	Yes	Yes	No	Yes
Russia	Yes	Yes	Yes	No	Yes
Serbia	No—non-gov strategy	Yes	Yes	No	Yes
Singapore	Yes	Yes	Yes	Yes	Yes
South Korea	Yes	Yes	Yes	Yes	Yes
Spain	No—non-gov strategy	Yes	Yes	No	Yes
Sweden	Yes	Yes	Yes	Yes	Yes
Switzerland	Yes	Yes	Yes	Yes	Yes
Thailand	No	Yes	Yes	No	Yes
Tunisia	No—in development	Yes	Yes	No	Yes
Turkey	No	Yes	Yes	No	Yes
United Arab Emirates	No	Yes	Yes	No	No
UK (England, Northern Ireland, Scotland, Wales)	Yes	Yes	Yes	Yes	Yes
Uruguay	No—non-gov strategy	Yes	Yes	No	Yes
United States	Yes	Yes	Yes	Yes	Yes

Notes:

According to the ADI (https://www.alz.co.uk/alzheimer-plans), a dementia strategy is generated by private, non-governmental groups, aiming to persuade governments to create plans, whereas a dementia plan is a statement, by which 'a government holds itself accountable for the accomplishment of specific objectives and policy changes', even if this depends on non-governmental collaborators.

European countries with dementia plans are Norway, Belgium, England, Scotland, Wales, Northern Ireland, Denmark, Finland, the Netherlands, Luxembourg, Switzerland, Greece, Ireland, Italy, and Malta. Draft plans exist in Slovenia, Bulgaria, Cyprus, and Portugal. In most of the countries, the plans were launched between 2007 and 2014 and had a duration of 4 years. This period in Scotland was 3 years, in Belgium 6 years, and in Norway 8 years. Like in France, a second plan has been launched in both Scotland (2013–2016) and Norway (2016–2020).

References

1. **Burns A (ed) (on behalf of European Dementia Consensus Network).** *Standards of dementia care.* New York, NY: Taylor and Francis; 2005.

2. **Prince M, Bryce R, Albanese E, Wimo A, Ribeiro W, Ferri CP.** The global prevalence of dementia: a systematic review and metaanalysis. *Alzheimer's and Dementia.* 2013;**9**:63–75.e2.

3. **World Health Organization.** *Dementia: a public health priority.* 2012. Available from: http://www.who.int/mental_health/publications/dementia_report_2012/en/ [accessed 21 August 2018].

4. **Alzheimer's Disease International.** *World Alzheimer's report 2015: the global impact of dementia.* 2015. Available from: https://www.alz.co.uk/research/world-report-2015 [accessed 21 August 2018].

5. **Brodaty H, Donkin M.** Family caregivers of people with dementia. *Dialogues in Clinical Neuroscience.* 2009;**11**:217–28.

Section 1

Africa

Chapter 1

Kenya

David M Ndetei, Erick S Nandoya,
Christine W Musyimi, Lucy W Kamau,
and Victoria N Mutiso

Summary

There is very little research conducted in Kenya on the prevalence
of dementia. Although there is no specific strategy on dementia
care in Kenya, the government of Kenya has made several
strides towards improving mental health service provision. In
1982, the Kenya government became one of the signatories to
the International Plan of Action on Ageing in Vienna, Austria.
Later on, it incorporated the rights of the elderly into the 2010
Constitution and recently launched a mental health policy to
address mental health issues in Kenya. While something has
been done by non-governmental organizations (NGOs) involved
in mental health, there is still a huge gap in increasing access
to mental health services, particularly dementia. This can be
overcome through massive research and collaboration between
the government and NGOs to detect dementia and support carers
for people with dementia.

Introduction

1. To promote the socio-economic aspects and the well-being of the elderly, the
   government put in place a social welfare programme like the cash transfer,
   National Social Security Fund (NSSF), and National Health Insurance Fund
   (NHIF) to meet their health needs, including dementia.
2. Kenya is moving towards the provision of free healthcare for special groups of
   people, including the elderly aged over 65 who mostly suffer from dementia.

3. Although there are no specific government policies or guidelines on dementia, there is a bill introduced in the senate as a guide on matters dealing with dementia service provision.

What needs to be done in future?

1. The government should allocate more funds to raise awareness on dementia by using posters placed in hospitals, billboards, and in other public places.
2. Collaboration within countries and with other countries should be increased in order to improve patient-centred care through evidence-based models and prioritize early treatment of acute symptoms.
3. Acknowledging the contribution of non-governmental organizations (NGOs), such as the Africa Mental Health Foundation committed to carrying out research to generate evidence and the Alzheimers and Dementia Organization Kenya (ADOK), a support group for people living with dementia in Kenya, will inform on the specific needs of the elderly and dementia care in Kenya.

The Kenyan context

Mental health problems in Kenya are categorized as: common mental disorders which include depression and anxiety; severe mental disorders such as psychosis, schizophrenia, and bipolar disorder; and neurological disorders comprising of epilepsy and dementia, childhood disorders, and alcohol and substance use disorders. In hospital reporting systems, epilepsy is listed on its own, while other mental disorders are reported as a single condition. There is also little or no research done in Kenya on the prevalence of dementia, as well as other mental disorders, making it very difficult to access epidemiological data.

Furthermore, most people in Kenya, including health workers, lack awareness of the condition and therefore commonly refer to dementia as the 'old people's disease'. As a result, families taking care of the elderly do not seek medical intervention for dementia because they are oblivious of the condition and feel that it is part of the ageing process or that the elderly have spent the most useful part of their life in their earlier years.

Although there are no specific guidelines on dementia care in Kenya, the Mental Health Act established in 1989 still exists. This Act, revised and gazetted in the Kenyan Constitution in 2014 [1] aims at decentralizing mental healthcare, thus making it possible for more people to access mental health services. Despite the good initiative taken by the Kenyan government to revise the Act, there was poor implementation. This is further aggravated by the fact that mental health is underfunded in Kenya, with an allocation of less than 0.5% of the national budget. This budget has been directed to very few psychiatric hospitals in Nairobi, including Mathari Hospital. This therefore further limits access of mental health services to people from other counties.

Only about 10% of people in developing countries receive mental health services. In Kenya, the ratio of patient to psychiatrist is 1:3–5 million people [2]. This means that the majority of people in Kenya are not able to receive mental health services, making it worse for undetected conditions such as dementia. Mental health services provided by mental health professionals, such as psychiatric nurses, are also limited to level 4–6 hospitals, with little or no access to psychiatric services for communities at levels 1–3. Healthcare workers who have little training on priority mental disorders during their school years are based at lower levels of care, thus exacerbating the situation. Evidence provided in the Kenyan health system shows that there is lack of preparedness with regard to human resources, delivery of services, and availability of medicines [2].

Currently, there are about 80 trained psychiatrists living and working in Kenya, while 20 are currently outside the country [2]. Most of the psychiatrists are located in the capital city of Kenya. Similarly, there are about 500 trained psychiatric nurses, of whom 50% are actively working in psychiatry and the rest are either retired, have left the country, are deceased, or have been deployed to work in other departments. There are few or seldom any trainees enrolling for mental health training. For instance, an average of six psychiatrists are trained per year in Kenya [2], and only one graduated in 2015.

Psychiatry training for a doctor in Kenya takes about 9 years. This is inclusive of 6 years of basic medical training and an additional 3 years for psychiatry specialist training. For psychiatric nurses, training takes about 6 years, including 3–4 years for a basic diploma/degree in nursing and 2 years' training for a diploma in psychiatry, usually at the Kenya Medical Training College (KMTC). It is therefore important for the government to establish basic psychiatric training for formal health workers to incorporate mental health in primary care for improved standards of mental health services at lower levels of care [3].

In 2005–2013, 3000 primary healthcare staff in public health, of a possible total of 5000, were trained in basic mental health. This was through a partnership between the Ministry of Health (MOH), the Kenya Psychiatric Association (KPA), the World Health Organization (WHO), and the Institute of Psychiatry, Kings College London, with funding from Nuffield Foundation. Another good example of this is training through the Africa Mental Health Foundation

(AMHF), with funding from Grand Challenges Canada (GCC), and in collaboration with the Global Mental Health Program; the Makueni County government has been able to train 45 formal health workers in the provision of intervention for mental disorders at the primary care level [4], using the WHO Mental Health Global Action Programme Intervention Guide (mhGAP-IG), designed for use by non-specialists in low- and middle-income countries (LMICs) [5]. A total of 161 community health workers, faith healers, and traditional healers were also trained in screening and referring people with mental health disorders, including dementia, to nearby health facilities [4].

There is still a very long way to go for Kenya in terms of delivery of mental health services, which will be guided by research. However, the Kenyan government is one of the signatories to the International Plan of Action on Ageing adopted in 1982 in Vienna, Austria, during the first World Assembly on Ageing. In addition, the Kenyan Constitution under the bill of rights supports the rights of the elderly (Article 57 of Kenya Constitution 2010), and the mental health policy that promotes universal mental health acknowledges that older persons lacking social protection and networks are vulnerable to mental disorders. The government has also put in efforts to provide social welfare programmes like 'cash transfer' for the elderly and the National Social Security Fund (NSSF) that helps to address social issues related to dementia. In addition, the elderly continue to be respected through councils for the elderly at village levels.

The way forward

Mental healthcare in Kenya should be included in primary healthcare, with most staff having basic training in mental health, so that healthcare settings provide epidemiological data for common mental disorders, rather than categorizing them as a single group of disorders. Moreover, the government should consider investing in strategies or campaigns to raise awareness of dementia and other mental disorders through the inclusion of dementia in Continuous Medical Education Sessions (CMES). There should also be community outreach programmes, medical camps, and health talks in places of worship that focus on mental health, especially dementia, in order to raise awareness and direct individuals to areas of specialized care.

The future of dementia care in Kenya is therefore bright. With the currently gazetted Mental Health Act (2014), the launch of the mental health policy, as well as training of primary healthcare staff in basic mental health, the future is very promising. This is not without forgetting the effort put in place by several organizations working in Kenya to ensure that mental health services are brought closer to the people. Through global collaborations and the work of the AMHF in mental health research, advocacy, and raising awareness, mental health services in Kenya are now being integrated into primary healthcare services to reach people living in both urban and rural areas in Kenya. Other organizations contributing to the provision of mental healthcare in Kenya include BasicNeeds Kenya, an organization that brings people together in setting up community-level services while raising awareness and petitioning for change, and the ADOK, a support group for people living with dementia and Alzheimer's disease (AD) in Kenya. There is also the Institute for Legislative Affairs which spearheads reforms for mental health policies and coordinates stakeholders in the civil society [6].

For a successful engagement, it is important to consider a multisectoral and multidisciplinary approach, as the medical profession alone would be overwhelmed by the needs of the country. The future of dementia care would require urgent studies in health, psychosocial, medical, economic, legal, and human rights needs, in order to provide a holistic approach to those in need of services.

References

1. **Government of Kenya.** *Mental Health Act 2014: No. 26 of 2014.* 2014.
2. **Kiima D, Jenkins R, Gureje O,** *et al.* Mental health policy in Kenya: an integrated approach to scaling up equitable care for poor populations. *International Journal of Mental Health Systems.* 2010;4:19.
3. **National Coordinating Agency for Population and Development (NCAPD) [Kenya], Ministry of Medical Services (MOMS) [Kenya], Ministry of Public Health and Sanitation (MOPHS) [Kenya], Kenya National Bureau of Statistics (KNBS) [Kenya], ICF Macro.** *Kenya Service Provision Assessment (SPA) 2010.* 2011. pp. 1–695.
4. **Africa Mental Health Foundation.** *Multi-sectorial stakeholder team approach to scale-up community mental health in Kenya: building on locally-generated evidence and lessons learned (TEAM).* Available from: http://www.africamentalhealthfoundation.org/project-team/ [accessed 28 October 2016].
5. **World Health Organization.** *mhGAP Intervention Guide for mental, neurological and substance use disorders in non-specialized health settings.* Version 1.0. Geneva: World Health Organization; 2010. pp. 1–65.
6. **de Menil V.** *Reforming Kenya's ailing mental health system.* 2013. Available from: http://www.africaresearchinstitute.org/newsite/blog/mental-health-in-kenya/ [accessed 28 October 2016].

Chapter 2

Mali

Mamadou Bengaly Minthe and Assyatou
Bobo Sow

Summary

In Mali, there are no specific official programmes for the medical
care of dementia. However, there is a law (decree 95-368/P-RM
du 13 octobre 1995) that stipulates the free nature of medical
consultations, with the elderly benefiting from a 50% reduction
in costs of medical care. The challenge in the future would be the
legislation for free treatment of psychiatric illnesses in general and
of dementia in particular. The therapeutic approach to dementia
care in Mali is multidimensional and includes spiritual, traditional
(medicinal plants), and social therapy, which is the most important
in the management of dementia. Daily recitation and teaching
of the holy book (Quran) is part of prevention and treatment
of dementia in current Sufi Islam. The cosmovision of Dogon
(worldview of a culture or civilization, especially its relationship
with the animated or environment) has its own method for the
prevention and treatment of dementia. This chapter describes
the sociological aspects, preventative measures, and traditional
therapy (Dogon ethnopharmacology) of dementia.

Introduction

One of the greatest intellectuals, the ethnologist, poet, and writer Amadou Bah
Hampate (1901–91) said: 'In Africa, when an old man dies, a library burns.' This
phrase defines the central role of the elderly in the organization and transmis-
sion of ancestral knowledge. Therefore, the preservation of the overall mental
health of the elderly is a primary objective of his as an individual, and of the
family and society in general. Perhaps this is still not a priority as part of government health programmes, since there are other pandemics like malaria and
HIV infection. However, it changes the order of importance if we give thorough
and methodical attention to the analysis of dementia.

There is no national health programme or register focusing specifically on dementia in Mali, and hence no reliable data on the prevalence or incidence of dementia. However, two recent studies [1] have estimated that the prevalence of dementia varies between 3.9% and 5.8%, respectively, based on a sample of 485 subjects from the capital city aged over 65, with these figures varying widely across different regions and ethnic groups in the country [2].

In Mali, dozens of different ethnic groups coexist, each with their history, idiosyncrasies, varied ancestral beliefs grouped into two trends today—those impregnated by monotheistic religions called the Islamic majority, especially the Sufi current, Malikite, and animist, especially in the central and southern geographical regions.

The aim of this chapter is to describe the characteristics of the different types of dementia care in Mali. For educational purposes, we will discuss the two main levels that are most commonly used by the general population.

Psychiatric semiotics in the tradition

In the Peul tradition (poular, foulfoulbe), one of the oldest in the country, the life of a man develops over nine periods, each period consisting of seven rainy seasons or years. The first period begins at birth until the age of 7 rain or lunar years (this corresponds to the number of years for each period of rain after birth, as the Gregorian calendar was not known to, and not used in, the Peul tradition), and the last period begins from 63 rain years to death.

The teraditerapeuta classifies mental illnesses into two syndromic groups. The difference between the two syndromic groups lies in the presence or absence of an altered level of consciousness and/or convulsions:

1. Djine bana: translated into another language, is defined as disorders or diseases of the devil or Satan, which have in common an altered level of consciousness and the presence or absence of seizures; they usually appear before the sixth or ninth decade age group.

2. Hakiliwili bana: a compound word which literally means Hakili (mind) wili (imbalance) and bana (disease or disorder). Suelen appears at any age but is very common from the sixth period or until the ninth age group (57–63 years); however, in women, it is not commonly present before the menopause. Its main features include usually the presence of typical symptoms of depression, delirium, hallucinations, mystical content, and the absence of altered consciousness, with subjects never presenting with seizures.

Psychosocial treatment of dementia in Mali

This is based on the bio-psycho-social nature and spirituality, as the core of an individual's life moves around with all other aspects of their existence. The cost of treatment is relatively cheaper than any other dependent care programme for dementia in the first world. The social model, based on an extensive, large family comprising two or more generations living under the same roof, makes this treatment method essential to any policies and strategies for healthcare in older people, and dementia is no exception here.

In the tradition and today, it remains in the collective consciousness that mental illnesses are almost always associated with ancestral explanations that include either a curse or guilt from ancestors, and which is dogmatic and mystical. Some historians describe the prohibition of marriage between some clans for fear of mental illness. However, there is a method of cross-selection among clans when there are high rates of mental illness.

Care for dementia and mental illnesses in general can be divided into three levels, which are not mutually exclusive and are often superimposed concurrently.

Level 1: scholars (Marabout)

This practice is based on the mystical and mystified interpretation of the scriptures, essentially verses of the Koran. This practice has its origin in Sufism, a tolerant and spiritual power of religion.

Prevention of dementia

From the point of view of these scholars (Marabout), the most important aspect of treatment is usually prevention through memorization and daily recitation and teaching of every chapter, or sura, of the Koran in the fourth and fifth prayers of the day. Also, in the first hour of the morning, the recitation and teaching are the most recommended by the sages. According to teachers at Koranic school, those who recite the holy book every day of their life never suffer from dementia. Although there is a lack of evidence from scientific studies, a low prevalence of dementia in small groups of individuals who have memorized the holy book may have a relationship between this fact and an adequate cognitive reserve. Also, the practice of meditation (dhikr), which consists of constant and repetitive recitations of a name or attributes of God, with or without the rosary, in the early hours of the morning, usually has an anxiolytic effect on those who practise it.

Scholar treatment method (Marabout)

The treatment of established dementia involves writing specific verses of the Koran on a bar usually of wood (see Fig. 2.1). The verses are usually written in the first hour of the morning on a specific day of the week, in general Friday or Monday, and are then washed with water mixed with other products, usually derived from plants, the name or properties of which remain a mystery

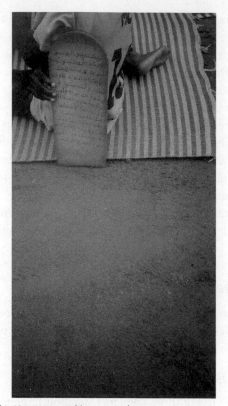

Fig. 2.1 Text from the Koran carved into wood.

for everyone else. The route of administration is generally oral (mixed with drinking water in the patient's food) or topical.

Level 2: animistic (Soma)

In the Dogon worldview and others, the image of each man is represented in the flora and fauna. For this reason, therapies often include slaughtering of animals and the use of mineral objects.

The therapeutic approach varies greatly across regions and ethnic groups in the country. The Dogon are the last people to resist the French invasion and conversion to Islam. They are part of the oldest ethnic groups, with the majority of the population ageing in mental and physical health. An old Dogon, who has probably met rains or 80 years, has a longilineo appearance, with a beard and white hair, a slightly bent back, and the characteristic smell of sweat reminiscent of a farmer. As a mark of respect, we carry his luggage, and once a relationship of trust is established, we receive from him 'the secret of ageing and good memory'. To grow old with good mental health, one must be born with it, must eat smart, must sleep like a rooster (which the sun never should leave while still in bed), and finally must sweat a lot.

Preventive measures of dementia according to the old Dogon

The old Dogon conveys in the form of ancestral wisdom the following tips to keep the mind healthy:

- Avoid promiscuity and forbid other women. This is because, apart from the fact that promiscuity is immoral, it can decrease one's memory capacity and encourage distraction.
- Eat breakfast every day with the inclusion of at least ten plants, mixed with honey and lemon.
- Eat in moderation. The mind is satiated before the stomach.
- Love and cultivate the land, and when one have no strength at dawn, one should walk with a cane.
- Have the young listen to stories in spring around a common fire. This was not new to us because our people spent our vacation listening to stories of the elderly. Every year, we repeated the stories without changing a phrase.
- Avoid loneliness. Know that one comes from the hands of a woman and one must die in the hands of others. Society is paramount to life, and loneliness is an attribute of Amma (meaning God in the Dogon worldview).

The Dogon treatment method

Promising data have been published in the *Journal of Ethnopharmacology* on the effectiveness of African Voacanga, a medicinal plant discovered in Sao Tome and Principe, in the treatment of neurodegenerative dementia [3].

The Dogon ethnopharmacology essentially comprises various medicinal plants, the use of which has precepts, rules, collections, preparations which are well defined and controlled by the therapist. The medicinal compound usually has a main plant mixed with other natural elements, such as honey and lemon, which plays the role of a catalyst of chemical reactions. Before commencing drug therapy, a spiritual washing ceremony is required, usually performed by a Dogon priest, and consists of offering animal blood to the gods. The cost of treatment for the patient or the family is usually in terms of the animals used in the offering. The therapist disclaims the treatment charges.

Level 3: modern medicine

This is concentrated only in the capital city and accepted by psychiatrists and neurologists, who are insufficient in number. Their efforts are limited by the lack of drugs and purchasing power of the population to buy them. It also reflects what little faith and confidence that the population has in modern medicine, specifically in this field.

Challenges and prospects of treatment of dementia in Mali

The challenges of care for dementia are multiple:

◆ Integration at public 2 levels described as part of non-pharmacological and pharmacological therapy through the creation of a box exchange of information and knowledge network.

◆ Promoting research in the treatment of dementia from the perspective of the Dogon ethnopharmacology, stimulating completion of end-of-study work in medical schools on this subject.

◆ Maintaining and promoting traditions and cultures that favour the maintenance of mental health.

◆ Perpetuating the values related to the elderly as a source of wisdom and as added value to the family and society in general.

Will the future treatment of dementia come from the Dogon ethnopharmacology?

References

1. **Guerchet M.** *Démences en Afrique Subsaharienne: outils, prévalence et facteurs de risque.* PhD thesis. Santé publique et épidémiologie. Limoges: University of Limoges, 2010.

2. **Paraïso Moussiliou N.** *Epidémiologie de la démence des personnes âgées de 65 ans et plus au Bénin (Afrique de l'Ouest).* PhD thesis. Limoges: University of Limoges; 2010. Available from: http://epublications.unilim.fr/theses/2010/paraiso-moussiliou-noel/paraiso-moussiliou-noel.pdf [accessed 5 September 2016].

3. **Currais A, Chiruta C, Goujon-Svrzic M,** *et al.* Screening and identification of neuroprotective compounds relevant to Alzheimer's disease from medicinal plants of S. Tomé e Príncipe. *Journal of Ethnopharmacology.* 2014;**155**:830–40.

Chapter 3

Nigeria

Olatunde Olayinka Ayinde and Adefolakemi
Temitope Ogundele

Summary

The burden of dementia and Alzheimer's dsease, the commonest
type of dementia in Nigeria, is expected to rise, necessitating
adequate health and social systems to meet the challenge. Late
presentation for orthodox care is the norm, due to poor public
awareness of the disease process and unfavourable cultural
beliefs. Orthodox care and psychotropic drugs are available
but remain largely inaccessible to the majority of people with
dementia. The preferred and predominant care model in late
dementia is one within the family, as opposed to institutional
care, which is largely unavailable. Family caregivers of the person
with dementia are often uninformed, unsupported, and heavily
burdened. There is no National Strategy for dementia care,
and social security for the elderly is almost non-existent. There
is an urgent need for policy formulation and implementation,
vigorous advocacy, and awareness creation, as well as adequate
social security for the person with dementia and psycho-social
interventions for their families and caregivers.

Introduction

Nigeria has a predominantly youthful population. However, with a gradual, but
relentless, reduction in crude mortality rate, both the proportion and absolute
number of the elderly population have been on the increase. For example, between 1991 and 2006, the proportion of those aged 65 years and older rose from
3% to 4.3%, while the total population rose from 93 million to 140 million.
A corresponding increase in the number of people with dementia in the near
future is therefore anticipated. Not only does dementia care involve specialized

medical care, but it also comprises an important social component and requires a coherent policy strategy where the roles of the different parties involved are clearly spelt out, as well as an adequate health system and an efficient funding mechanism. Although there have been advances in specialist geriatric care in Nigeria, as well as globally, there are various existing and emerging cultural, socio-economic, and socio-political factors in the country that act as barriers to dementia care. It is therefore pertinent to review the current state of dementia care in Nigeria, with a view to describing the practice environment, highlighting the challenges, and charting a course forward.

Epidemiology of dementia in Nigeria

Most of the epidemiological data on dementia in Nigeria come from two large studies: the Indianapolis-Ibadan Dementia Research Project (I-IDRP) [1] and the Ibadan Study of Aging (ISA) [2], the former being a prospective community survey and the latter a population-based follow-up survey conducted among the Yoruba from south-western Nigeria. The I-IDRP study reported an age-adjusted prevalence of dementia and AD of 2.29% and 1.41%, respectively. It also reported an age-standardized annual incidence of 1.35% for dementia and 1.15% for AD. The more recent ISA study estimated the prevalence of probable dementia to be 10.1% and the annual incidence of dementia to be 21.85 per 1000 person-years. AD is, by far, the commonest type of dementia in the Nigerian population, followed by vascular dementia. Across all studies, age and female gender were found to be associated with an increased prevalence, as well as incidence, of dementia. It is interesting to note that identified risk factors for incident dementia are mainly social, as opposed to lifestyle- or health-related factors reported in western countries. The I-IDRP study had earlier noted that vascular risk factors are of less importance among Yoruba Nigerians, compared to their African-American counterparts in Indianapolis in the United States. The ISA study reported later that living in rural areas, social isolation, and low socio-economic status are important risk factors in the onset of dementia. However, probably as a reflection of recent changes in societal lifestyle, lifetime alcohol use has been identified in a recent study as an emerging risk factor.

Dementia care

Transition from the well elderly to the elderly with dementia

The majority of the elderly population in Nigeria live in rural areas. In these communities, because of the multi-generational living arrangement and the extended family system, care of the elderly is a family affair and is often entrusted to, and shared among, the younger members of the family. However, for many families, care of the normal elderly person often segues into the care of the elderly person with dementia. Relatives initially either overlook or tolerate the cognitive and language problems early in the course of AD, in the erroneous belief that they are features of normal ageing. However, with increasing severity and near-total dependence on the family for daily activities, dedicated care becomes inevitable. It is often at this point that relatives of the person with dementia seek help. Late presentation to orthodox care facilities is the norm, and it is not unconnected with a lack of awareness of dementia in Nigeria, both among the general public and among policymakers. Even when gross behavioural abnormalities begin to dominate the picture, families of the person with dementia are reluctant to seek orthodox care because of the prevalent belief that dementia is caused by supernatural agents, and therefore not amenable to orthodox treatment. Caregivers are also often afraid of stigma and the embarrassment that the bizarre behaviours of relatives with dementia might cause them, with resultant delay in seeking help.

Orthodox care

Orthodox care for dementia is mainly at the tertiary healthcare level and is therefore far from the average rural-dwelling person with dementia. Baiyewu [3] noted that the hospital environment is anything but friendly. Service organization peculiarities and complex bureaucratic bottlenecks keep potential clients away. Out-of-pocket payment is still the main mode of payment for the majority of the population, and because of the often multiple medical and surgical comorbidities in the person with dementia, investigations can sometimes be unaffordable to the average caregiver. Cranial computerized tomographic scans are now available in many centres, but they are costly. Fortunately, psychotropic medications, especially cholinesterase inhibitors and memory-enhancing drugs, are becoming increasingly available. They remain expensive, however, in view of the economic realities of the average Nigerian.

Care in the later stages of dementia: community care versus nursing home care

Perhaps the cynical comment that 'most people with dementia live at home, this is where they want to live, this is where their families want them to live, and this is where the government wants them to live' [4] is truer in Nigeria than in many other places. In the later stages of dementia, well-coordinated community care and nursing home placement are the care of choice in many western countries. These models are supported by adequate medical and social welfare services. In Nigeria, many families continue to care for the person with dementia at home, long after it is clear that they are neither trained to do so nor equipped to bear the heavy financial, physical, and psychological burden.

Caregivers of people with dementia are often females (wives, daughters, daughters-in-law), who live with the patients, are largely uncompensated, and often have to cut back on paid employment to provide adequate care for the patient. The Nigerian constitution promises 'suitable and adequate' shelter, food, old age care, and pensions for all citizens, and the Social Policy promises that the care of the elderly shall be the duty of the three tiers of the government, who shall encourage the establishment of day care for the elderly and encourage home visits to the elderly while discouraging nursing homes. These promises have gone largely unfulfilled. There is a wide policy implementation gap for the care of the elderly, and there is currently no national policy or plan for dementia care. There is also no dedicated health insurance scheme or social security for the elderly, making institutional care almost impossible. The financial burden of care is therefore borne mainly by the family.

Although, at the last count, there are about 13 nursing homes dedicated to the care of the elderly in Nigeria, many of them are owned by private investors and religious bodies, and only those who are informed about them and can afford to pay patronize them. Among Nigerians, the general belief is that it is a taboo to 'abandon' one's parents in a home where the quality of care is feared to be inadequate since they would be cared for by 'strangers'. This fear of non-family caregivers is further reinforced by the concern that the bizarre behaviours in dementia might encourage abuse of the person with dementia by non-family caregivers.

Encouraging developments in hospital and community care

In recent years, stand-alone geriatric health facilities are beginning to see the light of day. One such health facility is the Tony Anenih Geriatric Centre at the University College Hospital in Ibadan in south-west Nigeria. It encourages an integrated approach to the care of dementia and associated medical comorbidities in the elderly. An optional in-house insurance scheme that covers consultations and basic medications is in place to support elderly clients.

As a more sustainable alternative to tertiary care, the Federal Government of Nigeria recently announced a policy redirection focusing on primary healthcare. Luckily, there had been ongoing efforts to integrate mental health into primary healthcare. One example of such efforts is the country's contextualization and piloting of the World Health Organization's Mental Health Gap

Action Programme (mhGAP), which introduces the concept of task sharing, that is, the involvement of non-specialist health workers in mental health service delivery in the primary care setting. One of the focus areas is dementia care. The mhGAP has since been adopted by the Federal Government, and it is hoped that it will become the foundation upon which a community care model for the care of dementia is built.

In the mid 1990s, the I-IDRP, a longitudinal, cross-cultural, transnational study that compared the epidemiology of dementia and AD between African-Americans and Yoruba Nigerians, commenced a modified community care model for dementia patients [5]. The patients were cared for by their families at home, but they were also visited at home by social workers and trained nurses who administered medications and called for more specialized care when needed. It also featured the empowerment of caregivers and regular meetings with them to recount and share experiences with other caregivers, as well as to get help from peers and specialists. This model, however, was part of a funded project, and its replication with locally sought resources is yet to prove that the model is sustainable.

Future of dementia care in Nigeria

Considering the anticipated growth in the number of elderly Nigerians and the concurrent rise in the number of people living with dementia, the disease is likely to cause a significant burden to the Nigerian society in the future, if more efforts are not made to improve the quality of care of dementia now. Although vascular dementia is the second commonest type, public health awareness of the vascular risk factors should be intensified to reduce the incidence of dementia. There is a rapid proliferation of both professional bodies and NGOs that are dedicated to promoting awareness of the care of the elderly and the person with dementia. However, there is still a need for vigorous advocacy at national and local levels.

The age-old reliance on the family might not hold out for much longer, as rapid urbanization takes its toll and young people move to cities to seek lucrative employment. Those who therefore remain behind to care for the person with dementia are in dire need of psycho-social interventions. There is an urgent need for community support services for the person with dementia and their caregivers in every primary healthcare centre to provide timely information, friendly counselling, and rehabilitative services, as well as respite care and financial support services. Ultimately, policy thrust towards well-coordinated community care models and institutional care, as well as infrastructural support around these, might be the way to go.

References

1. Hendrie HC, Ogunniyi A, Hall KS, *et al*. Incidence of dementia and Alzheimer disease in 2 communities: Yoruba residing in Ibadan, Nigeria, and African Americans residing in Indianapolis, Indiana. *JAMA*. 2001;**285**:739–47.

2. Gureje O, Ogunniyi A, Kola L, Abiona T. Incidence of and risk factors for dementia in the Ibadan Study of Aging. *Journal of the American Geriatrics Society*. 2011;**59**:869–74.

3. Baiyewu O. Dementia in Nigeria. *Archives of Ibadan Medicine*. 2005;**4**:21–2.

4. Graham N. Editorial: Dementia and family care: the current international state of affairs. *Dementia*. 2003;**2**:147–9.

5. Ogunniyi A, Hall KS, Baiyewu O, *et al*. Caring for individuals with dementia: the Nigerian experience. *West African Journal of Medicine*. 2005;**24**:259–62.

Chapter 4

Tunisia

Uta Ouali, Rabaa Jomli, Yosra Zgueb,
Fethi Nacef, and Saïda Douki Dedieu

Summary

This chapter provides an overview of the current situation and the
challenges Tunisia faces in the field of dementia care. Tunisia is a
country in full demographic transition, witnessing an ageing of its
population and an increase in dementia incidence and prevalence.
There is growing awareness that the healthcare system needs
to be better oriented towards this emerging problem. During
the last 10 years, a number of public and private initiatives were
implemented to improve diagnosis, treatment, training, and
research on dementia. Furthermore a number of public and private
institutions with focus on dementia care have been created.
However, family members remain the cornerstone of dementia
care in Tunisia. Currently, a National Dementia Strategy is being
developed in order to address the following challenges: (1) the
need for early diagnosis and intervention; (2) better coordination
of care circuits; (3) wider implementation of day care and
residential care with the concurrent establishment of rigorous
quality standards; and (4) financial and psychological support for
caregivers.

A country in demographic transition

Tunisia, situated in the extreme North of the African continent, has a population of about 11 million inhabitants. Since its independence in 1956, Tunisia has
initiated an ambitious programme of birth control, education, and health. As
a result of these policies, the country has entered a new phase of demographic
transition with ageing of its population. The percentage of the population aged
65 and over has risen from 3.5% in 1966 to an estimated 7.8% in 2015. Today's

life expectancy at birth is about 76 years (73.9 years for men and 77.4 years for women in 2014) [1]. Consequently, the incidence and prevalence of dementia is going to increase exponentially during the next years.

Limited data are available on the prevalence of dementia in Tunisia. An epidemiological study on a representative population sample conducted in 2001 found the prevalence of dementia in the subgroup aged 65 years and older (n = 482) to be 3.7% (4.6% of women and 2.8% of men) [2]. This low rate, compared to the more developed countries of Europe or America, could be explained by: (1) the lower life expectancy at birth in Tunisia, compared to developed countries, (2) the fact that dementia prevalence increases considerably with age, and (3) the small sample size of the study [3].

Based on the epidemiological study from 2001 and taking into account the current epidemiological data on dementia, Hajem *et al.* [2] made an estimate for 2012 and a projection for 2030. The prevalence of dementia of all types was estimated to be around 4.6% in the Tunisian population aged 65 and over in 2012, which equals 35,000 patients. Thus, the prevalence of dementia of all types has increased by 24% in just over 10 years. Their projection shows that in 2030, the number of seniors aged 65 and older with dementia would be around 58,000.

Current situation and challenges in dementia care

Tunisia's healthcare system comprises a public and a private sector. The public sector is represented by state-owned health facilities, with three levels of care: (1) primary healthcare centres, (2) district and regional hospitals, and (3) university hospitals. The public sector provides services to all Tunisian citizens and residents, which are entirely free of charge for a certain segment of the population. The private healthcare system in Tunisia has significantly expanded in terms of infrastructure, as well as capacity and healthcare personnel, during the last 20 years.

Tunisia has a national health insurance system covering more than half of the country's population. National health insurance pays up to 100% of the cost for each treatment, particularly in the case of certain severe and chronic diseases. This is especially true for services provided by the public sector, but a growing number of services in the private sector are also covered by health insurance.

In the past, dementia has not been a priority in the public health agenda. However, given the rising number of dementia patients, there is a growing awareness that the healthcare system needs to be more oriented towards the emerging problem of dementia.

The Alzheimer Centre is the first public medical institution entirely dedicated to dementia in Tunisia. To our knowledge, it is also the first institution of its kind in Africa and the Arab world. It is situated at the Razi University Hospital in Tunis. It was created through funding from private donors and was opened in September 2010. The Alzheimer Centre's mission is early detection, diagnosis and treatment of, and training and research in, dementia. It has a multidisciplinary team of neurologists, neuropsychologists, speech therapists, occupational therapists, physiotherapists, and nurses, all of whom are specialized in dementia. The centre comprises an outpatient department and a day clinic, with the aim of early diagnosis in patients with any type of cognitive impairment. Individual treatment plans are then elaborated with patients and their families. A department for cognitive rehabilitation, conceptualized as a day clinic, receives patients in the early stages of dementia. It offers physical and cognitive activities, as well as art and music therapy. Furthermore, family members, especially the main caregivers, receive psycho-education and psychological support. The centre also organizes training courses on the topic of dementia for healthcare professionals. Several research projects conducted by the centre's health professionals aim at exploring the epidemiological and clinical characteristics of dementia and the socio-cultural conditions in which dementia patients live in Tunisia. The results of these studies and, more generally, the experience of the Alzheimer Centre in terms of care might help to form the basis upon which to build in the years to come.

In the rest of this chapter, we describe the challenges in terms of dementia care in the public and in the private sector.

In the public sector, at the first level of care, there is insufficient awareness of the early signs and symptoms of dementia, and not enough knowledge about the diagnostic tools for early detection. This may lead to diagnostic delay or misdiagnosis. For example, prior to the Mecca pilgrimage (in which generally older people participate), a thorough health check-up is required. However, this check-up does not include a cognitive evaluation. In cases of unrecognized 'early-stage' dementia, this might expose the patient to a potential risk of acute aggravation or decompensation of dementia when they find themselves in an unfamiliar place. Indeed, there is a lack of specific training for most primary care doctors and nurses. Early signs of dementia, such as memory loss, are still often attributed to the normal ageing process.

Furthermore, there is a lack of coordination in the healthcare circuits for dementia patients. Many specialists (e.g. neurologists, psychiatrists, psychologists, speech therapists, nurses) in the field of dementia care work without networking. This makes it difficult for patients and their families to be aware of the various specialized services offered, especially in case of an emergency. Moreover, families are not sufficiently informed and guided through the institutions.

At the second and third levels of care, very few structures are adapted to the special needs of dementia patients. In recent years, geriatric units have been created within some departments of internal medicine, each containing a few hospital beds. However, these by no means cover the actual needs. For the time being, no department of geriatric psychiatry exists in Tunisia. In case of a psychiatric decompensation of dementia, the patient is admitted to a department of adult psychiatry and placed with patients suffering from schizophrenia or bipolar disorder. This kind of admission can be very unfavourable to dementia patients.

Furthermore, there are some public residential care facilities for elderly people without family support, but these facilities are not adapted to the special needs of dementia patients, and needs by far exceed demand.

In the private sector, many different facilities have emerged during the past 10 years, mainly day clinics and residential care facilities. However, most of these facilities are not specially designed for dementia patients. Moreover, the offerings are very confusing, and there are great variations in quality as nation-wide quality standards have not yet been established.

Another challenge is the financial burden of dementia for the family, as well as for society as a whole. So far, no study on the financial impact of dementia has been conducted in Tunisia. However, what we do know is that currently, families of dementia patients have to assume the main burden of the cost of the illness. Most types of dementia, in particular AD, are not included in the list of chronic severe diseases that are fully covered by national health insurance. This means that only partial coverage is granted, and this only for some medications. Professional help at home or in private care facilities are not covered by national health insurance.

The increasing difficulties faced by many families in providing care and the desire to raise public awareness led to the creation of the Alzheimer Association in 2006. This association is affiliated with Alzheimer's Disease International and aims, through education and lobbying, to improve the care for dementia patients.

Cultural specificities of dementia care in Tunisia

The care for dementia patients is mainly provided by family members. In the traditional Arabic society, members of the extended family live close together, with the elderly enjoying great respect. Until now, family care for the elderly and ill family members is considered a duty, and society does not accept that caregiving is performed by a person that is a 'stranger' to the family, even if these are neighbours or friends. Societal norms also reject placement of the ill family member into residential care; it would be perceived as neglect or rejection. However, with the adoption of more westernized lifestyles, the growing mobility of people, the changing working environment, and the formation of the nuclear family as the main family structure, looking after family members with chronic and deteriorating diseases becomes challenging. A study conducted in 2013 at the Department of Neurology and the Alzheimer Centre of the Razi University Hospital characterized the profile of the typical Tunisian caregiver of an AD patient [4]. It is a daughter or a daughter-in-law, in their fifties, looking after the ill parent between 12 and 24 hours per day. Two-thirds of caregivers did not have any other person with them to provide informal help, and only 5% of caregivers had professional help. Socio-professional consequences were common, with 65% of caretakers describing problems in their marriages and 35% having lost their jobs due to the care situation. The subjective burden of the Tunisian caregiver is very high. Compared to Western countries, the Tunisian caregivers are younger, are all family members, spend more hours per day caregiving, and have a burden at the upper end of the scores described in the literature. Indeed, 41% of caregivers wish to place their family member into residential care and deplore the absence of specially adapted residential care facilities in Tunisia.

Most families do not accept placing their family member into long-term residential care and prefer looking after them at home; however, they wish to utilize short-term residential care facilities in order to be able to recover from the constraints of caregiving or in case of an acute family problem if need be.

The future of dementia care in Tunisia

Given the current challenges in dementia care, there is a growing awareness of the need for coordinated measures provided by the government, as well as healthcare professionals. Indeed, a National Dementia Strategy is currently being developed. This strategy will evolve in several directions:

♦ To facilitate early diagnosis, optimize healthcare circuits, and improve services for dementia patients and their families.

♦ To develop training for healthcare professionals in order to acquire specific competencies in dementia.

♦ To anticipate the needs of patients and caregivers and improve their support in order to alleviate the moral and financial burden of the illness.

♦ To promote epidemiological and clinical research in the field of dementia.

In Arab and Muslim societies, the elderly are revered and are entitled to the best care from their families and society at large. This is why we are confident that a National Dementia Strategy will be implemented that would include significant progress in the field and be adapted to the cultural environment. This Strategy would incorporate considerable involvement of family members who should remain the cornerstone of the management of dementia patients.

References

1. **Institut National de la Statistique.** *Base de données.* Available from: http://dataportal. ins.tn/ [accessed 26 May 2016].
2. **Hajem S, Saidi O, Ben Mansour N, Mejdoub Y, Hsairi M.** [Épidémiologie des démences en Tunisie]. *NPG Neurologie—Psychiatrie—Gériatrie.* 2014;**14**: 326–33.
3. **Launer LJ, Anderson K, Dewey ME,** *et al.* Rates and risk factors for dementia and Alzheimer's disease. Results from EURODEM pooled analyses. *Neurology.* 1999;**52**:78–84.
4. **Ben Ghzaiel I.** [*Le fardeau des aidants naturels des patients atteints de maladie d'Alzheimer*] (unpublished dissertation). Tunis: University of Tunis-El Manar; 2014.

Section 2

Asia

Chapter 5

China

Huali Wang and Hengge Xie

Summary

With an ageing population, dementia care has become a great challenge in China. This chapter reviews the current major resources in dementia care in China. Memory clinics are the primary setting for diagnosis and management. Caregiver support groups and social media provide mainstream support to caregivers. This chapter also highlights the role of the community in dementia care. Community services are essential to health education, dementia screening, and home care support. In addition, the chapter discusses the role of collaborative research networks and point out that both research on services and dementia prevention are important. The chapter concludes by calling for action to address the priorities of dementia care.

Epidemiology and burden of dementia in China

By the end of 2014, the population of China aged 65 and above had grown to 137 million, accounting for 10.1% of the total population.[1] The prevalence of dementia in China has thus increased considerably from 1980s to 2010s [1]. It is estimated that approximately 9.19 million persons live with dementia in China [2]. Among the different types of dementia, AD is the commonest in China [3]. The 10/66 Dementia Research Group reported the incidence of dementia in China to be 24.0 [95% confidence interval (CI) 20.6–28.1] per 1000 person-years [4]. Although it is difficult to assess the contribution of dementia to mortality, the hazard ratio (HR) was calculated to be 3.02 (95% CI 2.13–4.28) in urban China and 3.59 (95% CI 2.47–5.21) in rural China [4].

---

[1] http://www.stats.gov.cn/tjsj/zxfb/201502/t20150226_685799.html

The journey of dementia care is challenging, with significant economic burden, caregiver distress, and increasing service demands [5, 6]. For example, the caregiver's time spent on personal activities of daily living (PADL) recorded using the Resource Utilization in Dementia (RUD) scale was 25 hours per month in mild cases and 172 hours per month in severe cases.

Service resources for dementia care

In China, people with cognitive impairment usually seek medical help from neurologists, psychiatrists, or geriatricians. Alzheimer's Disease Chinese (ADC), a member of Alzheimer's Disease International (ADI), is a leading non-profit organization that promotes dementia care in China. In 2014, the ADC Consensus on Memory Check-up proposed that screening for cognitive disorders be included in the annual wellness check-up plan [7]. The memory clinic is the optimal setting for comprehensive assessment and evaluation to enable diagnosis and management, as well as follow-up, in dementia care. More than 100 memory clinics have been set up in China, which could provide minimum service for people with dementia, including cognitive screening and assessment, neuroimaging examination, and medications. In major cities, such as Beijing, Guangzhou, Shanghai, and Hangzhou, medical professionals have also applied every effort to run dementia caregiver support groups. Lately, care support has often been provided via social media such as WeChat groups.

Building community-based care for dementia

In China, the current elderly care system primarily depends on family care and community-based social services. Commercially available care systems may not be affordable to the majority of the elderly population in China. The National Aging Committee has declared the importance and urgency of building elderly-friendly communities and a home care service system.[2] These strategies may, to some extent, urge society as a whole to be engaged in community-based services for the elderly.

The majority of people with dementia are cared for at home. As it is in Chinese tradition, as a sense of duty, and as an example to set for children, filial obligation and reciprocity are the two main philosophical underpinnings for caring for the elderly in China [8]. Thus, providing support to people living with dementia and their families is important for dementia care to be successful and effective. More specific strategies are, however, needed in order to

[2] http://shfl.mca.gov.cn/article/zcfg/zonghe/201610/20161000887130.shtml

build high-level readiness for dementia care in the community. For example, the quality indicators for community-based dementia care should be developed and validated in the Chinese context.

Community understanding and responsiveness are at the very initial stage, and public awareness of mental health problems is quite low [9]. In China, health education and promotion campaigns have had an impact on improving dementia literacy and raising public awareness. In many cities, public lectures and group consultations are commonly organized, particularly during World Alzheimer's Month, by health providers, social workers, and volunteers. Efforts to raise awareness of dementia have met with considerable public acceptance, including among community-dwelling elderly, nursing home residents, college students, social welfare staff, and the media.

Research on dementia care

In major cities, AD centres or collaborative networks have also been set up by well-established institutions such as the National Geriatric Mood and Cognitive Impairment Initiative led by the National Clinical Research Center for Mental Disorders (Peking University). Collaborative networks aim to explore the potential biomarkers for early diagnosis of AD and mild cognitive impairment (MCI), which may, in turn, be candidates for clinical trials on anti-dementia agents.

In addition, efforts to explore effective approaches to dementia care in the community have also received more attention from the local government. For example, an integrated care model in which social workers, community health workers, and memory specialists work together to promote cognitive screening, timely diagnosis, and post-diagnosis care support has been proposed. Evaluation of its effectiveness is currently under way.

Prevention of dementia remains a hot topic in public health. In China, MCI, a presumed pre-dementia state, affects nearly 20% of the elderly population [10, 11]. Addressing modifiable risk factors may be an important approach to reducing the onset of dementia. A multi-domain intervention of diet, exercise, cognitive training, and vascular risk monitoring may prevent cognitive decline in at-risk elderly people [12]. Whether the multi-domain intervention is culturally appropriate and able to reduce the conversion of MCI to dementia is being addressed in further ongoing investigations in China [13].

Future perspectives

With an increase in the ageing population and the number of people with dementia, more efforts should be made to address the grand challenge of dementia. First, we need to improve access to a timely diagnosis and post-diagnosis care support. Second, social and medical care should be integrated in multidisciplinary teams to provide comprehensive and holistic care for persons with dementia. Last, but not least, collaborative efforts from relevant stakeholders should advocate for policy development, e.g. development of a National Dementia Plan, and implementation, e.g. inclusion of specific action points in the National Mental Health Plan. Prioritizing dementia care on the policy development agenda will eventually pave the way for the implementation of the WHO Global Dementia Action Plan in China.

References

1. Jia J, Wang F, Wei C, *et al.* The prevalence of dementia in urban and rural areas of China. *Alzheimer's and Dementia.* 2014;**10**:1–9.
2. Chan KY, Wang W, Wu JJ, *et al.* Epidemiology of Alzheimer's disease and other forms of dementia in China, 1990–2010: a systematic review and analysis. *The Lancet.* 2013;**381**:2016–23.
3. Zhang ZX, Zahner GE, Roman GC, *et al.* Dementia subtypes in China: prevalence in Beijing, Xian, Shanghai, and Chengdu. *Archives of Neurology.* 2005;**62**:447–53.
4. Prince M, Acosta D, Ferri CP, *et al.* Dementia incidence and mortality in middle-income countries, and associations with indicators of cognitive reserve: a 10/66 Dementia Research Group population-based cohort study. *The Lancet.* 2012;**380**:50–8.
5. Wang G, Cheng Q, Zhang S, *et al.* Economic impact of dementia in developing countries: an evaluation of Alzheimer-type dementia in Shanghai, China. *Journal of Alzheimer's Disease.* 2008;**15**:109–15.
6. Wang H, Gao T, Wimo A, Yu X. Caregiver time and cost of home care for Alzheimer's disease: a clinic-based observational study in Beijing, China. *Ageing International.* 2010;**35**:153–65.
7. Xie H, Tian J, Wang L; ADC Expert Panel. ADC Consensus on memory check-up. *Chinese Journal of Internal Medicine.* 2014;**53**:1002–6.
8. Xiong Q, Wang H, Wang H, Chen B. Sociocultural beliefs on caregiver for the elderly in Chinese rural area. *Chinese Journal of Gerontology.* 2011;**31**:669–71.
9. Li X, Fang W, Su N, Liu Y, Xiao S, Xiao Z. Survey in Shanghai communities: the public awareness of and attitude towards dementia. *Psychogeriatrics.* 2011;**11**:83–9.
10. Jia J, Zhou A, Wei C, *et al.* The prevalence of mild cognitive impairment and its etiological subtypes in elderly Chinese. *Alzheimer's and Dementia.* 2014;**10**:439–47.
11. Ding D, Zhao Q, Guo Q, *et al.* Prevalence of mild cognitive impairment in an urban community in China: a cross-sectional analysis of the Shanghai Aging Study. *Alzheimer's and Dementia.* 2015;**11**:300–9 e302.
12. Ngandu T, Lehtisalo J, Solomon A, *et al.* A 2-year multidomain intervention of diet, exercise, cognitive training, and vascular risk monitoring versus control to prevent cognitive decline in at-risk elderly people (FINGER): a randomised controlled trial. *The Lancet.* 2015;**385**:2255–63.
13. Yu X, Wang H. Development and perspectives of geriatric psychiatry in China. *Chinese Journal of Psychiatry.* 2015;**48**:151–3.

Chapter 6

India

Santosh K Chaturvedi and Sundarnag Ganjekar

Summary

A number of traditional and socio-cultural factors are involved in the care of the elderly in general, as well as those with dementia, in India. Dementia care has attracted attention recently and is making rapid progress. There is no clarity on whether dementia care should be provided by psychiatrists, neurologists, or general physicians. Nursing care and home care are far from being well developed. Special clinics are few, and specialized centres for dementia care even fewer. Community care is still a distant dream. Family and social support, on the other hand, stands as a natural resource. Society and policymakers are now providing due attention to improving the care of the elderly with dementia, as well as their caregivers.

Growing older in Indian culture

In Indian mythology, the ancient Hindu scriptures categorize life into four phases: *Brahmacharya* (studentship, celibate), *Grihastha* (householder), *Vanaprastha* (retired), and *Sanyasa* (renunciation). Indian culture stresses upon growing older gracefully. Older people are given the highest rank in the family hierarchy. Their blessings and help are sought when taking decisions on important matters. Dementia is known as *vismriti* (loss of retention and memory). *Ayurveda* predominantly focuses on the prevention of dementia through various natural and traditional methods.

Dementia: problem statement in India

With the availability of better healthcare facilities and increasing life expectancy in India, the population of those above 60 years of age in 2016 was 103.9 million.

In recent times, India has witnessed a gradual, but definite, decline in the joint family systems, as a result of which a large proportion of the elderly population are neglected by their families, leaving the elderly exposed to a lack of emotional, physical, and financial support. There is no social security system for senior citizens.

Currently, it is estimated that 4.1 million people aged above 60 have dementia, with an expected rise to about 7 million by 2020 and rapidly escalating to reach 13–14 million by 2050. One in every 16 households with an elderly person has an elderly individual with dementia [1]. A 1-year prospective study found the incidence of dementia to be 5.34/1000 person-years [2]. Another study reported the incidence of AD to be 11.67/1000 population-years in those above 55 years and 11.54/1000 population-years in those above 65 years [3].

Efforts towards a National Dementia Strategy in India

A National Consultative Meeting of experts to develop a National Dementia Strategy was first held in 2009, organized by the Alzheimer's and Related Disorders Society of India (ARDSI), in association with the Centre for Physiotherapy and Rehabilitation Sciences. The ARDSI is a national voluntary organization dedicated to the care, support, and research of dementia. Three main areas needing to be addressed in India were discussed:

1. To raise better awareness of dementia among the general public and medical professionals.

2. To encourage early diagnosis and treatment.

3. To improve the quality of care of those affected and their caregivers.

Subsequently, the first *Dementia India Report* was released on World Alzheimer's Day in 2010 [1]. The ARDSI has been at the forefront of bringing to the government ministry's attention the needs of people with dementia. It is concentrating efforts in recognizing dementia as a disability of the elderly, so that the latter are placed on a par with people with other handicaps and resources are reallocated in a more equitable manner. As part of the next 5-year plan is the recognition of AD and other types of dementia as a disability. Memory clinics will be established at a district level for early diagnosis and management of dementia. Funds to support day care, respite care, long-term care, and home-based care for people with dementia, as well as for training of medical and allied healthcare professionals on dementia management, will be provided.

The Indian Government's Ministry of Social Justice and Empowerment has revised the Integrated Programme for Older Persons. The main objective of this revised scheme is to improve the quality of life of the older person by providing basic amenities like shelter, food, medical care, and entertainment opportunities and by encouraging productive and active ageing through providing support for capacity building of governmental organizations and NGOs, Panchayati Raj Institutions, local bodies, and the community at large. This or any other programme does not specify about a National Dementia Strategy in India.

There has been some research on 'dementia' in India, with PubMed listing 703 articles published in the last 5 years. The Indian Council for Medical Research (ICMR) has funded 53 extramural projects on the subject of 'geriatrics', of which 36 are clinical studies and the rest are molecular studies. Overall, it seems that research in the field of dementia is scarce, and an insufficient research output has failed to establish the need for a National Dementia Strategy in India.

Other reasons include: low awareness of dementia among the general public and medical professionals; early signs of dementia being neglected by family members who consider them as part of normal ageing; memory loss often being part of family humour; family members not seeking specialist consultation unless there are significant behavioural problems; and reversible causes of dementia not being treated early.

What are you particularly proud of in dementia care?

Social support

The traditional Indian joint family system is a great boon to the care of people with dementia. In a classical joint family system, more than three generations live together. This type of joint family system is highly essential where care is needed for a person suffering from dementia. The joint family system acts like a shock absorber.

Government support

The government of India provides a 'senior citizen card' to all individuals aged 60 years and above. Concessions and facilities are given to senior citizens by the government's different ministries. Specific programmes for the care of people with dementia are in development.

Non-governmental organizations

The role of NGOs is huge in the care of people with dementia in India. The ARDSI, Help Age India, Silver Innings, Nightingale, and many other NGOs provide support to people with dementia, including home-based care. Many families, especially in the states of Kerala and Tamil Nadu, have established self-help groups to care for people with dementia.

Role of complementary and alternative medicine

There are many forms of complementary and alternative medicine which place emphasis on the practice of healthy living. Yoga, meditation, naturopathy, and lifestyle modifications are widely practised by the elderly population in India [4]. Some methods using complementary and alternative medicines claim to treat and cure dementia; however, these claims have not been verified in modern clinical trials.

Clinical services for the geriatric population

Many public and private hospitals provide specialized care for the geriatric population. Most hospitals are disabled- and elderly-friendly. The first geriatric mental health department was established in 2005 at King George Medical University in Lucknow. Many other institutions have a geriatric clinic which runs either weekly or monthly. Since 2000, the Department of Psychiatry at the National Institute of Mental Health and Neuro-Sciences (NIMHANS) in Bangalore has been providing both inpatient and outpatient clinical services dedicated exclusively to old age. This specialized service at NIMHANS adopts a multidisciplinary approach, with neurology, psychiatry, psychology, and psychiatric social work teams working together in providing care for the elderly.

Manpower and resource development in geriatric medicine

The Geriatric Society of India and the Indian Association for Geriatric Mental Health (IAGMH) are registered NGOs dedicated to the cause of the elderly in India and publish the *Indian Journal of Geriatric Care* and *Journal of Indian Association for Geriatric Mental Health*, respectively. Geriatric medicine is developing as a specialized branch in the field of medicine, psychiatry, and neurology. The Indira Gandhi National Open University offers a Post-Graduate Diploma in Geriatric Medicine, and the King George Medical University now confers the degree of Doctor of Medicine (DM) in geriatric mental health. Moreover, the NIMHANS in Bangalore also offers Doctor of Medicine (DM) in Geriatric Psychiatry and a 1-year Post-Doctoral Fellowship in geriatric psychiatry.

Current challenges in dementia care in India and the way forward

The main challenges in dementia care in India are:

+ *Disability limitation in early and late dementia:* around two-thirds of India's population live in rural areas where resources are limited. Migration of younger generations to urban areas in seek of employment leaves the elderly population facing neglect, which, in turn, makes them psychologically weakened. If they develop an illness such as dementia, their medical condition will progress faster because of a lack of stimulation and treatment.

India has a very good healthcare system operating at the community level. The Accredited Social Health Activist (ASHA) workers make house-to-house visits in villages, covering a population size of around 1000. These workers need to be informed about dementia, its signs and symptoms, and how to make appropriate referrals to the nearest primary health centre. Manuals on home-based care and skills development should be made available at all primary health centres. Caregivers of the elderly experience considerable burden in their role, especially if the elderly is in the late stages of dementia [6]. It is therefore essential that caregivers are monitored periodically for stress and depression.

- *Early detection:* it is important to detect dementia in its early stages to mitigate its progression and prevent disability. Many young caregivers consider the early symptoms of dementia in the elderly as normal or they make fun of the elderly's forgetfulness, rather than taking them to the doctor.

One of the ways of increasing awareness of dementia is public education. Starting from primary education itself, the importance of geriatric health needs to be emphasized. Secondary education should focus on positive mental health of the elderly. Higher education should focus on the early signs and symptoms of dementia and preventive measures. At the community level, mass media and social media can play a crucial role. Caregivers should have the opportunity to set up self-help groups, which will provide them social and emotional support. Community-based care should be preferred.

- *At the level of policymaking:* in policymaking, all key stakeholders should be actively involved, including health providers, resource-allocating authorities, and intended recipients of the policy and representatives of the general population. NGOs should play an important role in bringing these key players together. A national dementia policy should provide direction to the government in designing appropriate health programmes, which can be implemented at a national level. Piloting the programme will give an insight into any implementation-related issues.

- *Prevention and specific protection:* India has a rich tradition of healthy lifestyle practices. There is huge scope for conducting relevant research, especially on identifying protective and preventive factors in dementia. Public awareness of the importance of lifestyle modifications in the prevention of dementia in the elderly needs to be emphasized. Currently, there are no specific evidence-based protective measures in dementia. Thus, further research is warranted to determine the specific protective measures in the prevention of dementia.

Future of dementia care in India

Prevention is vital. Health promotion, lifestyle modifications, and specific protective measures play a pivotal role in the prevention of dementia. Any symptom suggestive of memory deficits should be taken seriously and assessed by a doctor. Medical comorbidities, such as hypertension, diabetes, hyperchol-esterolaemia, vitamin deficiencies, and thyroid deficiencies, should be detected early and treated appropriately. Any possibility of neglect or abuse should be considered and investigated. This information about prevention and early de-tection of dementia should be made available across all forms of mass media (television, newspapers, radio), social media (e.g. Facebook, Twitter), and in-stant messaging services (e.g. WhatsApp). Public places and services should be made senior citizen-friendly. Early diagnosis and prompt treatment of de-mentia should be the key objective. Not only will it improve the quality of life of the elderly person, but it will also significantly reduce the caregiver burden. The family should be given help and support to spend time with the elderly with dementia. Stress is common among caregivers of dementia patients. Caregivers should be given the opportunity to meet each other and to use social media where face-to-face meetings are difficult. Caregivers should also be encouraged to share their difficulties [5]. In cases where the elderly with dementia has be-havioural disturbances, appropriate use of psychotropic medications, in con-sultation with psychiatrists, will help in managing the behavioural problems, as well as reducing the caregiver burden. Research should focus on early markers of dementia and how the disease can be prevented.

References

1. Shaji KS, Jotheeswaran AT, Girish N, et al. (eds.); on behalf of Alzheimer's and Related Disorders Society of India (ARDSI). *The Dementia India Report: prevalence, impact, costs and services for dementia*. New Delhi: ARDSI; 2010.
2. Raina SK, Pandita KK, Razdan S. Incidence of dementia in a Kashmiri migrant population. *Annals of Indian Academy of Neurology*. 2009;**12**:154–6.
3. Mathuranath PS, George A, Ranjith N, et al. Incidence of Alzheimer's disease in India: a 10 years follow-up study. *Neurology India*. 2012;**60**:625–30.
4. Verma V (ed). *Prevention of dementia with yogic and ayurvedic methods*. Occasional publication 18. New Delhi: India International Centre; 2015.
5. Chaturvedi SK. Quality of life of caregivers of people with dementia—report of an international collaborative study. Report from center in India. *Acta Medica Nagasakiensia*. 1999;**44** Supplement:18–20.

Chapter 7

Indonesia

Raden Irawati Ismail, Bastaman Basuki,
Martina Wiwie Setiawan Nasrun, and
Fidiansjah Mursjid

Summary

A comprehensive dementia service delivery is not well established
in Indonesia, even though geriatric teams have been in place
since 1997. Psycho-geriatric services are mainly provided by
departments of psychiatry, as well as the geriatric division
of internal medicine or neurology departments. Screening is
routinely performed using the Mini-Mental State Examination
and the Abbreviated Mental Test. In the near future, the division
of geriatric psychiatry in psychiatry departments will have
comprehensive services for dementia, from initial assessment
to cognitive and functional rehabilitation. This will comprise
screening, home visits, day care, home care, educational seminars,
and specific programmes tailored to the needs of the person with
dementia. Pre-dementia detection and any activities promoting
active ageing should be prioritized in Indonesia.

Background

Dementia is characterized by reduced memory ability and at least one domain
of cognitive impairment, including language, visuospatial, or executive functioning. It must cause daily activity impairment that affects the individual's
socio-occupational functioning. The two commonest causes of dementia are
AD and cerebrovascular disease [1, 2].

The condition of pre-dementia in ageing, which is a transitional condition
from a normal state to dementia, needs to be detected in people belonging to the
'brain-at-risk' group. Pre-dementia can progress to dementia within 5–6 years
and is characterized by 'forgetfulness', a decline in thinking and communication

ability, and difficulties with formulating ideas, decision-making, and anticipation of events [1]. The difference between dementia and pre-dementia is that the latter shows no impairment in activities of daily living. The Centre for Ageing Studies (CAS) of the University of Indonesia in Depok, Indonesia, conducts research, organizes joint activities for the elderly, and visits retirement homes across Indonesia.

In setting up primary services and health posts for health service provision, including mental health services to the elderly, transfer of knowledge was included as part of training. It was also important to demonstrate and emphasize the global burden of dementia to support the Ministry of Health's National Strategy for Dementia that was published in 2015 in Indonesia.

Dementia studies in Indonesia

We have carried out a number of studies in dementia, and a summary of these is given as follows:

1. A modified Hopkins verbal learning test detected 37% of respondents in Candi Borobudur, Central Java, Indonesia and 39% of Indonesian Hajj aged 60–74 years in Mecca and Medina. Pre-dementia was identified by using 'The Non-dementia Cognitive Disability Scoring Book'; comorbidity of pre-dementia and diabetes mellitus were detected in 54% of subjects. Thirty-four medical professionals (psychiatrists, doctors, mental health nurses) were trained in the use of the Cognitive Status Detection Module: Elderly in Rural Areas, to provide services to the elderly in the primary care setting.

2. Early detection of non-dementia cognitive disability in type 2 diabetes mellitus patients: the Clinical-epidemiological, Psychometric, and Magnetic Resonance Spectroscopic Approach Study was one of the studies conducted in the last 10 years in the Endocrine and Geriatric Integrated Clinic Cipto Mangunkusumo Hospital (RSCM). The sample population comprised a total of 199 patients aged 45–47 years. The proportion of pre-dementia patients was 45%, with a mean age of 56 years. A total of 48 patients (54%) were found to have comorbidity of pre-dementia and diabetes mellitus. Of the 199 patients, 7 (4%) had dementia. These study results should draw the attention of relevant stakeholders, especially those responsible for health management in the elderly [1].

3. Dementia screening for active ageing in Indonesia by using a reliable Dementia Questionnaire Study. This was a pilot study conducted in the Candi Borobudur area in Central Java, Indonesia and the Soeharto Heerdjan Mental Hospital in Jakarta, Indonesia, including 59 subjects, of whom 70% were women. The majority of subjects were aged 65 years (60–100 years), and

54% had a low educational level. This dementia questionnaire was found to clinically diagnose 71% of subjects as not having dementia (specificity) and thus has been shown to a reliable screening tool for dementia [3]. The aim of this screening questionnaire was to enable medical professionals in the primary care setting to easily and quickly make a clinical diagnosis of dementia.

4. Effectivity of Cognitive Status and Quality of Life of the Elderly Assessment Model in Primary Health Service in the Rural Area Study. This was conducted in the Candi Borobudur area in Central Java, Indonesia and included 113 respondents, with a mean age of 72.8 years (60–100 years), of whom 33% had a clinical diagnosis of dementia. This clinical diagnosis was used as the golden standard of reliability and validity testing of the modified Hopkins verbal learning test (HVLTm), which has been modified for the Indonesian population. The HVLTm showed validity with 70% sensitivity and 92% specificity, with a cut-off point of 14.5 (≤14 = dementia; >14 = non-dementia), and detected dementia in 37% respondents [2].

5. The quality of life was measured using the European Quality of Life-5 Dimension (EQ-5D), with Cronbach's alpha of 0.878. Health professionals in the primary care setting were trained and guided until they were deemed proficient to use the HVLTm and EQ-5D. The EQ-5D scores are as follows: 1 = no problem; 2 = few problems; 3 = major problem; the EQ-5D dimensions are given as: EQ-1 = mobility; EQ-2 = self-care; EQ-3 = daily activities; EQ-4 = pain/discomfort; EQ-5 = anxiety/depression. The results of this study are shown in Table 7.1.1.

6. The Application of Hopkins Verbal Learning Test by Hajj Health Officers to Detect Dementia in Elderly Pilgrims in Mecca and Medina Year 1436 H/2015 M Study. This was based on the 2013 database, including 22% of 156,466 Indonesian pilgrims aged over 60 years. Of note, in 2015, dementia was detected in a high proportion of Indonesian pilgrims. Through gradual transfer of knowledge (training, guiding, competence), Indonesia's hajj health officers (psychiatrists, GPs, and mental health nurses) were able to use

Table 7.1 Detailed scoring of each EQ-5D dimension

	EQ-1	EQ-2	EQ-3	EQ-4	EQ-5
Score 1	83 (73.5%)	101 (89.4%)	89 (78.8%)	37 (32.7%)	83 (73.5%)
Score 2	30 (26.5%)	11 (9.7%)	21 (18.6%)	66 (58.4%)	22 (19.5%)
Score 3	0 (0%)	1 (0.9%)	3 (2.7%)	10 (8.8%)	8 (7%)
Total	113 (100%)	113 (100%)	113 (100%)	113 (100%)	113 (100%)

the HVLTm to detect dementia in Indonesian pilgrims aged over 60 years. The setting of the study was in the Indonesian treatment hall and hajj service sectors in Mecca and Medina. As many as 101 individual HVLTm scores were collected, of which 39% were identified as dementia in the elderly group (60–74 years). These results demonstrated an easy, compact, and simple dementia detection tool that can be used by all Indonesia's hajj organizers [4].

Training of health professionals in the primary care setting and health cadres in health posts to assist health services for the elderly

The Cognitive Status Detection Module: for Elderly in Rural Area has been proven to be valid and reliable for use in the primary care setting [5]. In addition, a book on the Mental Health of the Elderly Module also gained appreciation from the Directorate of Innovation and Business Incubator of the University of Indonesia in 2015.

1. The Validity Test and Reliability of Cognitive Status Module: Elderly in Rural Area study. A total of 34 respondents, including psychiatrists, doctors, and nurses, were trained in the Cognitive Status Module: Elderly in Rural Area. Pre- and post-test item assessment showed Cronbach's alpha of 0.969, thus rated as reliable. The correlation range of an item to total items was 0.985–0.989, meaning that the pre-/post-test items are usable. Cognitive evaluation [mean pre-test 11.71 (8–15), mean post-test 17.24 (15–20)] showed a significant difference ($P <0.05$) [5].

Joint activities by the elderly in Indonesia

Social activities were organized by the CAS, including visits to retirement homes in several places across Indonesia. The CAS also sought funding from relevant resources and provided routine and scheduled health counselling, including counselling on 'stress and its prevention in the elderly', followed by discussions, conveying feelings ('curhat'), and consultation. Thus, the elderly had the opportunity to participate in sport activities together such as walking and attending physical gym and brain gym. These activities also included tea and snack breaks and ended with lunch [6].

Global description of the burden of dementia

Evidence is continuously needed for planning health services and health requirements and monitoring the mechanisms of dementia. Until now, there have been no systematic efforts for global data collection, including in Indonesia, as an effort to reduce the dementia burden. The efforts made so far have focused on reviewing and synthesizing the prevalence data on dementia globally. It is estimated that the prevalence of dementia in the world has reached 47 million and may reach 75 million by 2030 [7].

It is estimated that 60% of people with dementia live in middle- to low-income countries. This proportion is projected to increase within the next decade, which will widen the gap between the countries and their population [7].

The goal of the National Strategy of Dementia in Indonesia

To counter the development of AD and other types of dementia in the elderly is toward an emphasis for healthy and productive older population. In order to achieve this goal, the strategies used are: (1) to channel efforts to maintain a healthy brain for a productive older population, with a life cycle approach at each level on a national scale, (2) to improve the quality of services for cognitive and dementia disorders, and (3) to manage reinforcement in the efforts to optimally achieve a healthy brain [8].

The Seven Steps of Action

1. Conducting public awareness campaigns and promoting a healthy lifestyle.
2. Advocating human rights for people with dementia and families and caregivers.
3. Ensuring accessibility to, and information from, qualified health services.
4. Implementing early detection, diagnosis, and holistic management for cognitive problems and dementia.
5. Using a human resources reinforcement system professionally and continuously.
6. Having in place a cognitive health programme reinforcement system as the main driving force for educating the nation, with a life cycle approach.
7. Conducting research, and making use of research findings, in cognitive and dementia [8].

Future plan

The plan for the future in Indonesia is to implement the National Strategy of Dementia, collecting various research data on policies and providers and recipients of dementia services, as well as its negative and positive aspects, finding ways to address challenges and measure success, preventing and controlling dementia in Indonesia, and participating in consultations with the Global Dementia Observatory [7].

Conclusion

In this limited study, it can be concluded that: (1) in individuals aged 45–75 years, 45% had pre-dementia and 54% of type 2 diabetes mellitus patients had pre-dementia, (2) among those aged 60–100 years, 33% were clinically diagnosed with dementia, and (3) in Indonesian pilgrims aged 60–74 years, 39% were identified as having dementia using the HVLTm. Although only limited study findings and joint activities of the elderly were presented, this report marks the beginning of other reports on dementia in Indonesia. We expect there will be more reports, given the growing number of studies on dementia, which has become a national priority since it is written in the Ministry of Health's National Strategy.

References

1. **Nasrun MWS.** *Early detection of non-dementia cognitive disability in type 2 diabetes mellitus patients: clinical-epidemiological, psychometric, and magnetic resonance spectroscopic approach study.* Dissertation. Depok: Faculty of Medicine, University of Indonesia; 2007.

2. **Mursjid F.** *Effectivity of cognitive status and quality of life of the elderly assessment model in primary health service in the rural area study.* Dissertation. Depok: Faculty of Medicine, University of Indonesia; 2010.

3. **Ismail RI, Mansyur M, Fidiansyah, Marsubrin PMT, Rahardjo TB, Hogervorst E.** *Dementia screening for active aging in Indonesia by using a reliable dementia questionnaire.* Fukuoka Active Aging Conference in Asia Pacific 2010: Towards Age-friendly Communities, 30–31 October 2010. Fukuoka, Japan; 2010.

4. **Ismail RI, Mursjid F, Mawardi E, Ariffin S.** *The application of Hopkins Verbal Learning Test by hajj health officers to detect dementia in elderly pilgrims in Mecca and Medina year 1436 H/2015 M study.* Hajj Health Centre reports. Jakarta: Ministry of Health of the Republic of Indonesia; 2015.

5. **Ismail RI, Fidiansyah, Hogervost E, Rahardjo TBW, Agustin D.** *Validity test and reliability of cognitive status module: elderly in rural area.* The 8th Busan Active Aging Conference in Asia Pasific, June 2013. Busan: Indonesia; 2013.

6. **Ismail RI.** *Stress and its prevention in the elderly,* 13 December 2013. Depok: Centre of Ageing Studies, University of Indonesia; 2013.

7. **World Health Organization Global Dementia Observatory.** *A global dementia observatory: concept note.* Geneva: World Health Organization; 2015.

8. **Ministry of Health of the Republic of Indonesia.** *National Strategy. Countermeasures Alzheimer's disease and other dementias: towards the elderly healthy and productive.* Jakarta: Ministry of Health of the Republic of Indonesia; 2015.

Chapter 8

Japan

Yumi Shindo and Akira Homma

Summary

There are two strengths of dementia care services available in
Japan. One strength is the creation of the Integrated Community
Care System, which aims to provide various services that the
elderly might need within their areas of residence. It is the
responsibility of local governments to set up the ICCS, because
each community has different social resources, as well as
differences in the local population and the number of elderly
individuals. The other strength lies in the various educational
opportunities in dementia available to medical and long-term
care professionals. In 2001, the national government introduced
educational programmes for care workers in the field of dementia
care. In addition, educational programmes for medical doctors,
managers of facilities/service centres for people with dementia,
medical professionals working in hospitals, pharmacists, and
dentists are currently provided under the government's policies.

Introduction

In 2016, the proportion of senior citizens in the population of Japan was 27.3%
and is expected to reach 37.7% by 2050 [1]. Moreover, the number of people
above 65 years of age and suffering from dementia was approximately 5.17 million in 2015; this is projected to increase to 7.97 million in 2050, while the population in Japan is expected to decrease. Therefore, a shortage of professionals
involved in dementia care is set to become a major problem in the near future.

To tackle this problem, as well as to build communities where people with
dementia can live safely and independently, a national public campaign called
'Dementia Supporter' has been run since 2005. The purpose of this campaign
initially was to improve the public's understanding of dementia and to remove
the stigma associated with the disease. This has led to many supporters of the

campaign nowadays actively finding ways to support their community. Thus, the campaign has resulted in a process of building a social capital for people with dementia, giving them more opportunities to establish and maintain connections within their community.

To respect and reflect the ideas and suggestions from people with dementia has been the key pillar of the New Orange Plan. Examples include a local government working closely with a person with dementia in the creation of a booklet on dementia care pathways, and a day service centre providing various work opportunities for its members, all of whom have dementia.

This strategy will change the future of dementia care in Japan. People with dementia will no longer be regarded as 'people who need help'. Rather, they will become themselves policymakers and advocators who will build age- and dementia-friendly communities.

History of welfare policies for the elderly and the National Dementia Strategy

Since World War II, the population in Japan has increased rapidly, and the Japanese government has been promoting social welfare laws and policies for the elderly, according to the size of its elderly population. In reviewing the history of welfare policies for the elderly in Japan, particularly with regard to dementia care, three major periods are noted: (1) before implementation of the national Long-Term Care Insurance (LTCI) (before 2000) when the government established basic laws and regulations, (2) after implementation of the LTCI (from 2000 to 2014) when dementia care changed from institutionalized care to person-centred care, and (3) implementation of the National Dementia Strategy (after 2015) (see Table 8.1).

Before the implementation of the national LTCI, the government had established basic laws and regulations for the care of the elderly. In 1963, the Act on Social Welfare for the Elderly was enacted. Prior to this Act, shelters under the public assistance system were mainly responsible for the care of the frail elderly, including people with dementia. However, the Act on Social Welfare of the Elderly made provision for the introduction of various social services, including nursing homes and in-home services. In the 1980s, the rapid increase in the elderly population became a major issue, which prompted the Japanese government to launch in 1989 the Gold Plan (a 10-year strategy for the promotion of health and welfare of the elderly) to enhance the development of care facilities and in-home services for the elderly. In 1994, the national government revised the Gold Plan to the New Gold Plan (a new 10-year strategy for the promotion of health and welfare of the elderly). These plans thus enabled the

Table 8.1 The history of Japanese welfare policies

Year	Elderly population, % (year)	Major policies
1960s	5.7% (1960)	1963—the Welfare Law for the Aged enacted
1970s	7.1% (1970)	1973—Free Medical Care for the Elderly launched
1980s	9.1% (1980)	1982—the Health and Medical Service Law for the Elderly enacted 1983—Free Medical Care for the Elderly discontinued 1989—the Gold Plan (The Ten-Year Strategy to Promote Health Care and Welfare for the Elderly) formulated
1990s	12.0% (1990)	1994—the New Gold Plan (The New Ten-Year Strategy to Promote Health Care and Welfare for the Elderly) formulated
	14.5% (1995)	1997—the Long-Term Care Insurance Law enacted
2000s	17.3% (2000)	*2000—the Long-Term Care Insurance Law enforced*
	22.1% (2008)	2008—Emergency Project for Improvement of Medical Care and Quality of Life for Persons with Dementia
	25.1% (2013)	2013—the Orange Plan introduced
	26.7% (2015)	*2015—the New Orange Plan (National Dementia Strategy) introduced*

Source data from: Ministry of Health, Labour, and Welfare; National Institute of Population and Social Security Research.

establishment of in-home care, which many elderly citizens were able to receive. However, people with dementia were still sent to nursing homes and hospitals.

In 2000, the government implemented the LTCI, which aims to develop a community where the elderly can receive care and treatment in their residence area. Moreover, this programme allows the elderly and their families to choose care services relevant to their needs [2]. However, many of those with dementia remained unable to receive the benefits of the LTCI. In 2008, the Ministry of Health, Labour, and Welfare (MHLW) published the Emergency Project for the Improvement of Medical Care and Quality of Life for People with Dementia [3]. The project report stated that although the LTCI covered the majority of people with dementia, still many missed out on an early diagnosis of dementia and, along with their family members, experienced a lack of collaboration and cooperation between medical and long-term care services.

To change the culture that nursing homes and hospitals are responsible for the care of people with dementia, the MHLW introduced in 2012 the Five-Year Dementia Policy (known as the 'Orange Plan'). This plan clearly stated that people with dementia should not be sent to hospital for dementia care; rather, they should receive community-based care. To achieve this plan, the MHLW requested local governments to implement the seven pillars of the Orange Plan: (1) the development of a standard Dementia Care Pathway, (2) early diagnosis and intervention, (3) improved healthcare services to support living in a community, (4) improved long-term care services to support living in a community, (5) better support for daily living, as well as for family caregivers, (6) reinforcement of measures for those with younger-onset dementia, and (7) training of personnel engaged in care services.

In November 2014, Japan hosted the Global Dementia Legacy Event in Tokyo. Prime Minister Shinzo Abe asked the Minister of the MHLW to formulate a new policy programme for dementia as the national strategy for the fight against dementia. Taking advantage of this opportunity, the Japanese government revised the Orange Plan to the Comprehensive Strategy to Accelerate Dementia Measures (known as the 'New Orange Plan') in January 2015, with the involvement of 11 ministries [4]. This revised plan represents a milestone because various other ministries, including the Cabinet Office, the National Policy Agency, and the Ministry of Justice, worked collaboratively with the MHLW for its launch. The New Orange Plan is also underpinned by seven pillars (see Box 8.1).

Box 8.1 New orange plan

1. Advocate for a better understanding of dementia.
2. Provide appropriate medical and long-term care for people with dementia, based on their condition.
3. Enhance support for people with younger-onset dementia.
4. Provide support for caregivers.
5. Promote the development of dementia-friendly communities.
6. Promote research and development in prevention and diagnosis, along with the rehabilitation model and care model.
7. Respect and reflect ideas/suggestions from people with dementia and their families.

(January 2015)

Source data from Ministry of Health, Labour, and Welfare.

Strengths of dementia care in Japan

There are two strengths of dementia care services available in Japan: (1) the creation of the Integrated Community Care System (ICCS) and (2) the various educational opportunities in dementia available for medical and long-term care professionals.

The ICCS aims to provide various services that the elderly might need within their residence area. In the face of a super-aged society, the Japanese government plans to fully implement the ICCS by 2025, which is when the baby boomers would be 75 years old or older. It is the responsibility of local governments to set up the ICCS because each community has different social resources, as well as differences in the local population and the number of elderly individuals. To establish this system, the national government has addressed the following five aspects: (1) enhancing collaboration among healthcare professionals, organizations, and service providers, (2) improving and enhancing the capacity and flexibility of long-term care services, (3) promoting the prevention of long-term care, (4) ensuring advocacy and daily living support services such as meals on wheels and housework assistance, and (5) building and improving elderly-friendly housing (see Fig. 8.1).

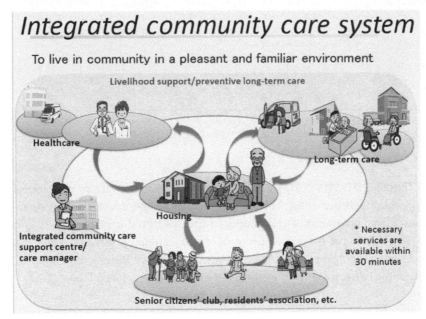

Fig. 8.1 The integrated community care system.
Reproduced from *Dementia-friendly community and ICT*, The Ministry of Health, Labour and Welfare (Presented by Yoshiki Niimi). Global Dementia Legacy Event Japan. Available at http://www.ncgg.go.jp/topics/dementia/documents/Topic3-6YoshikiNiimi.pdf. Accessed August 2016.

Table 8.2 Educational programmes for dementia care workers

Programme name	Who can attend	Curriculum
Practical Educational Programme for Dementia Care Workers	◆ Has basic knowledge of dementia care ◆ Has more than 2 years' experience in dementia care ◆ Works as a leader or promises to be a leader in the near future at the workplace	◆ Lectures/workshops (off-job training): 6 days ◆ Practice at the workplace (on-the-job training): 2 weeks
Advanced Practical Educational Programme for Dementia Care Leaders	◆ Works as a leader at the workplace ◆ Has more than 5 years' experience in dementia care ◆ More than 1 year has passed since the Practical Educational Program for Dementia Care Workers was completed	◆ Lectures/workshops (off-job training): 8 days ◆ Practice at the workplace (on-the-job training): 4 weeks ◆ Practice in the field (not at the workplace: on-the-job training): 5 days
Advanced Practical Educational Programme for Dementia Care Instructors	◆ Is nationally licensed ◆ Medical doctor, health nurse, maternity nurse, clinical nurse, assistant nurse, physical therapist, occupational therapist, speech therapist, social worker, certified care worker, or psychiatric social worker ◆ Works for an institution/service centre for the elderly and/or college/educational school/in the private sector on dementia care	◆ Lectures/workshops (off-job training): 200 hours ◆ Practice at the workplace (on-the-job training): 4 weeks ◆ Practices in the field (not at the workplace: on-the-job training): 3 days

Reproduced from *Meeting Materials regarding Dementia Policy*. The Ministry of Health, Labour and Welfare. Available at http://www.mhlw.go.jp/file/05-Shingikai-12301000-Roukenkyoku-Soumuka/02_3.pdf. (Japanese only) accessed August 2016.

The other strength of Japanese dementia care lies in the various educational opportunities in dementia available to medical and long-term care professionals. Educational programmes were developed after the introduction of the LTCI. In 2001, the national government introduced educational programmes for care workers in the field of dementia care, which is divided into three categories,[1] according to the participants' experience in dementia care (see Table 8.2).

---

[1] In 2016, the Japanese government introduced another educational programme for care workers who are new to working in the field of dementia care—'Basic Educational Programme for Dementia Care Workers'.

In 2005, the educational programme 'Dementia Support Physicians' was introduced. Participants in this programme learn how to work collaboratively with consultant physicians, the government, and municipal medical associations (support physicians' meetings) and also how to prepare and deliver lectures in educational sessions for primary care physicians. Moreover, in 2006, another programme—'Dementia Consultant Physicians'—was introduced to help participants improve their dementia care-related skills such as disease screening, management of dementia with primary care physicians, building a support network for people with dementia, and treatment of dementia once diagnosed.

In addition, educational programmes for managers of facilities/service centres for people with dementia and for medical professionals working in hospitals are also available. In April 2016, educational programmes for pharmacists and dentists were introduced to help them learn how to identify patients/clients with signs of dementia, as well as provide better services for people with dementia.

Challenges and solutions in dementia care

The proportion of senior citizens in the population of Japan was 27.3% in 2016, which is expected to reach 30.3% by 2025 and 37.7% by 2050 [1]. The proportion of people above 65 years of age and suffering from dementia was 15.7% (5.17 million) in 2015 and is projected to reach 19.0% (6.75 million) in 2025 and 21.8% (7.97 million) in 2050 [7]. These figures indicate that one in four persons aged 65 or above in Japan has dementia. Therefore, almost everyone in Japan is likely to be affected by dementia, either as someone with a diagnosis of dementia or as someone related to a person diagnosed with the condition. Thus, care provision for people with dementia is an issue that needs to be addressed urgently in Japan.

In addition, with negative population growth (–0.16, according to 2015 estimates) and zero immigration (zero migrants per 1000 population) [8], a shortage of healthcare professionals, such as certified care workers, medical doctors, clinical nurses, occupational therapists, and social workers, has become an important problem.

To address this problem, as well as build communities where people with dementia can live safely and independently, the MHLW, in collaboration with the Community Care Policy Network, launched a nation-wide public campaign called 'Dementia Supporter'. This campaign provides educational sessions to improve the understanding of dementia and to support people with dementia (see Fig. 8.2). As of 30 June 2016, the total number of Dementia Supporters had reached 7.6 million, and this number is constantly growing [9].

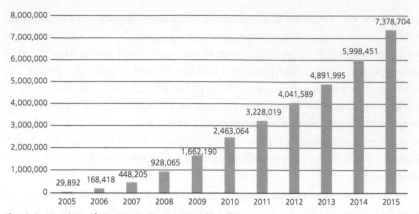

Fig. 8.2 Number of Dementia Supporters (total).
Source data from Community-Care Policy Network '*The number of Dementia Supporters*' (2016).

When the 'Dementia Supporter' campaign began in 2005, its main purpose was to help local residents understand dementia and to remove the stigma associated with dementia [10]. This has resulted in an increasing number of Dementia Supporters, with many willing to provide their support to people with dementia and their communities [11], e.g. by volunteering in their communities, opening community salons for people with dementia (called dementia cafés), involving people with dementia in agricultural work. In other words, this is a process of building a social capital for people with dementia, which will give them opportunities to establish and maintain connections within their community and thus help improve their quality of life and overall life satisfaction.

The future of dementia care: working together to build age- and dementia-friendly communities

As stated in the New Orange Plan, the government intends to respect and reflect the ideas and suggestions from people with dementia and their families in their policies. One example is the creation of a booklet on dementia and dementia care pathways by the government of Sendai, a city located in northern Japan with a population of more than 1 million [12]. In this process, the Sendai government worked together with a person with younger-onset dementia who was a Sendai resident whereby the latter shared their experiences of living with dementia, including when they were first diagnosed with the condition, actions taken since their diagnosis, their feelings and emotions, and their needs.

Another example is giving people with dementia the opportunity to keep active by, for example, working in day service centres. One such day service centre, called 'DAYS BLG!' located in Machida in Tokyo, provides various work opportunities to its members, all of whom have dementia [13]. For example, in one afternoon 'session', members are allocated to one of three 'job' groups: (1) washing cars at the Honda garage, (2) folding leaflets and delivering these to the local area, and (3) cleaning the barbecue that was used for cooking the members' lunch. Thus, although people with dementia can no longer remain in their previous jobs, they can still use their skills and abilities and contribute to their local community.

Therefore, with local governments now listening to the voice of people with dementia and taking into account their views and including their ideas and suggestions in newly formulated measures and policies, this new strategy will change the future of dementia care in Japan—people with dementia will no longer be regarded as 'people who need help'; rather, they will become policymakers and advocators. Thus, by having all key stakeholders working collaboratively together, including medical and long-term care professionals, local residents, Dementia Supporters, and people with dementia themselves, Japan will build age- and dementia-friendly communities for the future.

References

1. **Ministry of Health, Labour, and Welfare**. [*Health, Labour and Welfare White Paper 2012*] (in Japanese only). Available from: https://www.mhlw.go.jp/wp/hakusyo/kousei/17/dl/1-01.pdf [accessed 10 August 2018].

2. **National Institute of Population and Social Security Research**. *Social Security in Japan* (2014 edition). Tokyo: National Institute of Population and Social Security Research; 2014. pp. 33–6.

3. **Ministry of Health, Labour, and Welfare**. [*Emergency project for improvement of medical care and quality of life for persons with dementia*] (in Japanese only). Available from: http://www.mhlw.go.jp/houdou/2008/07/dl/h0710-1a.pdf [accessed 5 August 2016].

4. **Ministry of Health, Labour, and Welfare**. [*Dementia policy*] (in Japanese only). Available from: http://www.mhlw.go.jp/file/06-Seisakujouhou-12300000-Roukenkyoku/0000079008.pdf [accessed 15 July 2016].

5. **Ministry of Health, Labour, and Welfare**. [*Dementia-friendly community and ICT*] (presented by Yoshiki Niimi). Global Dementia Legacy Event Japan. Available from: http://www.ncgg.go.jp/topics/dementia/documents/Topic3-6YoshikiNiimi.pdf [accessed 8 August 2016].

6. **Ministry of Health, Labour, and Welfare**. [*Materials regarding dementia policy*] (in Japanese only). Available from: http://www.mhlw.go.jp/file/05-Shingikai-12301000-Roukenkyoku-Soumuka/02_3.pdf [accessed 10 August 2016].

7. **Cabinet Office, Government of Japan**. [*Annual report on the aging society 2016*] (in Japanese only). Available from: http://www8.cao.go.jp/kourei/whitepaper/w-2016/html/zenbun/index.html [accessed 5 August 2016].

8. **Central Intelligence Agency.** [*The world sactbook (Japan)*] (in Japanese only). Available from: https://www.cia.gov/library/publications/the-world-factbook/geos/ja.html [accessed 3 August 2016].

9. **Community Care Policy Network.** [*The number of dementia supporters*] (in Japanese only). Available from: http://www.caravanmate.com/web/wp-content/uploads/2016/07/H28.6index01.pdf [accessed 5 August 2016].

10. **Ministry of Health, Labour, and Welfare.** [*Dementia supporter caravan*] (in Japanese only). Available from: http://www.mhlw.go.jp/stf/seisakunitsuite/bunya/0000089508.html [accessed 10 August 2016].

11. **Community Care Policy Network.** [*Dementia supporter caravan activity reports*] (in Japanese only). Available from: http://www.caravanmate.com/reportlist/ [accessed 10 August 2016].

12. **Sendai City.** [*Dementia care pathways of Sendai City*] (in Japanese only). Available from: http://www.city.sendai.jp/fukushi/korei/ninchisho/1221818_2581.html [accessed 6 August 2016].

13. **DAYS BLG! Facebook page** (in Japanese only). Available from: https://www.facebook.com/DAYSBLG/ [accessed 5 August 2016].

Chapter 9

Maldives

Shanooha Mansoor and Ahmed Rasheed

Introduction

Maldives is a small island nation located in the Indian Ocean, comprising over 1192 islands, of which only 188 are inhabited. The country is spread over 90,000 km^2, with a land area of only 0.5% [1]. It is environmentally vulnerable, as the islands are less than 1.8 m above sea level. Maldivians are racially homogenous, and their main livelihood relies on tourism. Maldives has a literacy rate of 99.3%, and the official language is Dhivehi [1].

Maldives has a population of 344,023, with an almost equal sex distribution. The majority of Maldivians (45.5 %) are concentrated in urban areas, particularly in the capital Malé [2]. Life expectancy has increased to 77 years, which is almost by 9 years over the last decade [3]. Population studies revealed that the proportion of those above 65 years of age accounts for 5% of the population, and the elderly dependency ratio is 6.9%. The country is nearing the end of its demographic transition, with an average annual population growth rate of 1.65% [2], which means we are facing a future where the population will be older, with a higher number of elderly dependents [4]. Fig. 9.1 shows the population pyramids for 2006 and 2014 published in the most recent census report, showing an increased proportion of the population in older age groups as a result of declining mortality rates at older age in recent decades [5].

The country's economy has expanded significantly in the last 15 years, with a gross domestic product (GDP) per capita of $4,521, which represents an increase of over 60% over that time period [4]. As the country catapulted from being a low-income country to an upper middle-income (UMI) country, it also underwent the epidemiologic transition of burden of disease from communicable diseases to non-communicable diseases (NCDs). The proportion of the health budget of the GDP is 13.7%, with a total health expenditure of 9% of the GDP, which is mainly spent on curative healthcare and very little on preventive or rehabilitative care [6].

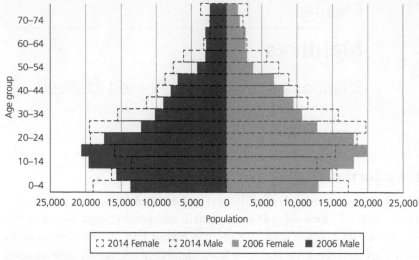

Fig. 9.1 Population pyramid of Maldives.
Source data from Census 2014, National Bureau of Statistics, Ministry of Finance and Treasury 2015.

Dementia in Maldives

Dementia is not a condition that is discussed in Maldives. Most dementia cases are often considered as normal ageing. Maldives has no formal research programmes on mental health or neurological conditions and therefore relies heavily on anecdotal evidence for prevalence data. In 2003, the Ministry of Health conducted a nation-wide survey to assess the magnitude of mental and neurological disorders. This survey reported that more than 29.1% of respondents reported that they had a mental health condition (with 22.3% reporting neurotic disorders, 1% psychotic disorders, and 6.1% epilepsy) [7]. However, there was no mention of dementia in this study. Maldives has a high burden of NCDs, including cardiovascular diseases, such as ischaemic heart disease, diabetes, respiratory diseases, and cancer, with a high risk factor profile of increased obesity, lack of physical activity, and smoking [6], all of which are likely to predispose to dementia—as observed in clinical practice. Despite the lack of formal clinical statistical data, dementia cases are often diagnosed during hospital admission as a sequale of a cerebrovascular accidents. Dementia cases also present to psychiatry outpatient or inpatient services as cases of depression, insomnia, and late-stage psychosis.

The health system in Maldives faces infrastructural and human resources constraints, due to limited availability, as well as geographical challenges. The country relies on a large workforce of expatriates for healthcare provision. National data revealed that Maldives has a total of two neurologists (one local) and six psychiatrists (three local), the majority of whom are concentrated in the capital Malé. Facilities for neuropsychiatric testing, rehabilitation, occupational therapy, and psychological support are unavailable in the government sector and can only be obtained in the private setting, with very limited availability and at high costs. In 2009, a Social Health Insurance scheme was established and became universal in 2013. It ensures that basic healthcare is provided to the population, which has possibly led to an increase in the detection of dementia cases and management [8]. Government-funded institutional care for vulnerable groups, including abandoned elderly persons, is provided at the Home for People with Special Needs, which has a limited capacity, just shy of 200 beds, the majority of which are occupied by patients with severe mental illness [9].

Provision of dementia care

Provision of mental and neurological healthcare is limited, and there are no formal legislations to address this. At this point in time, there is no national dementia strategy. The National Mental Health Policy (2015–2025) addresses mental health in old age and identifies the need for developing mental health-promoting strategies that covers an individual's lifetime, highlighting old age as a priority area [7]. The government has also highlighted its commitment towards health, with a special mention of mental and neurological conditions and healthy ageing. The Health Master Plan 2016–2025 also puts emphasis on older people's health and highlights dementia and cognitive impairment as conditions requiring long-term care [10].

For a country like Maldives, which is still in its infancy in terms of healthcare and struggling to establish a fully fledged healthcare system with Maldivians at its helm, the availability of free universal primary health services is a proud achievement. Medical consultations, investigations, and medications are available to each and every citizen through the Social Health Insurance scheme [10]. Through this scheme, patients can also be referred to specialist services available locally and abroad. As part of its commitment to the welfare of the elderly, the Maldivian government introduced a national programme which provides any citizen above 65 years of age a basic old age pension of US$3900 per annum [11]. Even though these are not directly earmarked for dementia care, these represent cornerstones for creating a dementia care programme. The passion and commitment of national NGOs, such as Aged Care, is commendable and has contributed to the provision of educational programmes and to skills development of families [12].

One of the major challenges in dementia care is a lack of awareness of the condition in the country, not only among the public, but also among healthcare providers and decision-makers. Dementia is often classed as normal ageing, so dementia cases do not reach healthcare providers and thus are not managed appropriately. This is where advocacy will play a crucial role and become instrumental in formulating a national strategy that will recognize dementia as a public health challenge and develop national programmes with a holistic approach. The lack of a national strategy is another obstacle to dementia care provision, including social support for people living with dementia and their caregivers. The third challenge is the lack of funds and coordination among the various government sectors, which should also be addressed when formulating a national strategic plan.

Maldives does not have any formal research or centralized database, which makes it hard for policymakers to prioritize their focus on dementia and highlights the importance of carrying out research. In addition, there is limited knowledge of dementia among healthcare providers. Even for specialized healthcare providers, the lack of formal neuropsychological testing or tools in a local language is an added obstacle. It is of utmost importance to detect dementia cases for early diagnosis and intervention, as the major causes of dementia have been found from clinical experience to be reversible, e.g. patients who present with dementia after a cerebrovascular accident. Even after diagnosis, care for dementia patients is limited, as the medications that are often required are unavailable in the country and have to be brought from abroad. There is also no rehabilitation and social support for people living with dementia or for their caregivers. In Maldives, the elderly are still cared for by the family, as there are no residential facilities or assisted living. This setup can, at times, lead to caregivers experiencing burnout which, in turn, can result in neglect and abandonment of the elderly.

Challenges and the way forward

The challenges that Maldives faces as a country are numerous, and the first step towards overcoming these obstacles is to raise awareness and educating the public, as well as the policymakers. The fact that Maldives is one of the countries participating in the WHO's Global Dementia Observatory gives hope for the future and is a strong step towards developing a strategic plan for dementia care. Government commitment is key in a country where medical services are provided by the government. The development of a National Dementia Strategy and its incorporation into the Mental Health Policy or Health Master Plan would be the next step. The development of such a national strategic plan would pave the way for instigating the necessary changes in dementia care provision, in terms of training, manpower, infrastructure, and coordination among the various government and private sectors and civil society stakeholders.

A measure of success would be formal commitment from the government to dementia care, with an active call for dementia to be recognized as a real public health issue and a dedicated unit or section for dementia in the Ministry of Health. Another measure of success would be initiating discussion about dementia among the public, as well as among the medical community and policymakers, and educating general health practitioners and equipping them with the necessary knowledge and tools to identify groups at high risk of dementia and with means of initiating appropriate care. Building manpower and infrastructure, including special dementia care units and residential facilities, would be the ultimate goal. A crucial step would be to conduct a population-based study which will help justify, as well as formulate, a holistic dementia care plan which ensures evidence-based treatment and improved quality of life.

Early identification of at-risk groups will facilitate patient (and public) education and immediate intervention. This would hopefully lead to a future where the diagnosis of dementia and treatment options are available and affordable to all. The recent development of sister policies and government's emphasis on old age care and protection of the elderly give hope for a time when dementia care will be an integral part of the new Maldivian healthcare framework. As Maldives takes its next steps as a developing nation into the world arena, it is also taking its first steps towards dementia care. The future is promising, and advocacy is central.

References

1. **National Bureau of Statistics**. *Statistical pocketbook of Maldives 2015*. Malé: Ministry of Finance and Treasury; 2015. Available from: http://statisticsmaldives.gov.mv/nbs/wp-content/uploads/2015/10/Statistical-Pocketbook-of-Maldives2015.pdf [accessed 11 October 2016].

2. **National Bureau of Statistics**. *Statistical yearbook of Maldives 2014*. Malé: Ministry of Finance and Treasury; 2018. Available from: http://statisticsmaldives.gov.mv/yearbook/ [accessed 23 July 2018].

3. **World Health Organization**. *Maldives: WHO statistical profile*. 2015. Available from: http://www.who.int/gho/countries/mdv.pdf?ua=1 [accessed 11 October 2016].

4. **May JF**. *Maldives' population dynamics: policy prospects for human growth and opportunity*. New York, NY: United Nations Population Fund; 2016. Available from: http://statisticsmaldives.gov.mv/nbs/wp-content/uploads/2016/07/Population-Dynamics-Report.pdf [accessed 11 October 2016].

5. **National Bureau of Statistics**. *Maldives: population and housing census 2014.* Malé: Ministry of Finance and Treasury; 2015. Available from: http://statisticsmaldives. gov.mv/nbs/wp-content/uploads/2015/10/Census-Summary-Tables1.pdf [accessed 11 October 2016].

6. **Planning and International Health Division**. *Maldives health profile 2016.* Malé: Ministry of Health; 2016. Available from: http://www.health.gov.mv/Uploads/ Downloads//Informations/Informations(73).pdf [accessed 16 July 2018].

7. **Ministry of Health**. *National Mental Health Policy 2015–2025.* National Mental Health Policy—Draft 2014-v3. Malé: Ministry of Health; 2015. Available from: http://www. searo.who.int/maldives/mediacentre/ental-health-policy-2015-2025.pdf [accessed 11 November 2016].

8. **Maldives Pension Administration Office**. *National pension scheme.* 2016. Available from: http://pension.gov.mv/dv [accessed 9 October 2016].

9. **Human Rights Commission of the Maldives**. *Activities addressing rights of persons with disability: a baseline assessment.* 2010. Available from: http://www.searo.who.int/ maldives/documents/Maldives_DisabilityReport13April2010.pdf?ua=1 [accessed 11 December 2016].

10. **Ministry of Health**. *Maldives health master plan 2016–2025: 'For our nation's health'.* Malé: Ministry of Health; 2014. Available from: http://www.nationalplanningcycles.org/ sites/default/files/planning_cycle_repository/maldives/proposed_draft_health_master_ plan_2016-2025.pdf [accessed 23 August 2018].

11. **Asian Development Bank**. *Republic of the Maldives: updating and improving the social protection index.* Regional–Capacity Development Technical Assistance (R-CDTA). 2012. Available from: https://www.adb.org/sites/default/files/project-document/76084/ 44152-012-reg-tacr-12.pdf [accessed 11 November 2016].

12. **International Federation on Ageing**. *Aged Care Maldives.* Available from: https://www. ifa-fiv.org/partner-profiles/aged-care-maldives [accessed 9 October 2016].

Chapter 10

Pakistan

Muhammad Nasar Sayeed Khan,
Muhammad Iqbal Afridi, and Afzel Javed

Summary

Pakistan is one of the largest and most populated nations of
South Asia and ranked sixth among the most crowded countries
in the world, with a population exceeding 196 million. Because
of a lack of research and the cultural setting, it is exceptionally
hard to obtain an exact number of individuals suffering from
dementia. However, the extrapolated prevalence of people with
dementia in Pakistan is around 200,000. Compared to developed
countries, only 4.2% of the Pakistani population are aged above
65 years, possibly due to an average life expectancy of 66 years
for both genders . Although no specific data on elderly people
with dementia in Pakistan are available, it is estimated that 8–
10% of the general population aged above 65 years suffer from
chronic memory loss. According to the latest 2014 World Health
Organization data, Alzheimer's disease/dementia-related deaths
in Pakistan reached a total of 1776 or 0.16% of total deaths.
Pakistan currently has the largest generation of young people
ever recorded in its history, who will be at risk for dementia and
Alzheimer's disease by 2050, at which time, life expectancy would
be expected to continue rising. Thus, the economic burden of
treating patients with Alzheimer's disease and other types of
dementia will increase considerably.

Introduction

Dementia is not merely a disease but also refers to a range of symptoms,
including a decline in memory, cognitive deficits, and eventually death, due
to progressive and irreversible brain damage. There are different causes for
various types of the condition, such as AD, vascular dementia, Parkinson's

disease, Huntington's disease, etc., of which AD is the commonest type of dementia. Disease entities comprising dementia primarily affect the geriatric
population.

Worldwide, there are around 900 million individuals aged 60 years and over
[1]. Rising life expectancy is causing a rapid increase in the elderly population,
along with increased prevalence rates of chronic diseases of adulthood such as
dementia. According to the World Alzheimer report, between 2015 and 2050,
the number of older people living in higher-income countries is forecast to
increase by just 56%, compared with 138% in upper middle-income countries, 185% in lower middle-income countries, and 239% (more than 3-fold
increase) in low-income countries. In 2015, the number of people living with
dementia worldwide was estimated to be 46.8 million. These numbers will almost double every 20 years, reaching 74.7 million in 2030 and 131.5 million
in 2050. It was estimated there would be 9.9 million new cases of dementia in
2015, equivalent to one new case every 3.2 seconds [2]. Therefore, dementia
constitutes a global disease burden in general, and particularly in the geriatric
population.

The prevalence of dementia is growing, which is associated with high economic and social burden. AD is often called a family disease, since being a constant witness to a friend or family member affected by the disease and their
gradual decline impacts on all close to the afflicted patient. AD is the sixth
leading cause of death in the world and the only cause of death among the top
ten that cannot be prevented, cured, or even slowed down [3].

Pakistan is one of the biggest and most populated nations of South Asia
and is ranked sixth among the most crowded countries in the world with a
total population of more than 196 million [3]. By 2050, Pakistan will turn
into the third most crowded country on the planet. In Pakistan, there is no
population-based study on neurological diseases, so dementia in Pakistan
has so far been under-investigated. Because of a lack of research and the
cultural setting, it is exceptionally hard to obtain an exact number of individuals suffering from the disease. However, the extrapolated prevalence of
people with dementia in Pakistan is around 200,000, which is predicted to
increase in future decades. Compared to developed countries, only 4.2% of
the Pakistani population are aged above 65 years. This may be because the
average life expectancy is 66 years for both genders in Pakistan [5]. Although
no specific data on elderly people in Pakistan suffering from dementia are
available, it is estimated that 8–10% of the general population aged above
65 years suffer from chronic memory loss. According to the latest World
Health Organization (WHO) data, published in May 2014, AD/dementia-
related deaths in Pakistan reached a total of 15,428 or 1.27% of total deaths

[4]. Pakistan currently has the largest generation of young people ever recorded in its history; 64% of the total population are below the age of 30 years, and 29% are aged 15 and 29 years, and they will be at risk for dementia and AD by 2050, at which time life expectancy would be expected to continue rising. Thus, the economic burden of treating patients with AD and other types of dementia will increase considerably.

Dementia strategy

Even after 69 years since its creation, Pakistan still has no National Dementia Strategy or plan despite the fact that there are an estimated 2 million people with dementia in the country—and this number is increasing. However, this alarming figure could be used as a springboard for planning and implementing dementia care services in Pakistan. Dementia not only has devastating effects on the sufferer, but it also has a huge impact on their families, their community, and the healthcare system. Therefore, it represents a public health issue with social and financial impacts.

Only about 15 years ago, dementia was not considered to be a problem in Pakistan and not discussed, and as a result has been under-treated. Like in most underdeveloped countries, there was a lack of awareness of dementia and its progressive course, as well as its treatment.

Memory loss may be pathognomonic of dementia. There is a continuous decline in memory with time and ultimately death due to brain atrophy and neuronal loss. Those most commonly affected are people in older age, usually above the age of 65 years. However, in Pakistan, dementia is not recognized early; patients usually present late—with associated complications [6].

Epidemiology and statistics

There are no specific epidemiological studies conducted on dementia. However, as Pakistan is the sixth most populous country in the world, it is estimated that there are about 8 million people suffering from dementia; however, this figure is likely to be considerably higher at present, given the recent population census showed the population growth to be much higher than previously predicted. Moreover, the Delphi consensus study reported the prevalence of dementia to be 1.9% in South Asia, so the estimated figures of people with dementia in Pakistan is 8–10 million [7].

Considering the economic, cultural, and healthcare provision implications of dementia in Pakistan, the burden of dementia care will escalate to a significant extent, to which will add the already massive problem of hepatitis (a prevalent medical problem in Pakistan) if not controlled or managed appropriately.

Recognizing dementia

There is limited knowledge of dementia among medical professionals. Physicians, in particular family doctors, have limited understanding of the illness and consider dementia to be a normal ageing process. A lack of early detection of dementia hampers appropriate subsequent management, since patients present with the disease late, usually with associated complications.

To raise awareness among the medical community of the differences between dementia and normal ageing and related complications, an extensive programme was launched by the Pakistan Psychiatric Society. However, physicians cannot be expected to be educated adequately through this programme alone. Collaborative efforts from national and international agencies and NGOs, as well as public and private partnerships, are needed to disseminate the necessary knowledge.

Dementia care

Alzheimer's Pakistan is an NGO working nationwide. Their fundamental aim is to work towards the welfare of individuals living with dementia and their caregivers. Individuals from different backgrounds have committed to this respectable purpose and to contributing to the organization's services. Alzheimer's Pakistan, in a joint effort with ADI and the International Psychogeriatric Association, has initiated a synergistic setup, called Global Improvement of Dementia Care, to enhance the lives of patients with dementia and their families by changing the human services framework through getting support from the government, healthcare professionals, community, and media.

Alzheimer's Pakistan and its branches run various administrations for people with dementia and their families. It currently supports around 400 people with dementia and their caregivers through its direct services like day care, home outreach services, support groups, and its telephone helpline. In addition, a huge number of people with dementia and their caregivers also benefit from its indirect services such as its website, information material, and training.

The goals of Alzheimer's Pakistan include:

◆ To raise public awareness of AD and related disorders through various awareness activities which are being run consistently throughout the year that include:

  • Events and lectures at different public institutions.

  • Seminars, workshops, and symposia.

  • Film shows and short recordings.

  • Stalls and leafleting at public events.

- To open the door to services, information, and optimized methods to maximize care and support for individuals with AD and their families.
- To train family caregivers and medical professionals.
- To prevent AD through spearheading efforts in research and treatment.
- To enhance care and support services for individuals and their families.
- To collaborate with other organizations and institutions on prevention, research, and treatment of AD and related disorders.

Alzheimer's Pakistan provides a resources section which contains educational materials tailored for family caregivers, healthcare providers, and the general public. Materials are available in Urdu (the national language) and English, and in hard (printed) and soft (online) formats. Resources materials and publications include:

- Booklet: *Help for caregivers* (translation by Alzheimer's Disease International Publications) (in English and Urdu).
- Booklet: *Alzheimer's Caregivers Guidebook* (in English and Urdu).
- Newsletter (in English).
- Fact sheets (in English and Urdu).
- Leaflet: *Is It Alzheimer's Disease?* (in Urdu).
- Leaflet: *Frequently Asked Questions About Dementia* (in Urdu).
- Leaflet: *Introduction to Dementia and Alzheimer's Pakistan* (in English).
- Website: http://www.alz.org.pk (in English and Urdu).

Alzheimer's Pakistan has teamed up with the government and also works in partnership with psychiatry departments in various government hospitals to organize training and provide information materials, and also to refer caregivers to relevant organizations for counselling and support. In 2013, Alzheimer's Pakistan formally signed a Memorandum of Understanding (MOU) with Mayo Hospital in Lahore, which is the biggest hospital in Pakistan, to establish the first dementia centre at the hospital. This dementia centre is manned by Alzheimer's Pakistan staff and provides services such as training, counselling, and support to families, awareness campaigns, etc. Alzheimer's Pakistan currently does not have the financial capacity to provide funding for dementia research, despite continuous efforts for funding availability. However, Alzheimer's Pakistan has developed a comprehensive dementia programme for the government, which includes, among others, proposals for allocating substantial funds for research. These proposals are in the process of being submitted to different provincial governments for approval. Also, considerable efforts are being focused on joint collaborations among different organizations to set up much needed dementia research projects. For example, a dementia research centre was opened in Lahore in collaboration with Alzheimer's Pakistan.

Two dementia clinics were established in university hospitals in Lahore and Islamabad in 2012. In addition, a national pharmaceutical organization is involved in recruiting doctors to review dementia patients in different urban areas in Pakistan, whereas general neurologists, psychiatrists, and family practitioners review dementia patients in their practices. The Department of Psychiatry and Behavioural Sciences of the Jinnah Postgraduate Medical Centre, which is a highly renowned institution in Pakistan, has also initiated its Golden Age Clinic, aimed specifically for the care of the elderly. This clinic was established with the aim of serving people who have devoted their lives to their families and country at large. Elderly people who are considered to be in their golden age, hence the name of the clinic, face limitations in terms of cognition, emotions, and physical mobility. It is our duty to help them cope with ageing issues, self-esteem, and well-being, in addition to their physical comorbidities. Therefore, a free-of-charge service would be a crucial step in providing free healthcare to the golden age group (old age people). In this process, improved transportation and better equipped environment, e.g. closed parking facilities near clinics, non-slippery floors, washrooms available in close proximity, building ramps to facilitate mobility and access, and safe furniture, are provided to patients.

The Edhi Welfare Trust (EWT) provides housing and shelter for elderly people who have been abandoned either by their children to be cared for by the EWT or by their family and relatives who are unable to provide care for the sick elderly individual due to socio-economic reasons. In addition, the Agha Khan Foundation has also established a senior citizen home for elderly people facing similar situations.

One of the finest aspects of our Eastern culture is that, in the majority of families, the young are taught respect for, and the sense of duty and filial obligation of taking care of, elderly family members. Senior family members are normally held in high esteem as they get older, and the rest of the family will endeavour to attend to the elderly's needs, thus making the latter feel they have their due place in the family, and not that they are a family burden.

Historical perspective

It has been estimated that in Pakistan, there are more undiagnosed cases of dementia than diagnosed cases. Initially, when dementia was still an 'unknown' topic of discussion in the country, its symptoms were not recognized, such that patients were not assessed for the disease. About 15 years ago, when a few

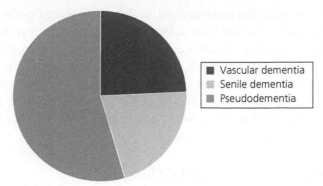

Fig. 10.1 Prevalence rates of vascular dementia, senile dementia, and pseudodementia in Pakistan.

psychiatrists began raising the problem of dementia in clinical settings, it was considered very odd as most psychiatrists and neurologists believed that there was no place for dementia in Pakistan and that it is a complicated problem of developed countries, and not developing countries like Pakistan. There was no dementia assessment for patients and hardly any appropriate treatment plans in place. However, after considerable persuasive efforts, a series of lectures on dementia were run across the country, aimed at informing and raising awareness among the medical community, including family physicians and neurologists. It became clear that dementia is a growing problem, especially in developing countries where life expectancy is increasing. According to the WHO, life expectancy in Pakistan 15 years ago was around 55 years and now it has risen to 67.5 years. With increasing life expectancy in the country, the proportion of elderly people with dementia in the population will also increase. Because of cultural difficulties and a lack of research, it is difficult to estimate the number of people suffering from dementia to date. Nevertheless, it has been reported that the prevalence of people living with dementia in Pakistan is around 200,000 [8]. As mentioned earlier, with a rising life expectancy and prevalence of dementia, the economic and social burden of the disease will also be set to increase.

A recent study reported that the incidence rate of dementia was 172.01 per 10,000 individuals. In addition, the prevalence rate of vascular dementia was 53.45%, senile dementia 46.23%, and pseudodementia 0.13% in the Pakistani population [6] (see Fig. 10.1).

Differentiating dementia

It is difficult for family physicians and general practitioners (GPs) to distinguish among the different types of dementia presenting to general clinics. The referral system needs to be systematized, so that these patients can be referred to specialist clinics. There is a dire need for the government, as well as the private healthcare sector, to realize the importance of timely and appropriate management of patients with dementia. Specialist clinics need to be set up in both tertiary and secondary healthcare systems in the country. The aim is for medical specialists to correctly assess for and diagnose the different types of dementia and make appropriate recommendations to family physicians, who then can take the lead in patient management.

Diagnosing dementia and differences from typical presentation

Dementia patients usually present to specialist clinics with behavioural and psychological symptoms of dementia (BPSD), rather than memory disturbances. A typical presentation is also disinhibition (i.e. where the elderly individual demonstrates increased sexual desires and wanting to have sex with their partner or making sexual advances to other women in the household) observed by family members or when the elderly person is adamant that they would make decisions related to the property in favour of family members.

Moreover, in the country, dementia cases are commonly identified by psychiatrists and neurologists as part of routine radio-neurological examinations for emergency physical presentations. However, these patients are also not appropriately managed for their dementia.

The commonest method used to assess for dementia is the Mini-Mental State Examination (MMSE). However, this tool is not clearly understood by many medical practitioners, and the translated and validated version is not accessible to the majority of physicians in the country. There are also discrepancies in the cut-off scores for a diagnosis of dementia. Taking into account the cultural and social context, this tool has its limitations. The psychometric tools used for dementia assessment, such as Mini-Cog and ADAS-Cog, are yet to be made available in tertiary care centres in Pakistan. This is due to a lack of awareness and funding, and most importantly due to bureaucratic barriers and a lack of political motivation.

Worldwide, there is much focus on the quality of life of people with dementia and on providing support to help improve their activities of daily living, as well as on the burden of care—which is a long way from where Pakistan is currently in terms of dementia care. The majority of patients with dementia still remain undiagnosed because of a lack of dementia screening in the country. There is no one single test to confirm a clinical diagnosis of dementia. As part of their patient evaluation, physicians rely on a detailed medical history (including assessing for any characteristic changes in the patient's thought processes and daily functioning, as well as any behavioural patterns associated with each dementia type), physical examination, laboratory tests, and screening tools, before they could reach a diagnosis of dementia with a high level of confidence. However, it is difficult to accurately identify the exact type of dementia, as the different dementia types share overlapping symptoms and brain changes. In some cases, a doctor may diagnose 'dementia', without specifying the type, in which case it may be necessary to seek the input of a specialist expert such as a neurologist or geropsychologist. Thus, it is crucial to have dementia screening tools readily available not only to enable a thorough patient assessment, but also to ensure early diagnosis and treatment—which, in turn, would help improve the overall quality of life of patients with dementia.

Cultural aspects in the management of dementia

The lack of awareness of dementia among family physicians and other medical professionals is another factor that needs consideration when addressing dementia care in Pakistan. In general, dementia is considered as a natural phase in old age, and not as a problem that needs to be addressed. It takes a lot of time before it is acknowledged that a patient is having some psychological or behavioural symptoms related to dementia.

Due to a small proportion of the gross domestic product (GDP) allocated to public health expenditure, there is resulting inadequacy in dementia care provision. At present, there are only a few elderly homes in Pakistan. Elderly homes are considered to be a taboo and not perceived favourably. The general sentiment is that it is disrespectful to the elderly in the family for them to be sent to an elderly home.

In Pakistan, most people who develop dementia remain with their families in the traditional joint family system and are usually cared for by their sons or daughters or a close relative or someone very close and dear to the family. Of note, care given to people suffering from dementia by their family is regarded as more suitable than care provided in nursing homes, which are still not well established in Pakistan—one nursing home, albeit private, opened very recently in the country, but its main scope is to offer respite care in cases where family caregivers need a break from their caregiving routine. Dementia is commonly known as a family disease, because the relentless stress of witnessing a loved one slowly decline as a consequence of dementia affects everyone related to that person. As mentioned earlier, the majority of elderly people with dementia remain in the comfort of their family home and are looked after by their family, with helpful input from appropriate services and medical professionals (e.g. psychiatrists, neurologists) for dementia screening, treatment, and education, should the family be able to approach and seek such help.

Caregiver burden

When dementia progresses to a point when physicians believe that no further medical intervention would help the patient, the entire burden of care rests on the caregivers. Thus, caregivers often experience burnout from intense pressure and stress, and they find it difficult to maintain a balance between their caregiving duties and their work routine. Only a couple of reports on caregiver burden in the context of dementia care in Pakistan have been published recently. These described very high levels of frustration among caregivers for the following reasons: not knowing what to do, how to provide care for the elderly, what interventions are required, what psychological support is available, and what educational resources are available to support them [9]. Therefore, caregivers should be educated about how to provide basic care for the person with dementia.

In the majority of cases, the burden of care is usually taken on by the women in the family, e.g. the daughter in law. This is because men are the sole bread earners in the family, so they are reluctant to also provide care to the person with dementia, including staying awake at night when needed. Such setup can compromise the outcome of caregiving by women, and in turn the dementia patient's prognosis, since female caregivers often are the sole caregivers in the family, as well as the person responsible for household duties such as cooking, laundry, cleaning, and other household chores.

Consequently, the psychological burden on female caregivers is often considerable. These women can experience burnout within months of caregiving, which can result in a decline in the quality of caregiving, along with poor compliance with treatment. In most cases, the need for psychological support for caregivers is not recognized. It would take much effort and persuasion for the importance of psychological help concurrently to both patients and their caregivers to be acknowledged.

Treatment

Only limited treatment for dementia was initially available in Pakistan. All anti-dementia medications are now available—and affordable to the majority of the population with the availability of their generic version [10]. Treatment for dementia depends on the type diagnosed, and psychiatrists emphasize on the importance of timely initiation of medical therapy, as well as appropriate care.

For mild cases of dementia, only limited medical treatment can be adequate. For moderate and severe cases, intensive therapy is required. Drug treatment helps to relieve the symptoms of dementia, e.g. depression and insomnia, but does not cure dementia itself. A specialist's input will help to alleviate the stress associated with dementia treatment and with how to manage the symptoms in a more informed manner [11], especially since families, in general, believe that drugs will cure the person suffering from dementia. However, as the majority of patients present at a late stage of dementia, with severe symptoms and significant atrophic changes in the brain, as observed on computerized tomography (CT) scanning and magnetic resonance imaging (MRI), treatment is usually difficult.

Challenges

Challenges that Pakistan faces regarding dementia care include:

+ Low awareness of dementia and the extent of care needed in the country.
+ The cultural context that contributes to the denial of the reality of the problem and to the stigma associated with dementia.
+ The general belief that dementia is not a disease, but a natural part of ageing.
+ Inadequate human and financial resources available to meet the care needs of people with dementia and, as a result, the constrained strategy for dementia care.
+ The estimated costs of dementia care in 2015 in Pakistan (according to data from the ADI 10/66 Dementia Research Group):
+ Inadequate training available to professional caregivers and lack of support for family caregivers.
+ The lack of legislation in Pakistan relating to 'mentally disordered' (a lawful term in Pakistan) individuals and their issues, apart from the Sindh Mental Health Act 2013 that was only recently enacted (http://www.pas.gov.pk/uploads/acts/Sindh%20Act%20No.L%20of%202013.pdf). This law makes provision for designating a 'Guardian' and a 'Manager of Property' for the person with dementia. However, this legislation does not apply to the three other provinces in Pakistan. Currently, there is no funding allocated to dementia care and no specific government plan for 'well-being support' as part of dementia care exists. Pakistan has no mandates set up for living wills, power of attorney, or medical services intermediary. There are no facilities in place in the country for assessing driving fitness in people with dementia. Pakistan has not defined any policy or made any arrangements to cater for the rapidly growing geriatric population. The Sindh Senior Citizens Welfare

Bill 2014 has been awaiting endorsement for a year, and yet a similar Bill has been resting in the rulers' halls of Islamabad since 2007.

◆ There is only one trained dementia specialist in Pakistan. There are no behavioural neurology, neuropsychiatry, or dementia modules as part of psychiatry or neurology degree programmes. There are as yet no neuroscience degree programmes available in Pakistan, both at undergraduate and graduate levels. The inclusion of neuroscience as a degree programme is currently being considered after Pakistan began collaborations with the International Brain Research Organization in 2007; a molecular research facility is being established. There are no research facilities or research groups dedicated to investigating the genetics of dementia, and hereditary testing for AD or other dementia types is not available. Brain banks are not yet available, and autopsies are not performed—which would otherwise prove useful for postmortem examinations, especially in the context of research. There is one dementia registry established at a tertiary healthcare facility in Pakistan that comprises a total of 60 patients to date. No epidemiologic studies in dementia in Pakistan have been conducted so far.

◆ In Pakistan, there is no research on cognitive psychology and psychometrics. In addition, there is a need for interpretation and approval of dementia screening tools accessible in Urdu, and efforts are being focused on the interpretation and approval of the MMSE.

◆ Brain MRI and CT scans are available at major hospitals, for which the vast majority of patients still need to pay, which is a massive impediment to accessing these imaging services. In the last 2–3 years, 18-fluoro-deoxyglucose positron emission tomography (FDG-PET) scans and medical cyclotrons have been introduced in three different hospitals in the country; however, they are primarily used for cancer imaging. Amyloid PET imaging and cerebrospinal fluid (CSF) biomarker studies (amyloid, tau, p-Tau, 14-3-3, neurone-specific enolase) are not performed in Pakistan.

◆ Unlike many developed countries, Pakistan has limited healthcare facilities for the elderly. There are no long-term care units or nursing homes for people with dementia, who are therefore cared for at home by their families. However, family caregivers provide dementia care spanning from the complex stages of the disease until death, without having access to support, e.g. counselling, social workers, case managers, or support groups.

◆ No clinical trials on dementia have been conducted in Pakistan, and there are no government policies for initiating any phase I clinical trials in the country.

◆ The elderly are treated either by GPs or by other medical specialists in Pakistan, because geriatric medicine is not considered as a specialty in medicine; this means patient management is often fragmented. There are a limited number of inpatient rehabilitation centres for patients with strokes, fractures, etc. Outpatient physical therapy services are, however, widely available, but their use is suboptimal.

◆ A lack of elderly-friendly transport facilities is also a major problem in Pakistan. Limited access to transport and poor affordability of travel costs to the elderly mean that elderly people find themselves confined to their home.

◆ Elderly people face an extensive range of upsetting life events—the passing of loved ones, loneliness, retirement, change in living arrangements, loss of financial well-being, reduced income, decline in physical energy, and physical limitations. In addition, the presence of medical conditions can result in substandard diets, insufficient exercise, smoking, excessive alcohol consumption, and so on. It has been observed that in Pakistan, the majority of the elderly population have poor nutrition with inadequate meat intake and lack of fresh fruits and vegetables [12].

◆ There is an increase in the number of young people who leave home to set up home with their own family. Once all their children have left, most parents experience empty nest syndrome with a feeling of loneliness and loss of meaning in life. Some elderly people also think of themselves as inadequate, as they are dependent on their children and even small arguments can result in a family crisis and create a situation of conflict and strain among family members. It appears that this idea is gradually making its way among the general public, which is a reason for caution.

◆ Pakistan has poor provisions for pensions. People primarily depend on the younger generation to provide for them upon their retirement. The legal retirement age in Pakistan is 60 years for men and 55 years for women. Except for some private sector employees and the organized sector workforce who are covered by funded pensions, a very large section of the population have no pension provisioning and are totally dependent on the joint family support system.

Pharmacological treatment

All anti-dementia drugs, including cholinesterase inhibitors and N-methyl-D-aspartate (NMDA) receptor antagonists, as well as other supportive drugs, including, for example, Inderal', baclofen, and quetiapine, are widely available in Pakistan, including remote areas, and are affordable. Importantly, family physicians and other relevant medical practitioners need to be educated about correct prescribing in dementia, including dosages and frequency .

Recommendations

Non-pharmacological interventions in dementia need to be well defined and made available at all levels to educate, as well as provide counselling support to, the patients and their family and caregivers. Where required and appropriate, non-pharmacological management can be supplemented by use of drugs such as antidepressants, antipsychotics, and mood stabilizers.

Patient safety issues

Patient safety is key in dementia management. Basic education regarding the safety of people living with dementia is crucial. If their memory is significantly affected, name tags need to be issued and properly attached to the person's clothes for identification. This is also necessary, since many patients with dementia find themselves involved in various criminal activities later in the disease course and are also sometimes charged with blasphemy. Such scenarios where patients with dementia are incapable of differentiating between right and wrong are unfortunately too common in the country—causing considerable anguish in both the patients and their family. The police, despite acknowledging the patient's background of old age and dementia, feel powerless in such criminal cases and are obliged by law to arrest and detain the patient with dementia, before the slow legal system investigates the case, often for years—during which time the patient is left in despair and sometimes even dies before justice is served by the judicial system.

Advance directives and the will

Families would usually suspect 'there is something wrong' and seek specialist advice in cases where an elderly family member refuses to divide their property among the legal heirs in the family and instead decide to donate their property to the mosque or charity. The legal battle to prove that the patient is suffering from dementia and needs treatment and care and that their decision-making capacity is compromised due to dementia is complex and tedious. Psychiatrists or other medical specialists usually tend to avoid being involved in the management of such cases, including giving their opinion on the diagnosis and initiating treatment.

Conclusions and future of dementia in Pakistan

Pakistan needs to set itself up for the rapidly increasing elderly population and its associated consequences by learning from other nations regarding capacity building, creating infrastructure, and management.

Awareness campaigns on dementia should be initiated to educate the public. Educational events, such as workshops, on dementia need to be organized for neurologists, therapists, and general physicians, all of which should be approved for Continuing Medical Education credits. Departments of neurology and psychiatry should include cognitive neurology and neuropsychiatry as subspecialties.

Neuropsychiatry should be included in residency and clerkship educational programmes in different medical specialties, e.g. family medicine and internal medicine, with the possibility to rotate for relevant clinical experience in dementia facilities. Exchange scholarship schemes/research projects and grants should be proposed by tertiary institutions and colleges in the field of neurosciences and neurogenetics. There should be joint collaborations among various organizations within Pakistan and also with its neighbouring nations, e.g. India and China—which are more developmentally advanced than Pakistan, yet face comparable social, financial, and administration issues—to share knowledge and information on innovative advances in dementia such as use of biomarkers and genetic testing applicable in the United States and Europe. A dementia research centre for dementia should be established in Pakistan. Cognitive psychology should be included in undergraduate and postgraduate curricula, and effective screening tools should be available for early detection.

An inpatient unit designed specifically to care for patients with dementia need to be established, and open approaches and appropriate legislation should be set up. Administrative and legal procedures to set up clinical trials need to be less complex, which will give new impetus to clinical research and collaborations. Doctors should acquire up-to-date knowledge of cognitive neurology, which should, in turn, encourage interest in new doctors.

There should be a multidisciplinary approach to dementia care, involving general physicians, psychiatrists, nurses, and social workers so to focus on both cognitive and physical (through promoting an active lifestyle) improvement. Telepsychiatry should be introduced for elderly patients with dementia who are house-bound. There should be improved access facilities for the elderly in public places such as shopping complexes, including ramps, low stair step heights, non-slippery floors, etc. Common safety issues for the elderly, such as sharp objects within reach, slippery floors, slippery floor mats, poor lighting, furniture with sharp edges, etc., should be addressed at every follow-up visit for patients with dementia. Although a good ambulance service is run by the EWT, there should also be transport facilities specifically for the elderly, as well as travel discounts at both domestic and international levels (trains, buses, planes, etc.). Utility services, including electricity, gas, and phone services, should be provided to the elderly at negligible charges. Costs of medical care should be controlled to encourage the elderly to seek, as well as improve their access to, medical care. Services which provide balanced cooked meals to elderly people who are not able to cook should be subsidized. Free meals for elderly people who have no financial means to support themselves would be a source of financial relief. Community health workers should be trained in old age nutrition and care, and they could make home visits. Falls are a major problem for the elderly, and to avoid the harmful, and potentially fatal, outcome of falls, security agencies could offer security medical alert facilities to the elderly. Pharmacies could provide call and delivery/auto-refill services which would enable the elderly to comply with their prescription regimen. Private companies could promote the concept of an inclusive society for the elderly in Pakistan by providing services at full charge for those who can afford to pay and at subsidized rates for those who cannot. For senior citizens, banks should provide credit facilities such as credit cards, car loans, and microfinance options, etc. For elderly people with limited finances, the government should pay them a monthly stipend by zakat or baitulmal funds.

The system of old age benefits scheme, set up under the guidance of the International Labour Organization (ILO), should be introduced in Pakistan for non-government employees. Vocational courses could be organized for those who enter retirement. In addition, when a diagnosis of dementia is communicated to the patient and their family, it is vital to discuss the issue of making advance directives and whether the patient should review and update their will before they lose their decision-making capacity about their wishes on these matters.

It is crucial to address all the discussed issues, rather than simply hoping for a treatment or cure for dementia in the future. Pakistan will face a huge dementia burden because of its increasing elderly population. As Pakistan is a developing nation, it has limited resources. Dementia affects the country at all levels—the individual, their family, the healthcare system, and the communities, and the country as a whole. A cohesive approach is required, including efforts focused on coordination of resources, better communication, raising awareness, and establishing vital links. Initiating all relevant measures should not be delayed if the burden of dementia in the future is to be tackled appropriately and in a timely manner—otherwise, dementia would result in a 'nightmare' situation for the elderly population and for the country. Collaborative work involving doctors, policymakers, and Pakistan's neighbouring nations would enable the country to achieve its objective of giving dementia patients and their caregivers the help they desperately need.

Improving access to services and facilities for the increasing number of elderly people with dementia can only be achieved by boosting capacity and enhancing the efficacy of care provision. Primary care facilities focused on dementia care are central to such care provision and need to be developed, with appropriate guidance and support from the relevant authorities [13].

References

1. **World Health Organization**. *Ageing and health*. Fact sheet. Geneva: World Health Organization. Available from: http://www.who.int/mediacentre/factsheets/fs404/en/ [accessed 28 June 2017].

2. **Alzheimer's Disease International**. *World Alzheimer Report 2015. The Global Impact of Dementia. An analysis of prevalence, incidence, cost and trends*. London: Alzheimer's Disease International; 2015.

3. **Shafqat S**. Alzheimer's disease therapeutics: perspective from the developing world. *Journal of Alzheimer's Disease*. 2008;**15**:285–7.

4. **Countrymeters**. *Pakistan population*. Available from: http://countrymeters.info/en/ Pakistan#population_2017 [accessed 30 June 2017].

5. **World Life Expectancy**. *Pakistan: Alzheimers/dementia*. Available from: http://www. worldlifeexpectancy.com/pakistan-alzheimers-dementia [accessed 28 June 2017].

6. **Shaukat U, Ahmad B, Shabbir MI**. A statistical and epidemiological analysis of dementia from population based survey in Pakistan. *Asian Academic Research Journal of Multidisciplinary*. 2016;**3**:1–14.

7. **Ferri CP, Prince M, Brayne C**, *et al*. Global prevalence of dementia: a Delphi consensus study. *The Lancet*. 2005;**366**:2112–17.

8. **The News**. *Number of people with dementia growing in Pakistan, say experts*. 2015. Available from: https://www.thenews.com.pk/print/63549-number-of-people-with-dementia-growing-in-pakistan-say-experts [accessed 25 July 2018].

9. **The Express Tribune**. *Strain on families: Neurologists worry about rise of dementia in Pakistan*. 2014. Available from: https://tribune.com.pk/story/764999/strain-on-families-neurologists-worry-about-rise-of-dementia-in-pakistan/ [accessed 25 July 2018].

10. **Alzheimer's Association**. *What is dementia?* Available from: https://www.alz.org/ alzheimers-dementia/what-is-dementia [accessed 24 August 2018].

11. **Ahmad A, Owais K, Siddiqui M, Mamun K**. Dementia in Pakistan: national guidelines for clinicians. *Pakistan Journal of Neurological Sciences*. 2013;**8**:17–277.

12. **National Council of Social Welfare**. Available from: https://cadd.gov.pk/national-council-of-social-welfare/ [accessed 24 August 2018].

13. **Dawn**. *Most of dementia patients in Pakistan undiagnosed*. 2016. Available from: https:// www.dawn.com/news/1285144 [accessed 25 July 2018].

Chapter 11

Singapore

Kua Ee Heok and Iris Rawtaer

Summary
The main caregivers of elderly people with dementia in Singapore are the family. In recent years, community services like day care centres, home care, respite care, and nursing homes have expanded. Non-governmental organizations are actively involved in providing a spectrum of services, ranging from medical, nursing, physiotherapy, occupational therapy, and counselling. General hospitals have set up geriatric and psycho-geriatric teams for dementia patients. There is now a focus on dementia prevention, and a successful prevention programme has been extended to three additional community centres. The challenge ahead is not only having sufficient dementia services, but also ensuring there are sufficient trained health professionals to provide the services. Current strengths in dementia care include strong emphasis on family care, increased availability of dementia community services like day care centres, and increased number of health professionals trained in dementia care. Future priorities include integrating hospital care into the community, keeping down the cost of dementia care, and creating dementia-friendly environments.

Introduction

There is growing concern in Singapore in recent years about caring for an increasing number of elderly people with dementia [1]. Not only is this concern due to an increasing number of elderly people with dementia, but also due to a diminishing number of family caregivers. Traditionally, caregivers have been women, but because of the social transformation of the Singaporean family, young couples prefer to live away from their parents and more women prefer to work outside of home. Another factor contributing to the decreasing number of caregivers is the reduction in family size—most families today have only one or two children. A study has shown that about 56% of family caregivers in Singapore had symptoms of anxiety and depression related to the stress of caring for an elderly with dementia [2].

Epidemiological studies of dementia in Singaporean elderly people aged 65 years and over living in the community indicated a prevalence of between 2.5% and 6% [3, 4]. However, the majority of cases are not detected, and under-diagnosis of dementia is partly because most doctors have difficulty in recognizing its early signs and symptoms. Medical students are often given clinical teaching in general hospitals or mental hospitals which have moderate to severe cases of dementia. In primary care practice, clinical presentations are usually mild and many elderly with early dementia do not seek medical consultation. Family members may ignore the elderly's complaints of poor memory, putting it down to 'normal ageing' and would only consult a doctor when the elderly shows behavioural symptoms of dementia such as agitation, insomnia, or a wandering tendency.

Dementia services

In many Asian countries, with the exception of Japan, there is a dearth of mental health services and dementia care is not considered a priority [5]. Many Asian elderly prefer to see traditional healers whenever they are unwell, avoiding psychiatric services because of the associated stigma. The mental health service in Singapore has emulated some aspects of the British National Health Service, including a large mental health hospital, a general hospital with psychiatric services, and recently the introduction of community services in psychogeriatric psychiatry [6]. However, there is always a human resource issue because geriatric psychiatry is not a popular subspecialty among mental health professionals, including psychiatrists and nurses.

In the last two decades, many NGOs and volunteer welfare organizations supported by funding from the government have taken an active role in providing day care centres, nursing homes, befriending services, home care, and respite care for dementia patients. To coordinate dementia services for the whole country, the Ministry of Health has set up an Agency for Integrated Care (AIC) to ensure links between hospital services and community care for the elderly with dementia. There is now an improvement in dementia services, and response from family caregivers has been very positive, especially regarding subsidized care for the poor.

A model of a dementia service in Singapore is the Geriatric Psychiatry Out-Reach Assessment, Consultation and Enablement (G-RACE) programme. This is a comprehensive programme that provides a broad range of services for the elderly in the community in the western region of Singapore. Care provision ranges from dementia screening and early detection and primary care partnership to providing quality home-based mental health services. The multidisciplinary team comprises geriatric psychiatrists, psychiatry residents in training, case managers, psychologists, nurses, and occupational therapists. The team meets weekly to discuss new referrals and challenging cases encountered by any team member.

The G-RACE Community Partnership is an arm of the service where the team equips and empowers elder care agencies—voluntary organizations or NGOs— with the necessary skills to identify psychological problems in the population that they serve. This is achieved through regular training workshops with both didactic and hands-on teaching sessions, as well as case consultations.

A primary care collaborative model has been established, with the aim of managing less complex cases of cognitive impairment or dementia at a polyclinic. A geriatric psychiatrist is involved in training physicians and nurses at the polyclinic and is available for consultation at weekly clinic sessions. Medical social workers are also involved in this shared-care clinic to assist with liaising with other community services and provide support for suitable cases. Stable cases of dementia with minimal neuropsychiatric difficulties are discharged from hospital care to be managed by the polyclinic.

Two other components of G-RACE services are the Allied Health Intervention (AHI) team, as well as the G-RACE Home Clinic (GHC). AHI receives referrals from both primary care and tertiary care physicians managing patients with dementia who are still ambulant and able to attend clinic visits but require home support by way of environmental modification, mobility aids, functional assessments, activity scheduling, behavioural interventions, and caregiver training and support. Case managers and occupational therapists would attend to these patients in their home and maintain close liaison with their primary physicians.

GHC is the domiciliary visit team. This model of care has a long history in the care of older adults and will be increasingly important as we see burgeoning numbers of elderly people with moderate to severe dementia living in the community. Elderly people referred to GHC typically have been diagnosed with a mental health problem but are housebound. The aim of GHC is to provide quality mental health services to the elderly who might otherwise not be able to access care. A multidisciplinary team conducts home visits and focus on three major areas: mental health of the older adult, the environment, and caregiver support.

The focus of dementia care in the future will still be on community care, as it is not in Asian culture to leave an elderly parent in an old age home for longterm care [7]. There is planning for a day hospital in the community which can be the nucleus of psycho-geriatric services, with doctors, nurses, physiother-apists and other health professionals working as a team. A combined geriatric medicine and psychiatry unit may be feasible to facilitate referrals, reduce costs, and allow for the integration of the two services. With referrals from the gen-eral hospital, the day hospital can provide step-down care facilities, which will alleviate the problem of bed shortage in many acute hospitals. Collaboration between health professionals and community workers in the health and so-cial sectors will expand community outreach and support for the elderly with dementia.

Training and education

In the past, many doctors, nurses, psychologists, and occupational therapists were sent to the United Kingdom for training. Recently, the National University of Singapore has organized training programmes with visiting experts from the United States, the United Kingdom, and Australia to teach local doctors, nurses, and psychiatrists in dementia care. A few psycho-geriatricians in Singapore and Australia have gone to neighbouring countries like Malaysia, Indonesia, Cambodia, and China to provide training programmes for dementia care—this project is one of the objectives of the Teachers of Psychiatry (TOP) club [6].

Public education through seminars, books, and mass media is important to ensure early referral, provide information on care, and de-stigmatize dementia. Using digital media, like apps for information on dementia and services, has now expanded [8].

A key feature in the provision of dementia care is the involvement of the community and community-based organizations. After attending training pro-grammes, many volunteers have given time to help in day care centres and pro-vided ideas for a dementia-friendly environment in the housing estates.

Research

Many existing clinical cognitive tests lack adequate normative data, reliability, and validity. A brief questionnaire is needed to screen for cognitive changes among elderly people in the community, clinic, and hospital. Currently, there are a few of these instruments, including the Mini-Mental State Examination (MMSE) [9], and the validity of these instruments would be doubtful in a dif-ferent cultural setting, especially where literacy is low. We have constructed a screening questionnaire called the Elderly Cognitive Assessment Questionnaire (ECAQ) [10] for the detection of dementia by the primary healthcare doctor or nurse. The ECAQ is a 10-item scale, and the items are culled from the MMSE and the Geriatric Mental State (GMS) schedule [11]. There is less bias on educational status, and the questionnaire can be completed in 10 minutes. It has been suggested that to assist primary care doctors to identify dementia, a screening questionnaire like the MMSE can be helpful. However, the MMSE is lengthy (takes 20 minutes) and is culturally or educationally biased—in most primary care clinics in Asia, doctors have only 10–15 minutes per patient. The ECAQ is more appropriate for those elderly who are less educated and can be administered in 10 minutes by a nurse or social worker.

With the rising tide of dementia, the Department of Psychological Medicine at the National University Health System (NUHS) has embarked on an innovative primary prevention programme targeting 'at-risk' elderly people living in the community at Jurong. This unique programme emphasizes preventive psychiatry in the community, by the community, for the community, with joint efforts from the private sector, NGOs, volunteers, and the NUHS research team. Every session begins with a 15-minute talk in Chinese on health issues, including controlling diabetes mellitus and hypertension with medications, diet, and exercise. After the talk, participants are divided into four groups for music reminiscence, art therapy, t'ai chi exercise, and mindfulness practice. After a year, a reduction in depression and anxiety scores and improvement in cognitive scores were obtained [12, 13]. This programme has now been extended to three more community centres, and this translational research will benefit the older generation with better physical health, mental health, and quality of life.

Conclusion

Asian caregivers tend to rely more on family support and less on psychogeriatric services for dementia care. Policymakers are increasingly aware of the fact that caring for an elderly at home has an economic cost. A cost analysis of care of dementia patients who attended the Memory Clinic showed the main bulk of the cost of care to be in medications and hiring a domestic helper [14, 15]. Caregivers incur numerous expenses, including home modifications, assistive devices, high utility costs, and the cost of foregoing paid employment. Because in Singapore, many retirees do not have pensions, they are financially dependent on their children.

The family and community will need to be given the necessary support, resources, and knowledge to care for the elderly at home. With appropriate information and good support from health professionals, family members will be more eager to take care of the elderly with dementia in their own home.

In future, caring for the frail elderly in Singapore will continue to rest on the family, but caregivers will need to seek help outside the home. Support networks typically have the family as the core but also include friends, neighbours, and home help. Community and governmental supports are necessary to alleviate the burden of dementia care on the family.

References

1. **Kua EH.** Alzheimer's disease–the rising tide. *Singapore Medical Journal*. 1999;**40**:722.

2. **Kua EH, Tan SL.** Stress of caregivers of dementia patients in the Singapore Chinese family. *International Journal of Geriatric Psychiatry*. 1997;**12**:466–9.

3. **Kua EH.** A community study of mental disorders in elderly Singaporean Chinese using the GMS-AGECAT package. *Australian and New Zealand Journal of Psychiatry*. 1992;**26**:502–6.

4. **Ng TP, Leong T, Chiam PC, Kua E-H.** Ethnic variations in dementia: the contributions of cardiovascular, psychosocial and neuropsychological factors. *Dementia and Geriatric Cognitive Disorders*. 2010;**29**:131–8.

5. **Tasman A, Sartorius N, Saraceno B.** Addressing mental health resource deficiencies in Pacific Rim countries. *Asia-Pacific Psychiatry*. 2009;**1**:3–8.

6. **Kua EH.** Focus on psychiatry in Singapore. *British Journal of Psychiatry*. 2004;**185**:79–82.

7. **Kua EH.** Elderly people with mental illness in South-East Asia: rethinking a model of care. *International Psychiatry*. 2010;**7**:34–6.

8. **Chan SWC (ed).** *A feasibility study on smartphone psychoeducation application for family caregivers of people living with dementia.* Cape Town: Sigma Theta Tau International's 27th International Nursing Research Congress; 2016.

9. **Folstein MF, Folstein SE, McHugh PR.** 'Mini-mental state'. A practical method for grading the cognitive state of patients for the clinician. *Journal of Psychiatric Research*. 1975;**12**:189–98.

10. **Kua E, Ko S.** A questionnaire to screen for cognitive impairment among elderly people in developing countries. *Acta Psychiatrica Scandinavica*. 1992;**85**:119–22.

11. **Copeland J, Kelleher M, Kellett J,** *et al.* A semi-structured clinical interview for the assessment of diagnosis and mental state in the elderly: the Geriatric Mental State Schedule: I. Development and reliability. *Psychological Medicine*. 1976;**6**:439–49.

12. **Wu DX, Feng L, Yao SQ, Tian, XF, Mahendran R, Kua EH.** The early dementia prevention programme in Singapore. *The Lancet Psychiatry*. 2014;**1**:9–11.

13. **Rawtaer I, Mahendran R, Yu J, Fam J, Feng L, Kua EH.** Psychosocial interventions with art, music, Tai Chi and mindfulness for subsyndromal depression and anxiety in older adults: a naturalistic study in Singapore. *Asia-Pacific Psychiatry*. 2015;**7**:240–50.

14. **Goh LG, Kua EH, Chiang HD (eds).** *Ageing in Singapore—the next 50 years.* Singapore: Gerontological Society; 2015.

15. **Kua E, Tan S, Lee K, Ko S, Tan C.** The NUH memory clinic. *Singapore Medical Journal*. 1997;**38**:112–15.

Chapter 12

South Korea

Cheolmin Shin and Changsu Han

Summary

In 2008, the first Dementia Management Plan was launched to focus on prevention and early diagnosis, the development of infrastructures and management, and raising awareness. In 2012, the Dementia Management Act was enacted. In addition, in 2008, Korea launched the Long-Term Care Insurance (LTCI) scheme, a social insurance scheme for elderly care and whose beneficiaries also include patients with mild dementia but who still need care. The third Plan launched in 2016 for the next 5 years (i.e. 2016–2020) focuses on investing in dementia research, setting up a robust dementia delivery system, and standardizing a dementia care pathway. The Korean healthcare system for dementia patients has universal health insurance coverage through the national health insurance. The national dementia policy in South Korea was announced as 'Dementia Comprehensive Management Measures' in September 2008, of which one of the primary measures is to provide early diagnosis of dementia through the establishment of dementia counselling centres in public health-improving centres. Furthermore, a comprehensive National Dementia Center was established and replicated in regional hospitals (base hospitals for dementia) to provide diagnosis of dementia, treatment, and consultation for BPSD. Korean Ministry of Health and Welfare published the second National Dementia Management Master Plan 2013–2015 In July 2012. The second dementia care plan includes the following four initiatives: early detection and prevention, tailored treatment, infrastructure for the management of dementia, and family support and improvement of social recognition. Recently (2014-2016), Ministry of Health and Welfare funded a few geriatric care centers to test the applicability of geriatric care hybrid model for dementia and depression to decrease increasing prevalence of depression and suicide of the old along with dementia.

National care plan for dementia in Korea

Korea is a rapidly ageing country among members of the Organization for Economic Cooperation and Development (OECD), and it has developed into an ageing society in early 2000. However, it is anticipated that Korea will become an aged society by 2019 and a super-aged society by 2026 [1]. Due to the rapid growth of the elderly population, it is estimated that the number of dementia patients will reach 1 million by 2024 and 2 million by 2041 (see Fig. 12.1). Since the early 1990s, epidemiological studies conducted in various communities in Korea have reported prevalence rates of dementia in elderly people over 65 years of age of 6.3–10.8% [2–5]. A systematic review of epidemiological studies on dementia in Korea reported a prevalence rate of dementia of 9.2%, which is much higher than in other Asian countries (4.19–7.63%) [6].

In 2015, the number of dementia patients in Korea was estimated to be around 650,000. As a result of care and treatment costs of dementia, which amounted to 22 million won (about US$20,000) per capita, the disease burden per year is estimated to reach 14 trillion won (about US$12 billion). In order to cope with the burden of an increasing number of dementia cases, the Korean government established the first and second National Dementia Plans in 2008 and 2012, respectively. The first Plan focused on the prevention and early diagnosis of dementia, development and coordination of infrastructures and management, and raising awareness. It also included the implementation of the National

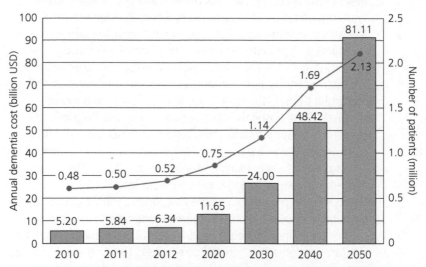

Fig. 12.1 Estimated rise in the number of dementia patients and care burden.
Source data from *The 2011 Nationwide Survey on Dementia Care in Korea*. The Ministry of Health and Welfare: Available from http://www.prism.go.kr/ [in Korean]).

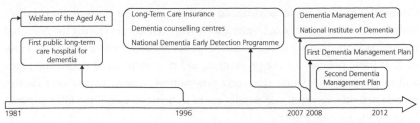

Fig. 12.2 History of key milestones in dementia care in South Korea.

Long-term Care Insurance (LTCI) scheme, which provides sufficient funds to ensure that each person has timely access to relevant services and support. The National Dementia Early Detection Programme was also introduced. This provides all elderly people in Korea with access to dementia screening and post-diagnostic services, including reimbursement for medications, if necessary. The second Plan focused more on supporting family members of dementia patients. In 2012, the Dementia Management Act was enacted to give a statutory status to the execution of the National Dementia Plans (see Fig. 12.2).

In 2016, the third National Dementia plan for the next 5 years was established. This Plan is based on comprehensive analyses of results from the first and second Plans, as well as the consideration of dementia management plans from other countries leading in dementia care. The aim of the third National Dementia Plan is to create a dementia-friendly society, wherein people with dementia and their caregivers can live well. This plan also focuses on dementia prevention and management, convenient diagnosis, and treatment and care for people with different dementia severities, while reducing the burden on caregivers and encouraging more dementia research.

The Dementia Management Act (enacted in February 2012)

Dementia has become a serious social problem for the government to address. Therefore, the Dementia Management Act was legislated in order to provide a systematic and legal status for implementing the National Dementia Plans. Furthermore, the National Institute of Dementia was established, in accordance with the Dementia Management Act. The delivery system for the dementia management programme, which is composed of, in hierarchical order, the National Institute of Dementia, metropolitan/provincial dementia centres, and dementia counselling centres in public health-improving centres, was also organized.

The Dementia Management Act states that the government should establish a National Dementia Plan every 5 years. The National Dementia Management

Committee was set up in accordance with the Act. The Committee together with the National Institute of Dementia are responsible for creating the National Dementia Plan. The Act specifies the contents of the National Dementia Plan, such as basic policies for the prevention and management of dementia, plans and methods for dementia screening programme, treatment and care for dementia patients, research and development in dementia, and specialist support in dementia management.

National Long-term Care Insurance (implemented in July 2008)

Increasing medical expenses for chronic diseases due to the growth of the elderly population have led to a need for a social insurance scheme for care provision. The Korean government introduced the national LTCI scheme in 2008 through a preparatory period of 7 years.

The LTCI scheme provides support services for physical activities or housework to people who experience difficulty with activities of daily living due to dementia or other geriatric diseases. Trained nurses and social workers visit and assess applicants in terms of their function with activities of daily living, as well as instrumental activities of daily living. LTCI recipients are categorized into five grades, according to the disability in activities of daily living. The recipient can access services either from their home or from an institution. Of note, grade 5 was added as a new category in 2013 and is regarded as a '*special grade for dementia*'. Prior to the introduction of grade 5, it was reported that the LTCI scheme did not provide adequate cover for patients with mild dementia only. With grade 5, dementia patients with slight limitations to their physical activities but who still need some support can be given access to more dementia-specific services, such as cognitive activity programme and medication management, through visiting nurse services. The LTCI scheme is regarded as the strength of the Korean dementia care plan because it enables the Korean society to become socially responsible for their dementia care and support.

With an ageing Korean society, the number of institutions of long-term care and home service centres has increased, and the number of beneficiaries of the LTCI scheme has also continuously increased over the last 8 years. As a result, Korea is now confronted with the challenge of maintaining the funds available in the LTCI scheme, while improving the quality of service provision at the same time.

Geriatric cohort studies on dementia

Large-scale elderly cohort studies on dementia have been conducted and supported by central and local governments. The Ansan Geriatric (AGE) study was designed to establish a prospective population-based cohort of subjects to study the prevalence, incidence, and related risk factors of geriatric diseases, as well as to obtain comprehensive information on public health and the functional status of elderly Koreans [7]. This cohort study was developed in Ansan, an urban area near Seoul, with the financial support from the local government. Unlike previous geriatric cohort studies in Korea, this cohort study used precise neuropsychological testing, recruited participants through population-based random sampling, and was designed as a prospective study.

The Korean Longitudinal Study on Health and Aging (KLoSHA) is another elderly cohort study that was developed in Seongnam [8]. This study was conducted with the aim to gather comprehensive data on the prevalence, incidence, natural history, and risk factors of common geriatric diseases and to establish a comprehensive database of the general health and functional status of the Korean elderly population. The study design focused on the use of comprehensive laboratory tests as the core of the study in order to achieve the study objectives.

Dementia care centres in Korea

National dementia service delivery system

Korea enacted the National Dementia Act in order to set up the National Institute of Dementia, as well as metropolitan/provincial centres nationwide. Until 2016, the National Institute of Dementia and 17 metropolitan/provincial dementia centres for dementia were established in Seoul and all metropolitan city and provinces in the country.

The National Institute of Dementia has the following roles: to predict demands for dementia research; to monitor for national and international research advances in the field of dementia; to formulate a dementia research plan; to set up proposals for public participation in dementia research projects; to evaluate and put forward dementia research project proposal applications; to provide support, education, and training to personnel involved in home dementia management services; to encourage public participation in dementia management; to be responsible for the collection, analysis, and provision of information and statistical data on dementia; to collaborate with national and international institutions in the field of dementia; and to introduce new technology for the prevention, diagnosis, and treatment of dementia.

The metropolitan/provincial dementia centres, in collaboration with the National Institute of Dementia and the regional government, is responsible for training healthcare professionals, establishing local infrastructures, and conducting research in dementia care and treatment. The regional centres have programmes locally tailored to the needs of each region. The centres run the Regional Dementia Council which provides advice and support to the regional government for the establishment and implementation of a regional dementia management plan.

Suwon Geriatric Mental Health Centre

Gyeonggi-do, one of the 13 provinces in Korea, independently established the Suwon Geriatric Mental Health Centre in Suwon. This centre runs geriatric mental health programmes, mainly on dementia and geriatric depression. Screening for mental health disorders is performed using various neuropsychiatric tools. In order to enhance knowledge of geriatric mental health, consultation and educational sessions for community members are provided. Furthermore, a cognitive rehabilitation programme can also be provided to high-risk members. Those with financial difficulties can receive support for medical expenses for the treatment of dementia, depression, and other psychiatric illnesses. Elderly people, who are at risk of wandering due to dementia, can be provided with an identification bracelet or tag in order to prevent them from getting lost.

Challenges in dementia care

Increasing elderly population and reduction in elderly income

The elderly population in Korea is continuously increasing. However, this increase has resulted in a reduction in the income of elderly people. In 2013, the poverty ratio of Korean elderly people over 65 years of age was 48.1% [9]. It far exceeds the average among the OECD member countries. As Korea appropriated social insurance funds for health expenditures, it is deemed possible that the reducing workforce and increasing elderly poverty can withstand the depletion of the health budget.

Lack of facilities and human resources

Although demands for dementia care have considerably risen, there is still a shortage of infrastructure and trained manpower. Infrastructure is particularly needed in local and rural areas. Human resources are scarce both in terms of medical professionals and healthcare workers. In addition, further development and appropriate distribution of resources are also needed.

Future of the dementia care plan

Investment in research and development for enhanced dementia prevention and treatment

In 2014, the Korean government allocated approximately US$35 million to support research and development in dementia, and the scale of such funding is set to be extended. There will be continued efforts in clinical research which will focus on developing novel imaging markers, biomarkers, and treatment agents for improved diagnosis and treatment of dementia. A large-scale elderly cohort will be established in order to collect valuable data on dementia and geriatric diseases. Moreover, analysis of results from previous dementia management programmes will be performed to gather evidence on outcomes of the dementia management policy.

Integration of dementia-related datasets

Currently, different dementia-related datasets are held by their respective institutions, e.g. national health insurance data and data collected by dementia centres. These need to be integrated into a central database containing all dementia-related data that can be shared and accessed by researchers, clinicians, and policymakers.

Improving the organization of the Korean dementia service delivery system

The existing dementia service delivery system should be more actively organized and managed. The issues of local infrastructure and manpower will be prioritized in the next National Dementia Plan. Moreover, a dementia specialist hospital will be set up in local areas to help fill the void in dementia care in local regions in Korea. The Regional Dementia Council will also have improved access to local resources for dementia.

Development of a standard dementia care pathway for appropriate care provision

One of the main issues in dementia care is that patient services should be provided appropriately, in a timely manner according to dementia phases. Currently, various medical and care services are provided to dementia patients in a 'generic' manner, i.e. the type of treatment and care is not tailored to the patient's dementia severity. In the near future, a standard dementia care pathway is expected to be developed in Korea—which will, in turn, enable the reorganization of existing services in dementia care and the allocation of service resources.

References

1. **Korean Statistical Information Service**. *Population projections and summary indicators for Korea*. Available from: http://kosis.kr/statHtml/statHtml.do?orgId=101&tblId=DT_1B35001&conn_path=I2&language=en [accessed 22 September 2016].
2. **Park J, Ko H, Park Y, Jung C**. Dementia among the elderly in a rural Korean community. *British Journal of Psychiatry*. 1994;**164**:796–801.

3. **Lee DY, Lee JH, Ju YS,** *et al.* The prevalence of dementia in older people in an urban population of Korea: The Seoul Study. *Journal of the American Geriatrics Society.* 2002;**50**:1233–9.

4. **Kim J, Jeong I, Chun JH, Lee S.** The prevalence of dementia in a Metropolitan city of South Korea. *International Journal of Geriatric Psychiatry.* 2003;**18**:617–22.

5. **Jhoo JH, Kim KW, Huh Y,** *et al.* Prevalence of dementia and its subtypes in an elderly urban Korean population: results from the Korean Longitudinal Study on Health and Aging (KLoSHA). *Dementia and Geriatric Cognitive Disorders.* 2008;**26**:270–6.

6. **Kim YJ, Han JW, So YS, Seo JY, Kim KY, Kim KW.** Prevalence and trends of dementia in Korea: a systematic review and meta-analysis. *Journal of Korean Medical Science.* 2014;**29**:903–12.

7. **Han C, Jo SA, Kim NH, Jo I, Park MH.** Study design and methods of the Ansan Geriatric Study (AGE study). *BMC Neurology.* 2009;**9**:10.

8. **Park JH, Lim S, Lim J,** *et al.* An overview of the Korean Longitudinal Study on Health and Aging. *Psychiatry Investigation.* 2007;**4**:84.

9. **Korean Statistical Information Service.** *Average monthly income and expenditure by age of household head.* Available from: http://kosis.kr/statHtml/statHtml. do?orgId=101&tblId=DT_1L9H020&conn_path=I2&language=en [accessed 22 September 2016].

Chapter 13

Thailand

Sookjaroen Tangwongchai, Chavit Tunvirachaisakul, Thitiporn Supasitthumrong, Kanitpong Phabphal, and Pichet Udomratn

Summary

Thailand has unique advantages and challenges in caring for people with dementia. Thailand is in the process of launching its National Dementia Strategy, based on the previously developed care and support policies for the elderly. Currently, care for people with dementia is provided through integrated community care by family and health volunteers, and care costs are covered by the Universal Coverage Scheme. The main challenges are to raise public awareness of dementia, to improve healthcare capacity, and to prepare for a long-term care system. There needs to be focus on innovative medical management and prevention strategies to tackle dementia in Thailand. In the future, Thailand expects to see an improvement in public education about dementia, an increase in specialist training involving multidisciplinary teams, the emergence of sustainable long-term community-based care, and the expansion of an accessible care system with adequate standards for the Thai population.

Introduction

Thailand is a developing country situated in South East Asia and classified by the World Bank as an upper middle-income country. It is the 51st largest country and the 20th most populous country in the world, with a population of approximately 66 million. The main healthcare scheme is the Universal Coverage Scheme, into which the state pays for predetermined costs of care. The increasing life expectancy and decreasing fertility rate of the Thai population resulted in the country turning into an ageing society in 2007. There were

10 million elderly Thai people in 2015, accounting for 15.8% of the total population of the country which is predicted to increase to 37.1% within the next 35 years. The country will become an aged society by 2021, with 20% of the total population aged over 60 years [1]. With the increasing number of elderly Thai people, a national policy has been launched to prepare the communities for an ageing society. However, few strategies and plans have focused on the prevention and care for people with dementia.

Current situation of dementia in Thailand

The prevalence of dementia in people aged over 60 years in Thailand in 2015 was estimated to be 2.35–3.30%, i.e. approximately 235,000–330,000 people with dementia [2–4]. No study has investigated the diagnostic rates and access to medical care in people with dementia in the country. Diagnosis and medical management of dementia are carried out mainly in large tertiary care hospitals, academic hospitals, or psychiatric hospitals, which have limited availability and accessibility. The majority of dementia patients are cared for by their family members, and less than 0.1% of the elderly population use long-term care facilities [5]. Public awareness and understanding of dementia is growing, possibly as a result of collaborations among various social and health organizations and the expansion of social media and the Internet. Urgent issues in dementia care in Thailand include emphasis on social and clinical research at all levels, preparation for an aged society, provision of comprehensive support for patients and their families, access to medical care, and improving the capacity of healthcare personnel. These require a combination of local innovative approaches and careful translation from western world practice to suit the Thai cultural context and economic status.

The Thai National Dementia Strategy

Currently, a specific National Dementia Strategy is still in its initiation phase. However, there are national policies in place that support the elderly population as a whole, which are important building blocks in dementia care in Thailand.

Important policies in response to an aged society have been put in place. These are reflected in various national plans and funding allocations to support the elderly in economic, social, and health areas. The Act on Older Persons 2003 [6] and the Second National Plan on the Elderly 2002–2021 [7], revised in 2009, were adopted and translated into comprehensive action plans focusing on social security of the elderly to promote independent living, with inclusive support from multiple levels of the government and society. Examples include monetary allowance, accessibility of public services, wide availability of elderly clubs, and elderly clinics in secondary care hospitals. In addition, several projects were initiated, as part of the National Plan on the Elderly, such as a long-term saving scheme, occupational training, use of assistive technology, housing modifications, and community-based long-term care. These action plans are well aligned with the United Nations' Madrid International Plan of Action on Ageing and the World Health Organization's policy framework Active Ageing in 2002. Dementia has been included as part of mental health and degenerative illnesses considered in these policies. It is acknowledged that dementia care would require considerable social and environmental support, in addition to medically focused support—which gives impetus to establishing a robust strategy of dementia care for the elderly population.

The problem of dementia is also recognized at a regional level. Accordingly, appropriate action plans have also been developed by academic institutions and NGOs in the healthcare sector, to prepare for, and alleviate, the increasing burden of dementia. These include organizing academic activities for healthcare personnel, setting dementia management recommendations, delivering educational programmes and support groups for caregivers, running regular public awareness activities, and conducting social and clinical research studies. These activities are supported by higher levels of regulatory and governmental bodies such as the Ministry of Public Health and national research agencies.

Dementia policies have benefited from strong advocacy. The Alzheimer's Disease and Related Disorders Association of Thailand (also known as the Thai Dementia Caregiver Association) published a policy recommendation for dementia management in Thailand in 2012 [8], which recommended multi-level cooperation for dementia prevention, diagnosis, and medical management, and short- and long-term care for people with dementia. At present, academic and governmental organizations are already working collaboratively for policy-making in dementia care. It is hoped that these efforts and recommendations will provide a solid foundation that would facilitate the successful implementation of the national dementia strategy in Thailand.

Role of the family and community in dementia care in Thailand

Family care and close community support are the main contributors to care provision for people with dementia in Thailand. The Thai family structure is overall distinct from that of western countries which is predominantly based on single or one-generation families. The majority of Thai people live harmoniously together in extended or multi-generational families. In Thai tradition, household members are responsible for taking care of each other, which stems from a family-based caring system characterized by strong bonds among all family members. For example, a daughter might take care of the activities of daily living of her mother who suffers from dementia, while her siblings take on the responsibility of providing financial and social support.

Local community also plays a significant role in caring for people with dementia. Many countries are promoting the development of community-based dementia care, although people with dementia are still facing social exclusion. However, the Thai culture is quite different in terms of community involvement in care provision. Community care, which includes care for dementia, chronic diseases, and disability, as well as health promotion, is led by village health volunteers. These volunteers help patients and their families by reinforcing basic healthcare and social support, with minimal input from healthcare professionals. This scheme not only reduces the amount of funding required for such care provision, but it also ensures inclusive services are specifically tailored to the needs and culture of the community. Thus, involvement of both the family and the community in caring for people with dementia helps to generate a positive outlook on dementia care overall, which will be complementary to care provision by professionals and dementia training of professionals and caregivers.

Challenges in dementia care in Thailand

Even though there are many healthcare sectors involved in the care provision for people with dementia in Thailand, an accurate, up-to-date prevalence of dementia in Thailand is still unknown. A national survey by Jitapunkul *et al.*, published in 2001, estimated the prevalence rate of dementia among the elderly population to be 3.3% [3]. Thus, the lack of accurate epidemiological data makes the national plan for dementia very difficult to achieve.

In Thai culture, great respect is paid to seniors, and memory lapses are usually perceived as a normal ageing phenomenon. Therefore, the lack of public awareness and knowledge about dementia needs to be addressed. A national campaign should be set up to raise public awareness of dementia and educate people that dementia is a disease, and not a normal ageing process.

The number of healthcare providers for dementia is another concern. Dementia specialists, including neurologists, psychiatrists, and geriatricians, in memory or dementia clinics in secondary or tertiary healthcare centres are in charge of dementia diagnosis and treatment. Although clinical practice and diagnostic guidelines for dementia are available in Thai language [9–11] and can be accessed online, all non-dementia specialists, internists, and primary care physicians are still reluctant to follow these guidelines in clinical practice.

The two main reasons include the lack of training in the detection and diagnosis of dementia in ageing patients and the lack of reimbursement for available treatments, even when a diagnosis of dementia is made. All anti-dementia medications, including cholinesterase inhibitors, and other cognitive enhancers are not included on the national essential drug lists. Pharmacological and non-pharmacological intervention programmes or day care services have been perceived as futile interventions from an economic point of view.

Long-term care is another issue that should be of concern because the Thai family structure will change in the next few decades. Currently, the majority of people with dementia are cared for at home. However, there is a trend towards a reduction in family size, as is the case in developed countries, which leads to a major concern on the future availability of family caregiving. Soon, caring for people with dementia by the family may not be possible or adequate, while the number of qualified long-term care institutions and professional caregivers and availability of assisted technology for patients with dementia still remain very limited, even in the major cities of Thailand, including its capital city. With the rapid growth of its ageing population, Thailand may find itself in the face of an inadequate long-term care system.

Quality of life in dementia and caregiver burden

Measurements of quality of life (QoL) and health-related quality of life (HRQoL) become more complex when assessing the HRQoL of a person with dementia while also taking into account the local culture and value systems. In Thailand, most healthy people who live in rural areas resign to a significant decline in cognitive ability and health status as a normal part of ageing. Research focusing on QoL or HRQoL in dementia-related disorders in Thailand is very limited. This is because, first, most patients with dementia present to medical professionals at an advanced stage of memory decline when their cognitive impairment is too severe to allow them to self-rate their QoL. This renders QoL assessment unreliable, as it relies on reports by proxy or on direct observation of the patient's QoL by their assessor. Second, with limited resources, QoL measurements that are compatible with Thai culture are still in development [12, 13].

Dementia is not 'one person's illness' only; there is almost always a 'second patient' affected—the family caregiver. In Thailand, the family bears the main responsibility for providing care to the elderly with dementia. Most patients continue to live at home until the end of their life. Patients with dementia can have a negative impact on a caregiver's physical, psychosocial, or emotional health, social life, and financial situation. Traditionally, in Thailand, the responsibility for caring for frail elderly people falls on their daughters or daughters-in-law

[14]. Muangpaisan *et al.* conducted a study on Thai caregiver burden in dementia and to identify services to support caregivers in their role [15]. The authors found that dependency of dementia patients for basic activities of daily living correlated with high caregiver burden. The top three caregiver's needs were: (1) caregiver education and training, (2) a telephone line for caregiver consultation, and (3) a special hospital system designed to provide rapid access for dementia patients to see a doctor. However, their study included caregivers who had no financial difficulties, were well educated, and had several years of experience in caring for their patients [15].

Future of dementia care in Thailand

It is important to determine the actual prevalence of dementia in Thailand for a clear picture of the true impact of dementia on the country. An epidemiological survey should be conducted to address this, which would serve as a guide in the planning of a national policy for dementia care. Moreover, the standard practice for dementia care should be reviewed according to the level of care needed. Primary physicians and non-dementia specialists should be trained in dementia screening and diagnosis, as well as in providing evidence-based pharmacological and non-pharmacological interventions which should be covered by the Universal Coverage Scheme. It is essential to create an efficient consultation and referral system to seek dementia specialist input in cases of uncertainty in diagnosis and treatment. In addition, given the lack of dementia specialists in Thailand, an extensive training programme should be set up to increase the number of geriatric psychiatrists, geriatric internists, and behavioural neurologists, hence to enhance the capacity of delivering specialized services in tertiary care. Moreover, there should be wider engagement in dementia research in response to the increasing prevalence of dementia in the country.

A national dementia campaign would aim to promote more active participation of the Thai society in raising awareness of dementia through the use of mass media and social networks. Thus, this would help to improve home care and empower the family by providing support through training courses, self-help groups, and access to resource centres. Training of professional caregivers to relieve the family's burden is another option for better care quality. However, as the Thai family structure is set to gradually change into a nuclear family, plans for establishing public long-term residential care and nursing homes are warranted.

Treatment of dementia is another challenge. Considerable research efforts worldwide have focused on finding novel disease-modifying agents for dementia. Certain traditional or herbal medicines, such as *Centella asiatica* [16] and *Bacopa monnieri* [17] that have been tested in healthy elderly subjects, may be effective in the treatment of people with dementia.

Dementia may be preventable, and intervention should be initiated as early as possible in at-risk middle-aged adults, as well as healthy elderly. A prevention strategy can be implemented as a multi-domain intervention to reduce vascular risk factors and promote a healthy lifestyle through a healthy Thai diet, active physical exercise, and cognitive-stimulating activities, which have been suggested as one of the major contributing factors for maintaining cognitive reserve. Cognitive interventions for normal elderly people are also relevant, as part of a positive psychiatric approach [18]. Practising Thai style meditation or following Buddhist-orientated mindfulness training may be helpful. All these measures will help the healthy elderly population, in an attempt to reduce the incidence of dementia in Thailand over the next few decades.

References

1. **Foundation of Thai Gerontology Research and Development institute.** *Report of Thai elderly situation.* Bangkok: Amarin Printing and Publishing; 2014.

2. **Ferri CP, Prince M, Brayne C,** *et al.* Global prevalence of dementia: a Delphi consensus study. *The Lancet.* 2005;**366**:2112–17.

3. **Jitapunkul S, Kunanusont C, Phoolcharoen W, Suriyawongpaisal P.** Prevalence estimation of dementia among Thai elderly: a national survey. *Journal of the Medical Association of Thailand.* 2001;**84**:461–7.

4. **Wangtongkum S, Sucharitkul P, Silprasert N, Inthrachak R.** Prevalence of dementia among population age over 45 years in Chiang Mai, Thailand. *Journal of the Medical Association of Thailand.* 2008;**91**:1685–90.

5. **Jitapunkul S.** *Current status of Thai older persons and national actions on ageing.* Bangkok: Chulalongkorn University; 2000.

6. **Bureau of Empowerment for Older Persons, Ministry of Social Development and Human Security.** *Older Persons Act, B.E. 2546.* Bangkok: The Publishing of the Agricultural Cooperate Federation of Thailand; 2005.

7. **The National Commission on the Elderly, Bureau of Empowerment for Older Persons.** *The Second National Plan on The Elderly.* Bangkok: Tanapress; 2009.

8. **Alzheimer's Disease and Related Disorders Association Thailand.** *Summary of report on policy development of prevention and management of dementia in Thailand.* Bangkok: The Graphico System; 2012.

9. **Prasat Neurological Institute.** *Clinical practice puideline of dementia.* Bangkok: Tanapress; 2003.

10. **Prasat Neurological Institute.** *Clinical practice guideline of dementia,* 2nd ed. Bangkok: Tanapress; 2008.

11. **Prasat Neurological Institute.** *Clinical practice guideline: dementia.* Bangkok: Tanapress; 2014.

12. Senanarong V, Harnphadungkit K, Poungvarin N, *et al.* The Dementia and Disability Project in Thai Elderly: rational, design, methodology and early results. *BMC Neurology.* 2013;**13**:3.

13. Buasi N, Permsuwan U. Validation of the Thai QOL-AD version in Alzheimer's patients and caregivers. *Australasian Medical Journal.* 2014;**7**:251–9.

14. Chunharas S. *Situation of the Thai Elderly 2007.* Bangkok: The Foundation of Thai Gerontology Research and Development Institute; 2007.

15. Muangpaisan W, Praditsuwan R, Assanasen J, *et al.* Caregiver burden and needs of dementia care in Thailand: a cross-sectional study. *Journal of the Medical Association of Thailand.* 2010;**93**:601–7.

16. Wattanathorn J, Mator L, Muchimapura S, *et al.* Positive modulation of cognition and mood in the healthy elderly volunteer following the administration of *Centella asiatica. Journal of Ethnopharmacology.* 2008;**116**:325–32.

17. Kongkeaw C, Dilokthornsakul P, Thanarangsarit P, Limpeanchob N, Norman Scholfield C. Meta-analysis of randomized controlled trials on cognitive effects of Bacopa monnieri extract. *Journal of Ethnopharmacology.* 2014;**151**:528–35.

18. Udomratn P, Nakawiro D. Positive psychiatry and cognitive interventions for the elderly. *Taiwanese Journal of Psychiatry.* 2016;**30**:23–34.

Chapter 14

United Arab Emirates

Amir IA Ahmed, Salwa Alsuwaidi,
and Abdullah Al Ali

Summary

In the United Arab Emirates (UAE), members of the extended
family play a key role in caring for people with dementia. Culture
has a strong influence on family caregivers' motivation, and
Emirati people believe strongly that it is their (religious) duty to
provide care for their parents and other family members, including
those with dementia. This setup contributes positively to keeping
elderly people living at home. However, maintaining health and
independence in old age will become increasingly challenging
in the future, with the increasing ageing population in the UAE,
which is expected to reach up to 11% by 2032. Currently, the UAE
has no National Dementia Care Strategy, and epidemiological data
on dementia in the country are scarce. However, Dubai is known
to have a more or less comprehensive system of care for geriatric
patients, including dementia care facilities. These dementia care
facilities are available free of charge to Emirati citizens.

Introduction

The United Arab Emirates (UAE) is a federation of seven emirates (Abu Dhabi,
Ajman, Dubai, Fujairah, Ras Al Khaimah, Sharjah, and Umm Al-Quwain) established in 1971. The UAE is situated in the South East of the Arab Peninsula in
the Arabian Gulf (North), bordering Saudi Arabia (South and West) and Oman
(East). In 2015, the UAE's population was estimated at over 9 million, according
to the World Health Organization (WHO) [1], comprising about 85% of expatriates and only 15% of Emirati citizens. Therefore, the country has a diverse
and heterogeneous population where cultural traditions and religions pervade
most aspects of life, including health and healthcare. Since the discovery of its

oil reserves, the country has experienced rapid economic growth and development, including in the health sector.

Ageing in the UAE

As a result of improved living standards in the UAE, life expectancy has increased significantly. Before the union of the emirates, life expectancy was estimated to be 53 years for both sexes, whereas in 2015, it was 76 years for males and 79 years for females, according to the WHO [1].

According to the Department of Economic and Social Affairs of the United Nations, 2.3% of the total population of the UAE consist of people aged 60 years and over, including immigrants [2], with the proportion of Emiratis over the age of 60 comprising around 4% of the total number of Emirati citizens. The high percentage of older Emirati citizens is attributed to the fact that the majority of expatriate workers are young adults. The percentage of older Emiratis is expected to increase to 6% by 2017 and 11% by 2032. Hence, with an ageing population in the UAE, maintaining health and independence in old age will become increasingly challenging.

Despite the economic prosperity and improvements in healthcare that have increased life expectancy in the UAE, there are few specialized geriatric services in the country, with only a few hospitals providing geriatric consultation. Moreover, the number of geriatricians and nurses specialized in geriatric care is very limited. Nowadays, only four of the seven emirates provide services for older people, all of which are free of charge, including:

1. Dubai: *The Family Gathering Centre* is a nursing home, established in 1993, with a capacity of 33 beds and has a day care centre for outpatients. In addition, Dubai offers two other services for older people through the Community Development Authority—the *Weleef Programme* which offers social home services for those who live at home, and the *Thukher Club* which provides social day activities for older people.

2. Ajman: the *Older Persons Care Residence* is a nursing home established in 1982.

3. Sharjah: the *Old People Home* is a nursing home established in 1986.

4. Ras Al Khaima: the *Ibrahim Bin Hamad Obaid Allah Geriatric Hospital* was established in 2009 and has 60 long-term beds.

Dementia care in the UAE

The UAE has no National Dementia Care Strategy, and epidemiological data on dementia in the country are scarce. A recent unpublished pilot study

(ElNoamani *et al.*, 2013) reported that 16.2% of study participants (*n* = 160) could be diagnosed with 'Probable Alzheimer's disease'. However, only 3% of diagnosed patients are formally registered in the medical records as having dementia.

Despite the paucity of dementia data, care for dementia patients in the UAE is one of the biggest challenges faced by healthcare providers and caregivers. However, the extended family structure which includes several generations from the same family living under the same roof is still preserved. This structure enables care for dementia patients to be provided by their family. Culture has a strong influence on family caregivers' motivation, and Emirati people believe strongly that it is their (religious) duty to provide care for their parents and other family members, including those with dementia. All these factors contribute positively to keeping older people living at home, maintaining the integrity of their social network, and reducing the need for their institutionalization.

Compared to the other six emirates, Dubai has a more or less comprehensive system of care for geriatric patients, including those with dementia. This include a specialized unit in Rashid Hospital that takes in acute and long-term cases, an outpatient geriatric clinic, a specialized memory clinic, a nursing home, and a day care centre.

Challenges in dementia care in the UAE

The UAE faces several challenges in dementia care that need to be addressed. These challenges include the following:

1. Over 95% of the UAE population is younger than 65 years. Therefore, government and public policies focus mainly on child and youth development. However, this focus needs to include also older people in general and, in particular, dementia patients.

2. The limited number of geriatricians and other geriatrics healthcare providers in the country could result in under-diagnosis of dementia and under-management of age-related issues. Geriatric care in the UAE is mostly provided by GPs and general internists who lack expertise in geriatric medicine.

3. There is a lack of specialized dementia diagnostic centres, as well as dementia organizations, such as Alzheimer's Association, to support healthcare professionals working with dementia patients and caregivers in the UAE.

4. The lack of awareness among caregivers of the symptoms of dementia could contribute to underdiagnosis of dementia. Most caregivers believe that memory problems and behavioural changes are a normal part of ageing and therefore do not seek medical help.

5. The majority of patients with dementia still live at home. Consequently, there is an increasing demand for home-based care; yet this service remains underdeveloped in the UAE.

6. The stigma associated with a relative being 'labelled' as having dementia may result in the family, out of shame or embarrassment, keeping their loved one at home and hence isolated from society. Patients and caregivers often seek treatment only when struggling at home with behavioural challenges many years after the symptoms of dementia first emerged.

7. The UAE, like many countries, faces the challenge of ensuring adequate infrastructure in place to support people with dementia, as well as their caregivers, when a diagnosis of dementia is made.

8. Epidemiological studies on dementia and a national register for dementia patients are lacking in the UAE. Therefore, there is a strong need for reliable and valid longitudinal data for the planning of population-based public health programmes.

Recommendations and future directions

Development of national policies in ageing and dementia care

Future policies should be developed by the federal government of the UAE for all seven emirates to improve the care for older people and dementia patients in the entire country. These policies should include educational and support programmes for patients, family members/caregivers, and service providers, to raise public awareness of dementia. In addition, older individuals and their families in the UAE have low awareness of the physical and mental effects of ageing [3]. Therefore, it is important that the design and delivery of educational and support programmes take into account the needs of the elderly individuals and their caregivers, as well as their convenience, to increase the likelihood of participation. Moreover, given the population demographics of the UAE, future national dementia care policies and initiatives should consider the socio-cultural, religious, ethnic, and educational diversity of the UAE society in the design, development, and implementation of local campaigns, interventions, and strategies.

Development of geriatric and dementia care facilities

In order to support elderly individuals and their families through ageing, the federal government of the UAE should play a proactive role in the development of geriatric and dementia care services. It is important that different types of geriatric services be made available and accessible in all seven emirates. These should include emergency medical and dental care, geriatric departments in hospitals, memory clinics, geriatric rehabilitation centres, specialized dementia units in nursing homes, and day care and activity centres.

Education and training of healthcare professionals

There should be adequate human resources in terms of trained healthcare professionals to improve the health status of patients with dementia. Currently, there is a shortage of specialist physicians and nurses in the field of dementia care. Furthermore, none of the medical schools in the UAE have a geriatric department, and very few offer courses in geriatrics for medical students. In the UAE, there is currently low incentive to encourage junior doctors or medical students to specialize in geriatric medicine—a situation that needs to be changed in order to ensure geriatric expertise and relevant knowledge among the healthcare workforce. In addition, primary care physicians should be educated about primary prevention, rather than secondary or tertiary prevention, of dementia.

Role of the family in the context of long-term care

Currently, the UAE government's healthcare and social policies for older people focus mainly on financial aid and subsidies allocated as social support. Families, including extended families, need to be supported not only financially in their long-term role as caregivers, but also by medical and social professionals specialized in geriatric care. Their legitimate concerns, worries, and needs should be acknowledged and addressed. Many elderly people from unsupported families are never diagnosed with dementia. Even those who are diagnosed with the condition rarely realize the true extent of planning and changes that are required as a consequence. Despite the availability of geriatric services, albeit limited, in the UAE, many caregivers are not aware of such services being accessible in their community. Therefore, future challenges in the UAE are to determine the types of support and services to cater for the needs of the elderly and their families, and how best to prepare for and develop these care plans.

References

1. **World Health Organization**. *United Arab Emirates: statistics*. Available from: http://www.who.int/countries/are/en/ [accessed 1 November 2016].
2. **Department of Economic and Social Affairs Population Division, United Nations**. *World population ageing 2015*. New York, NY: United Nations; 2015. Available

from: http://www.un.org/en/development/desa/population/publications/pdf/ageing/WPA2015_Report.pdf [accessed 1 November 2016].

3. **Aisha Zayed Al Ali**. *Aging in the UAE and services available for the elderly: structured interviews with experts in the field*. 2013. Available from: http://www.mbrsg.ae/getattachment/91a79863-e776-4b22-ae2c-9a7449b99f80/Aging-in-the-UAE-and-Services-Available-for-the-El [accessed 1 November 2016].

Section 3

Australia, New Zealand, and Oceania

Chapter 15

Australia

Henry Zeimer

Summary

Dementia is a major public health issue in Australia, with profound consequences for the healthcare system and society in general, with nearly 1.5% of the population living with dementia. It has wide-ranging effects on the Australian healthcare system and society and its prevalence is expected to increase significantly with the ageing of the population. Through the Medicare Benefits Schedule and the Pharmaceutical Benefits Scheme, the Australian government funds services for diagnosis and assessment, as well as subsidizing medications for the treatment of Alzheimer's disease. The government also funds community support groups and services to assist in the care, and improve the quality of life, of people with dementia. The Australian Health Ministers announced in August 2012 that dementia is a National Health Priority Area, the ninth medical condition to receive this important status. Commissioned by the Australian government, the Australian Institute for Health and Welfare in 2012 released Dementia in Australia [1], a comprehensive review of dementia, and from which statistics and information has been used in preparing this chapter.

Epidemiology

There are currently 322,000 people in Australia living with dementia. This represents nearly 1.5% of the total population, and of all Australians aged 65 and over, 9% have dementia. There are more women with dementia than men, with prevalence rates of 62% and 38%, respectively.

Estimates of prevalence by residency suggest that 70% of people with dementia live in the community, while the remaining 30% live in residential care facilities [1].

The *2015 Intergenerational Report: Australia in 2055*, released by the Australian Government Treasury, forecasts a significant change in size and structure of the population in the next 40 years. The number of Australians aged 65 and over is expected to more than double by 2055, compared with today [2]. As a result of the ageing of the population, the number of those with dementia is projected to triple to over 900,000 in 2050.

Burden of disease

The impact of dementia on healthcare and society is thoroughly covered in the *Dementia in Australia* report and is summarized here [1]. First, in disability-adjusted life year (DALY), a commonly used measure of disease burden, the burden of dementia in 2011 was projected to be 121,737 DALYs. This ranks dementia fourth in the leading causes of disease burden in Australia, while it ranks as the second leading cause of overall disease burden for people aged 65 and over (behind ischaemic heart disease).

General practitioners (GPs) play a vital role in the assessment and management of dementia. In 2011, it was estimated that about 552,000 GP consultations, or 0.5% of all GP visits, involved dementia care. In terms of hospitalizations, in 2009–2010, there were over 12,000 hospital admissions where dementia was recorded as the principal diagnosis (0.1% of all hospital admissions in Australia). These admissions accounted for nearly 217,500 patient days in hospital in 2009–2010, which equates to 0.8% of all patient days. This indicates that hospitalizations with dementia as the main diagnosis consume more patient days than average. Notably, the average length of stay for hospitalizations for dementia recorded as the principal diagnosis was over three times longer than the average length of stay for all hospitalizations (22 and 6 days, respectively). The number and proportion of deaths due to dementia have increased steadily over the last 15 years. In 2003, dementia was the sixth leading cause of death, and by 2014, it had risen to second place (behind ischaemic heart disease). The rise in death due to dementia exceeds the increase in prevalence over these interval years. Possible explanations for this are a greater awareness of dementia by medical practitioners, and updates in 2006 to the coding instructions in the International Classification of Diseases, tenth revision (ICD-10), which resulted in the coding of vascular dementia on death certificates that may have been coded as cerebrovascular disease previously. Currently, dementia is the cause of death for one in 19 female deaths and one in ten male deaths.

Finally, the total direct health and aged care system expenditure attributable to dementia was estimated to be around A$2.0 billion in 2009–2010, and this increases to A$4.9 billion if the total cost of care of people with dementia in residential care is included (rather than the proportion of cost of care that is attributable to dementia only). These figures do not include the expenditure for outpatient and emergency department visits, specialized mental healthcare services, and residential respite care, as well as indirect expenditure such as social and economic costs on caregivers and families, lost wages, and productivity.

Diagnosis and management

Assessment of patients for diagnosing dementia occurs in a variety of health services and settings. The commonest sites where the diagnosis is made are GP surgeries, government-funded outpatient clinics, and private specialist consulting rooms. Memory clinics, funded by state health departments, are the best resourced service for dementia diagnosis and have essentially adopted a team-based multidisciplinary approach to the assessment of cognitive impairment. These clinics are available to everyone nationally, although they are usually located in the major cities and larger regional centres. There has been a progressive increase in the use of telehealth in major centres to provide diagnostic services to those in remote rural areas who have difficulty accessing a memory clinic. Although the level of resources vary from clinic to clinic, they are typically staffed by specialists (geriatricians, neurologists, psycho-geriatricians), nurses, social workers, neuropsychologists, and occasionally other allied health practitioners (occupational therapists, clinical psychologists, speech therapists). Memory clinics are not only involved in the diagnosis and initial management of dementia, but also provide links to other service providers such as aged care services, community care providers, and community support groups.

An overview of all Australian memory clinics identified by key specialists working in dementia assessment services was published in 2009 [3]. The first memory clinic was established in 1985, and at the time of publication, 23 clinics were operating across Australia. However, this number has most likely increased since then. Most patients (59%) were referred by their GP and 16% by other doctors, and 12% were self-referrals. Unlike other specialty clinics, patients, families, and allied health practitioners can make referrals to memory clinics.

In terms of the diagnostic workup for dementia, most investigations are covered in the Medicare Benefits Schedule (MBS) and are available to patients free of charge. CT brain scanning is widely available and covered by Medicare. Medicare funding for MRI scanning requires the investigation of specific clinical conditions approved by Medicare Australia. AD and dementia are not included on the approved list for MRI brain scanning, but trauma, stroke, and toxic, metabolic, or ischaemic encephalopathy are. Hence, a request for MRI brain scanning in someone suspected of having AD must include a condition such as stroke or multiple infarcts as a differential diagnosis, in order to be funded under Medicare. Also, MRI scans can only be requested by specialists (not GPs) to be funded under Medicare. Functional imaging with single-photon emission computerized tomography (SPECT) scans for diagnosing dementia is Medicare-funded but is only available at tertiary referral hospitals. Positron emission tomography (PET) and dopamine transporter scans are not Medicare-funded for dementia. However, whole-body PET (including brain) is covered by Medicare in those with a history of certain cancers (colorectal, melanoma, lymphoma) for purposes of re-staging but, once again, is only available in larger centres. Efforts are being made by key opinion leaders to lobby the government to increase funding in order to make MRI and functional imaging more available in dementia diagnosis.

Approved medications for dementia, namely acetylcholinesterase inhibitors and memantine, are available for the treatment of AD at a subsidized price under the Pharmaceutical Benefits Scheme (PBS). In order to obtain the PBS subsidy, the diagnosis must be made by, or in consultation with, a specialist. Acetylcholinesterase inhibitors (donepezil, rivastigmine, galantamine) are all available for mild to moderate AD patients with MMSE scores of 10 or above. Memantine is available to moderate to severe AD patients with MMSE scores of 10 to 14 inclusive. The PBS will not subsidize dual therapy, but patients may elect to pay full price for one of these drugs while receiving the other drug at the PBS-subsidized price. In order to continue on subsidized medication beyond 6 months, the PBS requires a doctor's assessment that the patient has achieved a clinically meaningful response during the first 6 months of therapy. Also, risperidone and first-generation antipsychotics are subsidized for the management of behavioural and psychiatric symptoms of dementia.

In the 2009–2010 financial year, over 392,000 subsidized prescriptions for dementia-specific medications were dispensed, which equate to 0.2% of all subsidized medications dispensed that year [1]. The number of prescriptions dispensed for AD has increased steadily, with a 74% increase from 2002–2003 to 2009–2010.

Community supports and research

As mentioned, dementia has been given the status of a National Health Priority Area. As a result, the Australian government, mainly through the Department of Social Services, funds a number of activities to support people affected by dementia. Under the umbrella of the National Dementia Support Program (NDSP), the government has put in place a range of services and resources to primarily improve the quality of life and provide assistance for dementia patients and their caregivers in the community. With the rising prevalence of the disease, further initiatives and re-structuring of the NDSP are in the planning stages.

Alzheimer's Australia is the national peak body for people with dementia, their families, and caregivers. It is predominantly government-funded but also receives funds through charitable donations. It has branches in all states and territories and provides educational, social, and counselling services, raises awareness of this important condition, and has an advisory role with the government in planning community programmes. Another of its main roles is to establish and maintain the National Dementia Helpline. This service is available across Australia on a toll-free number during business hours on Monday to Friday. It is staffed by trained, experienced professionals and provides support, practical information, advice, and information about services that are available to people with dementia and their caregivers.

The Dementia Behaviour Management Advisory Service (DBMAS) is also a government-funded nationwide telephone service, established to provide advice to families and caregivers of people with dementia who experience behaviours of concern. Caregivers or healthcare professionals can contact the service 24 hours a day, 7 days a week. In the 2013–2014 financial year, DBMAS provided 6715 episodes of service, of which 45% were referrals from residential care facilities. In February 2015, the government announced that Severe Behaviour Response Teams would be established to augment DBMAS and provide assistance to residential care facilities with residents experiencing severe dementia-related behavioural disturbance. The first phase of this programme was launched in late 2015.

In order to improve the quality of care and enhance the dementia care skills of health professionals, the government in 2006 established Dementia Training Study Centres in each state and territory. These centres coordinate educational programmes and activities to transfer evidence-based knowledge to healthcare professionals involved in the day-to-day care of those with dementia. In 2012, the New South Wales–Australian Capital Territory training centre launched *The Australian Journal of Dementia Care*, Australia's first and only multidisciplinary journal for healthcare workers dedicated to dementia care. The journal disseminates news, latest research developments, and practice and training issues from Australia and around the world to its subscribers.

In Australia, the National Health and Medical Research Council (NHMRC) is responsible for distributing funds for health-related research on behalf of the government. In 2015, the NHMRC's total expenditure for research grants was over A$8.8 billion, of which only A$35.1 million was allocated to dementia research [4]. This was the third lowest allocation of the National Health Priority Areas and represents less than 0.5% of the total research expenditure. Despite this imbalance in research funding, dementia research in Australia is thriving and is producing high-quality outcomes that influence practice. An example of this is the internationally renowned Australian Imaging Biomarkers and Lifestyle Study (AiBL), which is one of the largest cohort studies assessing risk factors for developing AD. Alzheimer's Australia continues to actively lobby the NHMRC to increase expenditure for dementia research in future grant allocations.

References

1. **Australian Institute of Health and Welfare**. *Dementia in Australia*. Canberra: Australian Institute of Health and Welfare; 2012. Available from: http://www.aihw.gov.au/publication-detail/?id=10737422958 [accessed 27 July 2018].

2. **Commonwealth of Australia**. *2015 Intergenerational Report: Australia in 2055*. Canberra: The Treasury; **2015**. Available from: https://treasury.gov.au/publication/2015-intergenerational-report/ [accessed 27 July 2018].

3. **Woodward MC, Woodward E**. A national survey of memory clinics in Australia. *International Psychogeriatrics*. 2009;**21**:696–702.

4. **National Health and Medical Research Council**. *Research funding and statistics data*. Available from: https://www.nhmrc.gov.au/grants-funding/research-funding-statistics-and-data [accessed 27 July 2018].

Chapter 16

New Zealand

Jane Casey and Gary Cheung

Epidemiology and health funding

The New Zealand (NZ) population is living longer and becoming more ethnically diverse. At the time of our last census in 2013, 14.3% (607,032) of the NZ population were aged 65 years and over [1]. The 65+ population in 2013 has nearly doubled since 1981; and by 2063, people aged 85 years and over will also be doubled. In the 2012–14 period, the average 65-year-old woman could expect to live another 21.3 years, and the average 65-year-old man another 18.9 years.

The population of our older NZ indigenous Māori people is predicted to grow. Between 2011 and 2026, the older Māori population will grow by 7.1%, double the growth expected for non-Māori, to 9.8% of the total older population [2]. However, the long-standing issue of inequalities in health between Māori and non-Māori has not improved in the last few decades [3]. In 2013, life expectancy at birth was 73.0 years for Māori males and 77.1 years for Māori females, which was 7–8 years less than their non-Māori counterparts [2]. Auckland is now home to the largest Pacific Islands population in the world. The incidence of ischaemic heart disease, stroke, and diabetes is higher in Pacific people than other ethnic groups [4]. They are also exposed to higher levels of lifestyle risk factors such as obesity, smoking, and poor nutrition. Māori and Pacific peoples are also disproportionately represented in lower socio-economic areas and have lower incomes and higher levels of unemployment. Meanwhile, almost one out of eight people living in NZ are Asian, and nearly two-thirds of Asian people live in the Auckland region where over one in five people are of Asian ethnicity.

There is one previous study examining the prevalence of dementia in a rural centre in NZ where 7.7% of those aged 65 years and above suffered from dementia [5]. A 5-years cohort study of Māori aged 80 to 90 years and non-Māori aged 85 years found that dementia was present in 26% of the participants 'at some time' in the study and there is no significant difference in prevalence between Māori and non-Māori, nor between women and men [6]. The incidence and prevalence of dementia in Pacific and Asian people living in NZ is unknown, although there is some evidence to suggest that Pacific people with dementia presented to a specialist memory service at a younger age and with more advanced cognitive symptoms than NZ Europeans [7]. It was estimated that 52,509 New Zealanders had dementia in 2014, an increase from 48,182 people in 2011. By 2050, 147,359 New Zealanders will have dementia—over 2.6% of the population, and more than triple the current numbers [8].

NZ health services are primarily funded by the central government, based on a community-oriented model. There are 20 district health boards (DHBs) of varying sizes. For example, Canterbury DHB has the largest age 65+ catchment of 72,195 people, while West Coast DHB has the smallest catchment of 5184 older people. DHBs are responsible for providing or funding the provision of health services in their district to meet local, regional, and national needs, including primary and secondary care services. The demographic changes in NZ will certainly have a significant influence on how future gerontology health and social services are structured and delivered in a manner that would meet the needs of our culturally diverse communities in both rural and urban settings.

NZ National Dementia Strategy, the NZ Framework for Dementia Care, and Improving the Lives of People with Dementia

In 2010, Alzheimers New Zealand launched the National Dementia Strategy 2010–2015. This was replaced by a new Strategic Framework in 2014, which is aimed to challenge all organizations in the dementia community to focus on a vision of 'towards a world without dementia', with five shared goals: (1) a dementia-friendly NZ, (2) good brain health, (3) early recognition and assessment, (4) living well with dementia, and (5) high-quality services. However, neither the Strategy nor this Framework were formally adopted by the government.

In 2013, the NZ Ministry of Health published their own NZ Framework for Dementia Care informing the development of cognitive impairment care pathways in each of the 20 DHBs [9]. These pathways were expected to be implemented in the DHBs by the end of the 2013/14 financial year. The NZ Framework for Dementia Care is underpinned by three main principles: (1) following a person-centred and people-directed approach, (2) providing accessible, proactive, and integrated services that are flexible to meet a variety of needs, and (3) developing the highest possible standard of care. Fig. 16.1 shows an earlier version of the cognitive impairment pathway developed for the Northern Region.

In addition, the Ministry of Health published the *Improving the Lives of People with Dementia* document in August 2014 [10]. Through this document, the Ministry will support action in nine key areas to improve the quality of life for people with dementia:

♦ Implement a nationally consistent approach to dementia care.

♦ Increase dementia awareness.

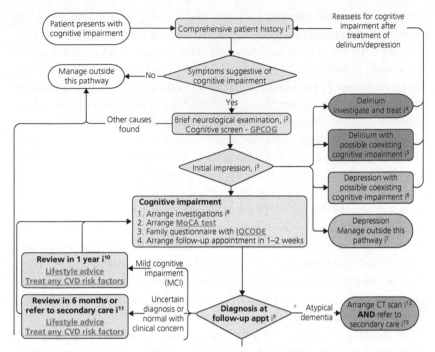

Fig. 16.1 An earlier version of the cognitive impairment care pathway in the Northern Region of New Zealand.

Reproduced from Comprehensive Care. Source data from: Canterbury HealthPathways Cognitive Impairment http://canterburyinitiative.org.nz and the waltermata DHB pathway.

- Reduce the risk of dementia.
- Increase access to a timely diagnosis of dementia.
- Provide navigation of services and increase the quality of information and education.
- Increase the ability of people with dementia to remain living at home.
- Increase the quality of information and education for the workforce.
- Develop dementia-friendly health and social support services.
- Provide respectful and supportive end-of-life care.

Snapshot of current services and innovations across NZ

The existing dementia services that are well developed are mainly based in urban settings. A feature of many of these services is an established primary care-based cognitive impairment pathway with support from secondary care-based specialist services. Many old age psychiatry services have established memory services, day hospital assessment clinics, and working inter-relationships between specialist services such as geriatric medicine and neurology. There is progress in public hospitals to establish 'dementia champions' to raise the profile of the needs of people with cognitive impairment and to ensure at-risk groups, such as those over 75 presenting with falls or delirium, are captured in the acute hospital setting. The 'Better Brain Care' pathway is such an example aimed to provide routine cognitive screening, assessment, early intervention, and follow-up for older people admitted to Auckland City Hospital. The concept of a 'dementia navigator' for education, advice, and coordination of care and for providing a point of continuity is in the early phase of uptake, with the centre of care beginning to shift to the primary healthcare team. The relationship between secondary services and primary healthcare teams is well established in NZ, with ongoing education and shared care approaches to management. Likewise, the interface and collegial working relationships with NGOs, such as Alzheimers New Zealand, Age Concern, Carers NZ, and Aged Residential Care, are strong. There is a wealth of NZ-centric information available on the Internet. Some regions have produced person-centred booklets held by the person and the family such as the Northern Region's *Living Well with Dementia Plan*.

The 'Walking in Another Shoes' programme for caregivers is small-group experiential training developed to promote a person-centred approach to dementia care and to behaviours that challenge [11]. It was developed in Canterbury for caregivers working with people living with dementia in the residential care setting in the region. The success of this programme has resulted in its rollout via the South Island Dementia Initiative, and like other innovations, it is cited in the NZ Framework as a 'Good Practice' example. Currently, there is also work on translating and implementing Cognitive Stimulation Therapy, an evidence-based psychosocial intervention for mild to moderate dementia developed in the United Kingdom, in a small number of secondary services, Alzheimer's societies, and aged residential care facilities [12].

The New Zealand Dementia Cooperative (NZDC) was established in 2011 with the vision to 'co-operate and collaborate with like-minded people who are passionate about advancing knowledge of approaches to dementia care in NZ' (https://nzdementia.org). It now is approaching 1000 members, the majority of whom are individuals who work in the sector, provider organizations or funders, and government departments. This successful innovation has linked sectors across the country, channelling knowledge and expertise via the website, regional network groups, and the biannual Knowledge Forum. The NZDC, with the goal of improving standards of care and support for people with dementia and their families, functions as a collective voice in the development of both policy and practice in dementia care in NZ.

The future and dementia care in NZ

Significant progress has been made in raising awareness of the needs of persons with dementia and their family and whānau. The concept of 'Dementia-Friendly Communities' has been spearheaded by Alzheimers New Zealand; a national bank has developed the first dementia-friendly bank in the country, and Bupa in the Aged Residential Care sector has also adopted the philosophy. In Christchurch, the 2010/2011 earthquakes created a unique opportunity for local researchers, in partnership with people with dementia, to promote the design of a dementia-friendly model of a new physical environment with the progressive re-build [13].

Educational advertisements now screen on national television, and there is an increase in readily available resources, education, and training for people with dementia. However, there is a long way to go to address the negative social stigma—to demystify the disease and enable early diagnosis and treatment, so as to effect the longer-term goal of communities where New Zealanders can indeed live well with dementia.

The future challenges of dementia care include the increasing need for early diagnosis, improved primary healthcare involvement, and easier access to well-coordinated, culturally appropriate services. There is ongoing development aimed to up-skill primary care clinicians in the diagnosis and management of dementia. For example, in 2017 the University of Auckland Goodfellow Unit released a free e-learning dementia educational resource for GPs and practice nurses (https://www.goodfellowunit.org/courses/dementia).

The fragmentation and duplication of assessment and services require addressing across both the health and social sectors. The role of both informal and formal caregivers needs to be valued, aiming for increased stability in the residential care workforce and improved education and training. There need to be increased accountability at the local and regional governance level where measurable outcomes are developed to evaluate new models and pathways in dementia care. The lack of national consistency in funding streams and benchmarking for specialist services remains an obstacle to identifying gaps and ensuring improvements in caring for people with dementia care in NZ.

Research and evaluation will continue to underpin the development of dementia strategy and management in NZ, along with the identification of biomarkers and risk and protective factors associated with cognitive decline in a longitudinal study through the newly established Dementia Prevention Research Clinics in Auckland, Christchurch, and Dunedin. Work is currently underway to examine the validity and/or feasibility of the 10/66 dementia assessment protocols in our main ethnic groups (Māori, Tongan, Samoan, Chinese, Indian and NZ European) [14]. The findings will be used to inform a future dementia prevalence study in NZ. Finally, a suite of tools for dementia assessment and management focused on Māori people is in development to meet the cultural needs of our indigenous people.

References

1. **Statistics New Zealand**. *2013 Census QuickStats about people aged 65 and over*. Available from: http://www.stats.govt.nz/Census/2013-census/profile-and-summary-reports/quickstats-65-plus/population-overview.aspx [accessed 20 October 2016].

2. **Ministry of Health**. *Ngā mana hauora tūtohu: Health status indicators*. Available from: http://www.health.govt.nz/our-work/populations/maori-health/tatau-kahukura-maori-health-statistics/nga-mana-hauora-tutohu-health-status-indicators/life-expectancy [accessed 20 October 2016].

3. **Dyall L**. Dementia: continuation of health and ethnic inequalities in NZ. *The New Zealand Medical Journal*. 2014;**127**:68–81.

4. **Statistics New Zealand and Ministry of Pacific Island Affairs**. *Health and Pacific peoples in New Zealand*. Wellington: Statistics New Zealand and Ministry of Pacific Island Affairs; 2011.

5. **Campbell AJ, McCosh LM, Reinken J, Allan BC**. Dementia in old age and the need for services. *Age and Ageing*. 1983;**12**:11–6.

6. **Kerse N, Lapsley H, Moyes S, Zawaly K, Hayman K, LiLACS NZ 2017**. Dementia: Supplementary Findings from LiLACS NZ for Section Five, 'Service Use and Common Health Conditions' in the report 'Health, Independence and Caregiving in Advanced Age'. Auckland. School of Population Health, The University of Auckland.

7. **Cullum S, Mullin K, Zeng I, Yates S, Payman V, Fisher M, Cheung G**. Do community-dwelling Māori and Pacific peoples present with dementia at a younger age and at a later stage compared with NZ Europeans?. International journal of Geriatric Psychiatry. 2018; May 15.

8. **Alzheimers New Zealand**. *Dementia economic report 2012*. 2012. Available from: http://www.alzheimers.org.nz/news-info/nz-information/dementia-economic-report-2012 [accessed 20 October 2016].

9. **Ministry of Health**. *New Zealand framework for dementia care*. Wellington: Ministry of Health; 2013.

10. **Ministry of Health**. *Improving the lives of people with dementia*. Wellington: Ministry of Health; 2014.

11. **Gee SB, Scott-Multani M**. Walking in Another's Shoes: encouraging person-centred care for people living with dementia in NZ. *World Federation of Occupational Therapists Bulletin*. 2015;**70**:15–17.

12. **Cheung G, Peri K**. *Cognitive stimulation therapy: A New Zealand pilot*. Auckland: Te Pou o Te Whakaaro Nui: The National Centre of Mental Health Research, Information and Workforce Development; 2014.

13. **Smith K, Gee S, Sharrock T, Croucher M**. Developing a dementia-friendly Christchurch: perspectives of people with dementia. *Australasian Journal of Ageing*. 2016;**35**:188–92.

14. **Prince M, Ferri CP, Acosta D, Albanese E, Arizaga R, Dewey M, Gavrilova SI, Guerra M, Huang Y, Jacob K**. The protocols for the 10/66 dementia research group population-based research programme. *BMC Public Health*. 2007;**7**:165.

Section 4

Europe

Chapter 17

Belgium

Eric Salmon

Summary

Although, in Belgium, there is no national Alzheimer's plan, several national initiatives are in place for promoting care for patients with dementia and supporting their caregivers. There are strict rules for reimbursement of the cost of dementia drug treatment, which also includes neuropsychological evaluation in the early stages of dementia. Memory clinics provide cognitive rehabilitation to adapt daily activities to help preserve the independence of patients with dementia and also to help support caregivers facing daily difficulties in their caregiving role. Belgium also has legislation in place relating to euthanasia and relating to impaired mental capacity and advance directives. The main challenges in dementia care in Belgium lie in care planning, ensuring the involvement of patients and their chosen caregivers, and the comprehensive assessment of prevention programmes.

Is there a Belgian National Dementia Strategy?

Belgium has the particularity of comprising three regions and three national languages. Although there is no national Alzheimer's plan, numerous national, regional, and local initiatives concerning dementia care are in place for both patients and their relatives. There are also several National Dementia Strategies which are very useful. This chapter is based on multiple reports issued from different groups of actors interested and involved in discussion on dementia in Belgium [1].

What can Belgium be particularly proud of in dementia care?

In Belgium, there are relatively strict rules for reimbursement of costs of drug treatment for AD (acetylcholinesterase inhibitors, without or with memantine) by the national health services. The first criterion is a diagnosis of dementia, as certified by a neurologist or geriatric or psychiatric specialist. The MMSE is used, with a cut-off score of 24 and lower confirming cognitive impairment, while a complete neuropsychological assessment is required for MMSE scores higher than 24. Reimbursement is possible for only one neuropsychological assessment if deterioration due to a neurocognitive disorder is confirmed. Moreover, additional evaluations are required to determine the global severity rating (such as Clinical Dementia Rating) and to assess activities of daily living (basic and instrumental) and psychological and behavioural symptoms (such as the Neuropsychiatric Interview). Neuroimaging investigation must also be carried out to exclude possible causes of dementia other than AD. The cost of positron emission tomography imaging (currently FDG-PET) can be reimbursed for patients with MMSE scores of 24 and higher and with cognitive impairment confirmed by formal neuropsychological assessment. Care planning for patients and their relatives must be initiated upon the initial request for drug cost reimbursement. A follow-up visit is required after 6 months to assess the patient, using the MMSE score and Clinical Global Impression of Change, to determine whether to continue treatment. Subsequent follow-up visits are conducted once every year to monitor and adjust the patient's treatment according to their clinical response. The cost of combined treatment with acetylcholinesterase inhibitors and memantine is reimbursed for MMSE scores in the range of 10–14. Reimbursement is not allowed for MMSE scores below 10.

A memory clinic has been established in each province to provide cognitive rehabilitation and psycho-social support for patients with early-stage neurocognitive disorders and to help patients and caregivers adapt the activities of daily living. The programme duration is 1 year, with reimbursement for the cost of 25 sessions. Sessions comprise several evaluations, initially to set up a personalized therapeutic programme, and also at 3 months and 1 year after programme completion. Programmes are tailored to patients' and caregivers' requirements and needs by neuropsychologists and occupational therapists and comprise readaptation techniques (such as spaced retrieval and errorless learning) and environmental adaptations (e.g. diary and written procedures). Social help is provided by nurses and social workers. Programmes are run either at home or at the memory clinic, and any acquired adaptation is always transferred into the patient's environment [2].

Professional caregivers can be hired by nursing homes to encourage social participation of residents according to their level of cognitive ability. A function of 'referent people for dementia syndrome' has been described, allowing for better recognition of specific difficulties associated with neurocognitive disorders. Help for basic activities of daily living can be provided at home by the health system. Nursing homes often also have daily care centres which provide patients with social activities. Family associations offer information and counselling.

A law on mental incapacity and for the protection of people and their property has been revised [3], clearly stating the role of all stakeholders. Thus, two options are available: (1) a representative may be appointed by the patient, or (2) legal protection may be requested by either the patient or their caregiver. For legal protection, incapacity/competence is confirmed by medical evaluation, as well as taking into account the patient's functioning in daily life and the consequences on their property management.

In Belgium, there is legislation in place relating to euthanasia [4], which, in summary, states that there is no penalty against a medical doctor (MD) involved in cases of euthanasia if the patient has reached the age of majority and has mental capacity and awareness when requesting euthanasia, if the patient's request is voluntary and well considered and made repeatedly without external pressure, and if the patient feels their physical or psychological suffering cannot be alleviated due to their serious and untreatable illness. The MD must inform the patient of their clinical status and treatment options and must consistently record the patient's suffering. The MD must be certain that the patient has discussed their request with any individual they wish to contact. The request for euthanasia must be written, dated, and signed by the patient. A second doctor (who is a specialist in the patient's pathology) must be consulted to confirm the patient's suffering and their considered wish for euthanasia. An anticipatory statement requesting euthanasia (which is valid for 5 years) can be written by people, in the event of a serious accident occurring, with untreatable clinical sequelae, including loss of consciousness, and no reversal possible. A person of confidence is designated in the anticipatory statement, who will witness the patient's will. The euthanasia request must be registered with a national registry.

The King Baudouin Foundation is a non-profit Belgian organization that is active in addressing societal issues. For example, the Foundation encourages discussions and initiatives that focus on ensuring the place of people with dementia in society.

What are the current challenges in dementia in Belgium?

Recent epidemiological studies suggest that prevention of dementia and AD through early control of vascular and lifestyle risk factors is an important goal. However, this remains to be validated by careful evaluation before implementation into the healthcare systems.

Creating a dementia-friendly environment is an important challenge in our society. Information and education should be provided to the public so they can help as informed neighbours or even as informal caregivers for people with neurocognitive disorders. Such programmes are currently under way in Belgium, as well as through European inter-regional initiatives, and are supported by Belgian family organizations.

There is evidence for sustained effectiveness of psycho-social interventions in managing the functional, behavioural, and psychological symptoms of dementia, as reported by many well-conducted randomized studies. Basic processes involved in psycho-social interventions should be better identified to optimize their implementation, and further research is warranted to determine the most efficient procedures, their mechanisms of efficacy, and modulating factors.

Recommendations have been made in Belgium regarding assessment of competence in daily activities. A person diagnosed with AD should not be automatically considered as lacking capacity; indeed, people with early stages of dementia have full capacity to make their own decisions and to give consent, although their ability to communicate their wishes regarding daily life experiences is highly tenuous at very advanced stages of the disease. The competences must be assessed on a case-by-case basis, and this assessment must be repeated for all major decisions regarding treatment or care provided to the patient. Assessing a person's capacity to make decisions about their care and treatment must be performed by a trained and qualified healthcare professional. When assessing individual competencies, contextual factors must be considered, including medical, psychological, and social factors. Further research is necessary on the development and validation of effective and practical tools for competence assessment in AD.

How might these challenges be addressed and how can success be measured?

Prospective studies on prevention are in progress. These should help determine the effectiveness of prevention programmes that would be accessible to the majority of the population. For example, prevention measures can include promotion of physical activities or changes to dietary habits, and cognitive function can be evaluated in subjects participating in these prevention programmes compared to those not on these programmes.

Plans for creating dementia-friendly environments are being established. Strengths and weaknesses of such setups should be assessed that allow their application in different contexts, with quality of life and participation in social activities as possible measures of success.

One particular trend in Belgium is to develop care diagnosis and care planning. Meeting care needs corresponds to providing a fair compromise that takes into account the patient's wishes, their relatives' wishes, and what the healthcare professional considers as possible and/or necessary. When an individual with dementia experiences difficulties with defining their own care wishes, it is possible that people close to the patient may understand their wishes and thus provide some care. Care diagnosis is tightly related to illness diagnosis and forms an integral part of the diagnostic process. Care diagnosis aims at enabling timely care planning to ensure optimized quality of life for both the patient and their informal caregiver. Information sharing via communication between the GP, specialists, and health service providers is vital. Assessing the patient's needs includes regularly evaluating the following: the impact of disclosing the diagnosis on the patient, their mood, how they perceive their quality of life and how it can be improved, their functioning with activities of daily living and instrumental activities of daily living, their personal identity and individuality (including their profession, beliefs, purpose, values and norms, and spirituality), their driving abilities, advance care planning, their wishes for the future, their views on institutionalization, the legal aspects of patient representation, and any declaration of intent regarding care provision in case of legal incapacity. When assessing the needs of informal caregivers, attention should be given to care burden and capacity when providing support (mental and social well-being), their personal experience of care burden, with possible referral for psycho-education and coping strategies, and their physical health and emotional stress.

What does the future hold for dementia care, in particular, treatment and prevention?

Basic and *in vivo* imaging studies on the pathological processes of dementia remain of utmost importance to understand the evolution of the disease.

Moreover, research on cognitive reserves and brain health prevention programmes to be made available in a timely manner has gained increasing importance in recent years. There is much emphasis on the importance of early prevention to maintain brain function, which can be prospectively studied by population comparisons.

Adaptation of daily activities, personal and public environment, and life conditions to preserve capacities of patients with dementia and their caregivers is an absolute necessity. Participation of patients in family and social activities will be a major objective.

The issue of advance directives concerning possible occurrence of disease, particularly dementia, may be challenging. The main principle rests on an individual's autonomy, and consequently, nobody can be forced to draw up an advance directive. Considerable attention is given to what the individual considers to be their wishes, which should be determined rationally. Advance directives should preferably be accompanied by a personal statement explaining about what is important and meaningful in the life of the person who has drawn up the directive. Wishes may be dependent on circumstances at the time and subject to subsequent changes. Wishes expressed in an advance directive need to be understood by the physician responsible for the individual's care and achievable. Writing down one's wishes is a difficult task that requires considerable cognitive, emotional, as well as relational, input. The individual should establish a dialogue with others (including family members, GP, etc.), so they can gradually formulate their own wishes before putting them down formally in writing, and also preferably appoint a person who will be able to provide an verbal explanation of, and interpret, their written wishes. Advance directives should be integrated into the advance care planning model, so to include comprehensively the patient's wishes regarding their future. This model ensures that there is a continuous communication process between the patient and all those who, in a positive way, are concerned with their well-being (family members, caregivers, etc.). Such a context allows for a growing awareness of the care that is best suited for patients reaching the end of life.

References

1. **Superior Health Council.** *Dementia: diagnosis, behaviour management, ethical issues.* Advisory Report of the Belgian Superior Health Council No. 8890. 2016. Available from: http://www.health.belgium.be/en/advisory-report-8890-dementia [accessed 27 July 2018].

2. **Adam S, van der Linden M, Juillerat AC, Salmon E.** The cognitive management of daily life activities in patients with mild to moderate Alzheimer's disease in a day care centre: a case report. *Neuropsychological Rehabilitation.* 2000;**10**:485–509.

3. **Moniteur belge.** *Loi réformant les régimes d'incapacité et instaurant un nouveau statut de protection conforme à la dignité humaine du 17 mars 2013* [in French]. **2013.** Available from: http://www.ejustice.just.fgov.be/cgi_loi/change_lg.pl?language=fr&la=F&table_name=loi&cn=2013031714 [accessed 27 July 2018].

4. **Moniteur belge.** *Loi relative à l'euthanasie du 28 mai 2002* [in French]. 2002. Available from: http://www.ejustice.just.fgov.be/cgi_loi/change_lg.pl?language=fr&la=F&cn=2002052837&table_name=loi [accessed 27 July 2018].

Chapter 18

Croatia

Ninoslav Mimica and Marija Kušan Jukić

Summary

For many years, dementia care in Croatia was provided traditionally by the family, without no organized support, and many people with dementia were undiagnosed. Treatment for people with dementia presenting with serious behavioural and psychiatric symptoms was provided on psycho-geriatric wards in psychiatric hospitals. Alzheimer Croatia, founded in 1999, provides information, support, and education to caregivers, as well as to health professionals including psychiatrists, and neurologists, and also raises public awareness of Alzheimer's disease. The continuing voluntary work of Alzheimer Croatia has helped to encourage the development of other types of services for people with dementia in Croatia. We are proud in dementia care in Croatia in following three key points. First, the activities and continuous work of Alzheimer Croatia since 1999 in raising awareness through public activities, education, counselling, support, negotiation with authorities about Alzheimer's disease and especially about the needs and problems of people with dementia (PWD) and their carers. Second, we would like to emphasize the activity of Croatian Alzheimer Alliance (31 professional and NGO organizations) in preparing content of National strategy to combat Alzheimer's disease and other dementias in Croatia. Third, introduction of first Day hospital for PWD, the first state specialized public nursery unit and first palliative beds were established and become available for people living with Alzheimer's disease and other dementias in Croatia. We presume that National strategy to combat AD in the next years will become the powerful instrument in negotiation with policy makers in Croatia is term to ensure the better treatment and care for PWD equally in the different regions of Croatia.

Current dementia care

In Croatia, there are great differences in the availability of early diagnosis, treatment, and care for people with dementia in different regions of the country. The current goal of the 31 professional societies and NGOs gathered together under the Croatian Alzheimer Alliance (CAA) is to work actively on the content, development, and implementation of a National Strategy in the fight against AD. The priorities of the National Strategy are: (1) timely diagnosis of AD, (2) availability of pharmacological and non-pharmacological treatment, and (3) establishment of a coordinated support system for people with dementia and their caregivers in the community. Appropriate steps forward have been taken already in the field of palliative care service provision for people with dementia and in institutions with specialized care.

The first psycho-geriatric ward was established at the Psychiatric Hospital Vrapče in Zagreb in 1959. During the following decades, similar psycho-geriatric wards were opened in other psychiatric hospitals, all with the aim of providing specialist treatment to people with dementia in Croatia.

The 'decade of the brain' saw an increasing interest worldwide, as well as in Croatia, among neurologists, psychiatrists, and basic neuroscientists in the aetiology, early diagnosis, and treatment of AD and other dementia types. In 1999, the Croatian association for AD—Alzheimer Croatia (AC)—was founded on the initiative of the Dajčić and Šljivarić families. The purpose of AC is to help families of people with AD caring for the patients through providing education and counselling, organizing self-help groups for caregivers, and introducing the families to health and social rights. Also, AC runs campaigns to raise public awareness of the growing problem of AD and its destigmatization, as well as educational programmes for health professionals and social workers. Moreover, AC works to influence changes in legislation to ensure better care for people with dementia (e.g. accessibility of nursing homes for the elderly and disabled to people with dementia, access to orthopaedic equipment, granting disability status). As a result of its continuing activities, as well as its constant presence in the media, AC has become known to families of people with dementia, who turn to the association for help and advice, including via its SOS-telephone, often even before consulting health professionals. Therefore, the mission of AC is to expand knowledge of AD, clarify misconceptions, destigmatize the disease, thus extending its reach to the general population, and influence healthcare and social welfare institutions, all in the best interests of people with dementia. A particular feature of AC is that it works actively with a range of health professionals (including neurologists, psychiatrists, and GPs) who, through AC, offer their expertise to people looking for help regarding AD. We are proud that AC is a full member of the international umbrella organization ADI since 2006 and a full member of the European organization Alzheimer Europe (AE) since 2012.

Dementia care policy

Since 2012, AD/dementia have been declared a public health priority worldwide. An increasing number of countries are working on developing their own national strategies and plans specifically to tackle this problem. Croatia is still among those countries with no clear AD/dementia strategy. The draft proposal of the 'Croatian Strategy to Combat Alzheimer's Disease (2015–2020)' was put forward by members of the Croatian Society for AD and Old Age Psychiatry and AC, acknowledging the national specificities, as well as using existing plans from other countries and taking into account the recommendations and advice from international organizations (ADI and AE). The draft was published in the supplement issue of the scientific journal *Neurologia Croatica* and was presented and discussed for the first time during the Round Table at the Croatian Congress on AD (CROCAD-14) with international participation. To continue developing and implementing the National Strategy, the CAA was established in 2014. The CAA now consists of 31 members, professional societies, and NGOs, which have all pledged to jointly advocate for a National Strategy in the fight against AD and other dementia types. The three main goals of the Croatian National Strategy are: (1) timely diagnosis of dementia [1], (2) availability of treatment with anti-dementia drugs as well as proven non-pharmacological therapies, and (3) establishment of a coordinated support system for people affected by AD, their families, and caregivers to improve the quality of treatment and care. To achieve these three goals, implementation of the National Strategy includes the following proposed ten action plans: (1) timely diagnosis of dementia, (2) availability of pharmacological treatment (anti-dementia drugs and other psychopharmacotherapies) and non-pharmacological therapies [repetitive transcranial magnetic stimulation (rTMS), cognitive training] [2], (3) support of research in the field of AD, (4) setting up of a register of people with dementia, (5) access to social benefits and services, (6) development of systematic support for those suffering from AD and their families/informal caregivers, (7) equivalent development of regional centres for the diagnosis and treatment of AD, (8) equivalent development of regional nursing homes for the elderly and disabled, with specialized accommodation units for people with AD in full-time residential living and day stays, (9) development of palliative care services for people with dementia, and (10) destigmatization of dementia.

Shortly after the presentation of the first draft proposal of the National Strategy, a second public discussion took place at the Round Table of the 6th Croatian Psychiatric Congress, with international participation. This was followed by several meetings among representatives of the CAA, which—unexpectedly and very surprisingly—is composed of a large number of members. All members of the CAA, including the names of the president and representatives of individual associations or societies, are listed in Table 18.1. The concept of the structure of the CAA and the contents of the updated and published draft of the Croatian strategy to combat AD and other dementia types in 2015 were presented to the national, European, and international professional community [3]; the draft has received approval, support, and acclaim. In the past 2 years, work has continued with open public discussions at different meetings to define the strategy. It is anticipated that the final version of the National Strategy will be published soon and handed over to the authorities for its approval and implementation.

Volunteering sector

We are particularly proud of the continuous volunteering work of AC, as well as the CAA, in building a National Strategy in Croatia. Also, it is important to emphasize that Croatia is making progress in dementia care; the first specialized units for the care of people with dementia in nursing homes were opened in 2015 in Zagreb, with a capacity of 12 beds, and this move was soon followed by other nursing homes for elderly people (relevant legislation was even put in place, stating that 7% of beds in nursing homes should be reserved for people with dementia). In addition, an increasing number of health professionals are being provided with education on AD through international congresses (nine times, biennially), educational conferences (e.g. EdukAl 2015, 2016, 2017 and 2018 held in Zagreb), and various educational workshops and lectures across the country. Moreover, the Alzheimer Café is well accepted in Croatia, which brings social, cultural, artistic, and educational dimensions to people with dementia and their caregivers. More than 50 Alzheimer Café meetings have been organized so far in various towns in the country.

In Croatia, it is estimated that there are 3000 new patients diagnosed with dementia every year, of which 70% are caused by AD, and there are around 250,000 family caregivers (which represents 1/15 of the total population of Croatia) providing care to a family member with dementia. To support people with dementia and their caregivers, there has been a significant shift in the organization of palliative care services for people with dementia in the last 2 years. Palliative care beds for people with dementia have been included in the bed network of the Croatian Institute for Health Insurance (CIHI). Psychiatric

Table 18.1 Croatian Alzheimer Alliance (CAA)

Founding members (name in Croatian and English)	President/head	Representative
Hrvatsko društvo za Alzheimerovu bolest i psihijatriju starije životne dobi, HLZ (Croatian Society for Alzheimer's Disease and Old Age Psychiatry, CroMA)	Prof Ninoslav Mimica, MD, MSc, DSc, Prim	Marija Kušan Jukić, MD, DSc Paola Presečki, MD, DSc
Hrvatska udruga za Alzheimerovu bolest (Alzheimer Croatia)	Prof Ninoslav Mimica, MD, MSc, DSc, Prim	Morana Ivičić, MD, MSc
Members (name in Croatian and English)	**President/head**	**Representative**
Centar za palijativnu medicinu, medicinsku etiku i komunikacijske vještine, Medicinski fakultet Sveučilišta u Zagrebu (Centre for Palliative Medicine, Medical Ethics and Communication Skills, School of Medicine, University of Zagreb)	Prof Veljko Đorđević, MD, DSc, Prim	Assistant Prof Marijana Braš, MD, DSc
Društvo nastavnika opće/obiteljske medicine (Association of Teachers in General Practice/Family Medicine)	Prof Biserka Bergman Marković, MD, DSc	Miroslav Hanževački, MD, DSc
Hrvatska udruga socijalnih radnika (Croatian Association of Social Workers)	Štefica Karačić, grad soc worker	Ljiljana Vrbić, grad soc worker
Hrvatska udruga za neurointervencije u cerebrovaskularnim bolestima (Croatian Association for Neurointervention in Cerebrovascular Diseases)	Assistant Prof Branko Malojčić, MD, DSc	Assistant Prof Marina Boban, MD, DSc
Hrvatsko društvo farmakologa (Croatian Pharmacological Society)	Prof Mladen Boban, MD, DSc	Prof Nela Pivac, DVM, DSc
Hrvatsko društvo umirovljenih liječnika, HLZ (Croatian Society of Retired Medical Doctors, CroMA)	Prim Peter Brinar, MD, MSc	Prim Peter Brinar, MD, MSc
Hrvatsko društvo za biologijsku psihijatriju i psihofarmakoterapiju, HLZ (Croatian Society for Biological Psychiatry and Psychopharmacotherapy, CroMA)	Prof Miro Jakovljević, MD, DSc	Assistant Prof Bjanka Vuksan Ćusa, MD, DSc

(*continued*)

Table 18.1 Continued

Founding members (name in Croatian and English)	President/head	Representative
Hrvatsko društvo za EEG i kliničku neurofiziologiju, HLZ (Croatian Society for EEG and Clinical Neurophysiology, CroMA)	Prof Sanja Hajnšek, MD, DSc	Prof Fran Borovečki, MD, DSc
Hrvatsko društvo za gerontologiju i gerijatriju, HLZ (Croatian Society for Gerontology and Geriatrics, CroMA)	Prof Zijad Duraković, MD, DSc, FB & HA	Nada Tomasović Mrčela, MD, DSc
Hrvatsko društvo za kliničku farmakologiju i terapiju, HLZ (Croatian Society for Clinical Pharmacology and Therapy, CroMA)	Prof Dinko Vitezić, MD, DSc	Prof Dinko Vitezić, MD, DSc
Hrvatsko društvo za liječenje boli, HLZ (Croatian Society for Pain Treatment, CroMA)	Prim Mira Fingler, MD	Prim Mira Fingler, MD
Hrvatsko društvo za neuroznanost (Croatian Society for Neuroscience)	Prof Ivica Kostović, MD, DSc, FCA	Prof Goran Šimić, MD, DSc
Hrvatsko društvo za palijativnu medicinu, HLZ (Croatian Society for Palliative Medicine, CroMA)	Vlasta Vučevac, MD	Vlasta Vučevac, MD
Hrvatsko društvo za zaštitu i unapređenje mentalnog zdravlja, HLZ (Croatian Society for Protection and Promotion of Mental Health, CroMA)	Prof Veljko Đorđević, MD, DSc, Prim	Prof Veljko Đorđević, MD, DSc, Prim
Hrvatsko farmaceutsko društvo (Croatian Pharmaceutical Society)	Darko Takač, MSc, mag pharm	Maja Jakševac Mikša, DSc, mag pharm
Hrvatsko katoličko liječničko društvo (Croatian Catholic Medical Society)	Prof Ana Planinc-Peraica, MD, DSc	Petar Bilić, MD, DSc
Hrvatsko neurološko društvo, HLZ (Croatian Neurological Society, CroMA)	Prof Silva Butković Soldo, MD, DSc	Assistant Prof Nataša Klepac, MD, DSc
Hrvatsko psihijatrijsko društvo (Croatian Psychiatric Society)	Prof Vlado Jukić, MD, DSc, Prim	Prof Vlado Jukić, MD, DSc, Prim
Hrvatsko psihološko društvo (Croatian Psychological Society)	Josip Lopižić, mag psych	Assistant Prof Slavka Galić, DSc, mag psych
Hrvatska udruga koncesionara primarne zdravstvene zaštite (Croatian Association of Primary Health Care Concessionaries)	Josipa Rodić, MD	Sanja Klajić Grotić, MD

Table 18.1 Continued

Founding members (name in Croatian and English)	President/head	Representative
Palijativni tim LiPa (Palliative team LiPa)	Goran Čičin Radin Sarajlić, MD	Ljerka Pavković, MA
Psihijatrijsko društvo Hrvatske udruge medicinskih sestara (Psychiatric Society of Croatian Nurses Association)	Zinka Bratuša, MA	Tatjana Horčička, MN Senka Repovečki, MN
Sekcija za gerontostomatologiju Hrvatskog društva za gerontologiju i gerijatriju, HLZ (Section for Gerontostomatology of Croatian Society for Gerontology and Geriatrics, CroMA)	Prof Adnan Ćatović, DDM, MSc, DSc, Prim	Dunja Kuliš, DDM
Referentni centar Ministarstva zdravstva za Alzheimerovu bolest i psihijatriju starije životne dobi (Referral Centre of Ministry of Health for Alzheimer's Disease and Old Age Psychiatry)	Prof Ninoslav Mimica, MD, MSc, DSc, Prim	Assistant Prof Suzana Uzun, MD, DSc, Prim
Sindikat umirovljenika Hrvatske (Retired Persons' Trade Union of Croatia)	Jasna A Petrović, grad soc worker	Prof Nikola Mandić, MD, DSc
Udruga 'Zajedno' (Association 'Together')	Assistant Prof Igor Filipčić, MD, DSc	Assistant Prof Igor Filipčić, MD, DSc
Udruga za psihosocijalnu pomoć i rehabilitaciju 'Zagreb' (Association for Psychosocial Help 'Zagreb')	Domagoj Vidović, MD, DSc	Domagoj Vidović, MD, DSc
Udruga za unapređenje kvalitete življenja 'Medveščak' (Association for Protection Quality of Life 'Medveščak')	Krasanka Glamuzina, grad soc worker	Krasanka Glamuzina, grad soc worker
Zagrebački institut za kulturu zdravlja (Zagreb's Institute for the Culture of Health)	Prof Veljko Đorđević, MD, DSc, Prim	Filip Đerke, MD

Assistant Prof, Assistant Professor; CroMA, Croatian Medical Association; DSc, Doctor of Science; DVM, Doctor of Veterinary Medicine; FB & HA, Fellow Bosnian & Herzegovina Academy; FCA, Fellow of the Croatian Academy; grad soc worker, graduate social worker; HLZ, Hrvatski liječnički zbor; MA, Master of Arts; mag pharm, magister of pharmacology; mag psych, magister of psychology; MD, medical doctor; MN, Master of Nursing; MSc, Master of Science; Prim, Primarius; Prof, Professor.

hospitals that also include psycho-geriatric wards have also become part of this network, and currently there are 62 contracted beds for palliative care patients in psychiatric hospitals, with priority given to patients suffering from dementia. Our goal is to make palliative care services available to people with AD and other types of dementia who are living at home or in elderly homes [4].

Anti-dementia drugs

We are proud of our battle to ensure the availability of anti-dementia drugs to people with dementia in Croatia, although this 'battle' is not over yet. Donepezil, rivastigmine, and memantine are now registered in Croatia and are on the additional 'B list of drugs' (e.g. with only 25% of costs reimbursed) of the CIHI. A Croatian algorithm for the pharmacological treatment of AD was defined in 2006, revised in 2010, and finally introduced in 2011 [5]. These guidelines recommend donepezil as the first-line treatment in mild to moderate AD; if a satisfactory therapeutic response is not achieved, the second-line pharmacotherapy is either rivastigmine or galantamine, and if a satisfactory treatment response is still not obtained, memantine may be recommended. In moderate to severe AD, memantine is the treatment choice and may be combined with donepezil, especially in moderate dementia. Studies have shown that these drugs slow the progression of dementia and delay the patient's loss of independence, as well as their institutionalization [6]. Anti-dementia drugs also reduce the need for additional psychotropic drugs such as antipsychotics and mood stabilizers, which can cause serious side effects in elderly people. Thus, anti-dementia drug treatment not only reduces the cost of patient care, but importantly also significantly improves the quality of life of people with dementia and their families. Our goal is the inclusion of anti-dementia drugs (donepezil, galantamine, rivastigmine, and memantine) on the basic 'A list of drugs' (hence with full cost reimbursement) of the CIHI, because these drugs represent the standard pharmacological treatment of AD in accordance with professional guidelines based on pharmaco-economic principles. In addition, people with AD can suffer from mood disorders, insomnia, psychosis, delirium, and/or manifest behavioural disorders, including aggressiveness and disorganized behaviour, at different stages of the disease. Treatment with psychotropic drugs (antipsychotics, antidepressants, mood stabilizers, hypnotics, and anxiolytics) for treating particular symptoms in people with dementia should also be made accessible through the CIHI, with careful monitoring of their possible side effects.

Another great challenge in Croatia lies in the legislation in place for people with dementia. Currently, in Croatia, people with dementia, including those with moderate dementia, cannot be included in clinical trials. According to a new family law, published in the official gazette *Narodne Novine* (NN 103/

15), which was in use from 1 November 2015 in article 258, paragraph 8—'The decision to participate in biomedical research', every person/patient, including people with dementia, participating in biomedical research (including clinical trials) should sign and date their own informed consent. Informed consent should be written in lay language and be understandable by lay people. The person participating in biomedical research may withdraw their consent at any time during the trial. The problem faced by people with dementia is that their guardians are not allowed to sign on their behalf to provide consent to research participation. Therefore, many people with dementia in Croatia, particularly those with moderate to severe dementia, do not have the possibility to participate in clinical trials as a result of this new law.

Conclusion

There are so many challenges in the field of dementia care in Croatia, but of these, we would underline the inclusion of anti-dementia drugs on the CIHI's 'A list of drugs' and education of GPs for early recognition of symptoms of cognitive disorders and early diagnosis of AD, as well as recognition of the role of, and financial compensation for, informal caregivers for informal caregivers. We believe that the systematic approach based on the goals of the National Strategy to combat AD and also on the detailed action plans with set deadlines and measurable outcomes represents the right way forward to improve dementia care in Croatia. Therefore, our efforts in the next year will be focused on implementation of the National Strategy and negotiation with authorities on behalf of people with dementia and their families.

References

1. **Boban M, Malojčić B, Mimica N,** *et al*. The reliability and validity of the Mini-Mental State Examination in the elderly Croatian population. *Dementia and Geriatric Cognitive Disorders*. 2012;**33**:385–92.
2. **Mimica N, Klepac N.** Person-oriented approach to people with dementia. In: **Đorđević V, Braš M, Miličić D** (eds). *Person in medicine and healthcare—from bench to bedside to community*. Zagreb: Medicinska naklada; 2012. pp. 215–19.
3. **Mimica N, Kušan Jukić, M, Presečki P,** *et al*. [Hrvatska strategija borbe protiv Alzheimerove bolesti i drugih demencija—prijedlog nacrta uz nadopune]. *Medix* 2015;**XXI**(117):111–18.
4. **Kušan Jukić M, Mimica N.** [Palijativna skrb o oboljelima od Alzheimerove bolesti i drugih demencija]. *Medix*. 2016;**XXII**(119/120):179–83.
5. **Mimica N, Presečki P.** Current treatment options for people with Alzheimer's disease in Croatia. *Chemico-Biological Interactions*. 2010;**187**:409–10.
6. **Mimica N, Presečki P.** How do we treat people with dementia in Croatia. *Psychiatria Danubina*. 2010;**22**:363–6.

Chapter 19

Czech Republic

Iva Holmerová

Introduction

The Czech Republic has a total population of 10,543,000, of which 18.6% (1.96 million) are represented by people aged 65 years or above, including 4.1% (447,000) of seniors aged 80 years or above. The current life expectancy is 81.5 years for women and 75.5 years for men. There are approximately 156,000 people with dementia in the Czech Republic, the majority of whom are women (105,000 women, 51,000 men). Demographic ageing is set to accelerate over the next decades by the transition of cohorts of people born in the 1940s and 1950s—and at a faster rate than in other European countries. The population of those aged 75 years or over is projected to increase from 10% to 17%, representing a 2.3-fold increase, between 2013 and 2050, and from 2% to 6%, representing 3.5-fold increase, for those aged 85 years or over. These projected figures will, in turn, influence the number of people with dementia in the country.

Dementia has become an important topic of public discussion, and the National Action Plan on Alzheimer´s Disease and Similar Disorders (NAPAD) was approved by the Czech Government in 2016. The Czech Alzheimer Society (CALS) has been playing an important role over the last two decades by raising awareness, promoting a better quality of care, introducing practical tools, and helping in case finding and organizing other activities. The Alzheimer Foundation has been supporting young scientists, as well as useful projects on improvement of care. However, there is still much to do for people with dementia and their family caregivers. The goals of the NAPAD set the trends in the right direction, but they need to be implemented with the official support of institutions at different levels and also by the allocation of relevant funding [1].

History of dementia research in Prague and recent history of health and social care

There has been a long history of valuable research conducted in the field of dementia in Prague. In 1892, Professor Arnold Pick, head of the Department of

Neuropsychiatry at Charles University (known as Karl-Ferdinands-Universität at the time), described a case of frontotemporal dementia. In 1907, Dr Oskar Fischer, who was working in Professor Arnold Pick's department, published an important paper presenting the pathological changes in the brain of people with senile dementia, while comparing these findings with a control group of subjects without dementia. However, Oskar Fischer remains largely unknown in the field of dementia research, despite publishing his findings in the same year as Alois Alzheimer. Until the 1980s and 1990s, AD and dementia had been considered rare conditions, although patients with 'arteriosclerosis praecipue cerebri' were being increasingly reported in different hospital departments, the majority of whom had undiagnosed advanced dementia. It was only in the last decade that the societal challenge presented by dementia was first highlighted by professionals and later became a topic of public discussions. This time was also marked by the launch and beginning of activities of the CALS, as well as collaborations among professional organizations, followed by other subsequent developments such as drug reimbursement [2].

Social care

The recent development of social care in the country has been influenced by nearly five decades of totalitarian systems (1939–1945 and 1948–1989). The socialist state (post-1948) declared that it would take over the care of 'all people in need' and directly controlled social and healthcare provision. Social care institutions (which formed the basis of the social care system) were created from expropriated mansions and castles, mostly located in remote places. People with disabilities and dependent seniors were thus segregated from the 'normal' population. Following many partial changes in the social care system, in 2007, a new legislation on social services, which enables their decentralization and development, was enacted. The Act on Social Services [3] provides definitions of different modern types of ambulant and semi-mural services, residential care, counselling, etc. It also defines residential services (including homes for seniors and homes with specific care regimes for people with chronic disease, e.g. those with AD and reduced independence). Recently, a new law was passed that stipulates that residential care homes are obligated to ensure their residents' healthcare. The aim is to improve the situation of family caregivers and dependent seniors who are entitled to care allowance. However, paradoxically, this has also led to problems relating to funding of social care. Many people, instead of purchasing formal social services, prefer to save their allowances for themselves and especially for their families. This situation was predictable and known to scientists and informed professionals. Despite these issues, the new legislation on social services has ensured the implementation of important measures in social care, quality control, and also the assessment of independence. Thus, citizens of the Czech Republic have the right to being assessed for their status and level of independence. People who are dependent are entitled to a care allowance (in cash) that covers the costs of care provided at home (by informal caregivers) or by registered social care providers. The levels of dependency (and corresponding monthly allowances—for adults) are categorized as follows: (1) mild dependency—800 CZK (€31.5), (2) moderate dependency—4400 CZK (€173.2), (3) severe dependency—8800 CZK (€346.5), and (4) total dependency—13,200 CZK (€519.7). The allowance is higher for people aged below 18 years. Care allowance is financed from the state budget (tax-funded) and is not means-tested. It represents the main source of funding of care, both at home and in institutions. People who receive a care allowance may receive care either from their family caregivers or from registered social services. Social care providers are required by law to register with the regional authorities, according to the Act on Social Services. The Act on Social Services and other related legislation ensures appropriate assessment of their level of independence for people with frailty and dementia (which is an important improvement, compared to the above-mentioned previous standards). In practice, however, these assessments are sometimes performed by social workers who have inadequate knowledge of geriatric syndromes, including dementia. Despite the above-mentioned (and other) issues, it is clear that the change in legislation related to social care was necessary and that the new system has potential for improvements.

Residential care

Currently, there are two types of institutions in the social care system that are in line with the definition of 'nursing home' [4]: (1) homes for seniors and (2) homes with special care. Of a total number of 47,834 places in these institutions, 11,784 are available in homes with special care, and 36,050 in homes for seniors. According to the Act on Social Services, these homes should provide 'social services', as well as ensure healthcare provision, for their residents. According to our research figures in 2013, the proportion of people with dementia among residents in homes for seniors was about 66%, and 97% among residents in homes with special care [5]. Moreover, preliminary results from our recent research on a representative sample of nursing home residents in Prague and the Central Bohemian region showed that 54% of the residents in these institutions were composed of people with dementia.

The interface between healthcare and social care

Despite the fact that the health status of nursing home residents is often very complex, the Act on Social Services does not stipulate for healthcare issues to be part of the formal system of quality control in these institutions. Skilled nursing personnel is not considered necessary in residential 'social-type' institutions, even though these residential homes are, in fact, nursing homes which provide care for dependent and sick older people. In the Czech Republic, one of the reasons behind poor care continuity in general (and not only in institutional care) is the fact that the health and social care systems operate separately, with poor communication between them—the Ministry of Health is responsible for healthcare, and the Ministry of Labour and Social Affairs for social care. While social care services do not manage complex health needs of residents, healthcare services, on the other hand, do not recognize the fact that patients with chronic health conditions need continuous healthcare, as well as long-term care and support. People with dementia are one of the most vulnerable groups of residents in long-term care institutions. They often have more complex medical backgrounds and more significant care needs, compared to other residents or people with dementia who live in the community. Despite these challenging conditions, there are many local initiatives and various departments for people with dementia in nursing homes that provide good-quality care [6].

Home help is provided by different agencies and municipalities. It is the commonest type of social services. However, its development depends on the availability of local support, e.g. from the municipality, the regional authorities, charities, etc. Therefore, in some regions and municipalities, these services are well developed, whereas in others, there is a scarcity, or even a total lack, of home help.

Day care units, or similar facilities, are extremely limited in number because the system of funding for social services does not support such facilities. Therefore, these can be found usually in cities or as part of institutions run by charities which provide co-funding for these units.

Similarly, *other social services* for people with dementia (including personal assistance, morning or late night help, night stays, etc.) are very rare.

People with dementia and their families also *need information, support, consultations, self-support groups*, etc., all of which are provided mainly by contact points (or collaborating centres) of the CALS. However, there is inadequate coverage and limited availability.

Other *good practice examples* also include Alzheimer Cafés, home assistance, respite care at home provided by the Czech Alzheimer Society, and various other activities for people with dementia. These activities are usually organized by charities or some social care providers.

Healthcare services

During the socialist period, the healthcare system was hierarchical and state-controlled (National Health Service). The National Plan of Care for the Aged and Chronically Sick (1982) was approved by the government, and geriatric medicine became an independent medical specialty. The aim of this National Plan of Care was to establish places for part-time geriatric nurses in each general practice. By 1989, there was a geriatric nurse working on a half-time basis in almost each general practice (300–400 older people). These nurses were involved in prevention and in providing care and home visits for seniors [7]. Following the political changes in 1989 and in later periods, the National Health Service was significantly decentralized and privatized. Most general practices and specialist outpatient departments, as well as home care agencies, have been purchased either by private companies or individuals. The system of geriatric nurses was abolished. Currently, healthcare costs are reimbursed by the general healthcare insurance, and according to the Constitution, healthcare is free. However, there have also been some co-payments—and these have remained a hot topic for political debates.

Home nursing care is provided by nurses, mostly from home care agencies, the majority of which are private-owned and a few run by non-profit organizations (e.g. Charita, Diakonie, Czech Red Cross, etc.). Some home care agencies also provide physiotherapists, while others offer a certain amount of home help as a paid service, depending on clients' needs and choices.

GPs for adults (most of whom are private) provide care for all adults, including seniors, as well as home visits for patients when necessary. The care provided by GPs is reimbursed by the healthcare insurance on a per capita basis (capitation), according to age groups. However, this system disadvantages people with chronic diseases (including those with dementia) who have high care and support needs, especially people with dementia. Unfortunately, there are insufficient incentives and quality control in place, and it depends on the individual GP.

Rehabilitation care, long-term care, aftercare, and long-term nursing care are provided by various types of healthcare facilities. Specialized dementia care units in the healthcare system are extremely rare across the whole healthcare system. Neither discharge planning nor transitional care formally exists. These might be provided by some geriatric or psychiatric facilities, but such services are equally very rare. Therefore, the situation of people with dementia receiving care in hospitals and other healthcare institutions is very problematic.

Regarding *specialist care*, neurologists, psychiatrists, and geriatricians are entitled to prescribe anti-dementia drugs. Specialist care is available to patients with dementia upon their referral by a GP (with the exception of psychiatric care), although many patients consult a specialist without being referred by their GP. Patients with neuropsychiatric symptoms are usually treated by psychiatrists, older patients with multimorbidity and frailty by geriatricians, and younger patients and atypical cases requiring an accurate diagnosis by neurologists. Home visits are conducted by specialists in exceptional cases.

Psychiatric or mental care nurses work as nursing specialists. The majority are based in psychiatric hospitals and centres, focusing on psychoses—and usually not dementia.

In hospitals, there is a total of 48,903 acute care beds, including 391 acute geriatric beds. In post-acute care, there are 28,683 post-acute beds in the healthcare system. There are currently 72 aftercare hospitals or departments, with a total of 7200 beds (we can assume that 30–60% of patients consist of people with dementia), and a smaller number of psycho-geriatric departments (with approximately 80–90% of patients with dementia) with 2500 beds.

The Czech Alzheimer Society (CALS) and its activities

The CALS began its activities in 1996, and in 1997, it was established as a registered charity. Currently, it has over 30 contact points (collaborating centres) in all 14 regions. The CALS is active in running various activities, including communication, education, advocacy, and publication. It also participates in what can be considered as innovative initiatives. One such initiative is the development of tools for cognitive training, as well as brochures describing tasks that focus on training of cognitive functioning. In addition, the 'Memory Days' project focuses on case finding of people with memory problems and dementia. It is a low-threshold project for cognitive function testing. For the last 5 years, there have already been 7000 assessments performed with use of a battery of tests. One of the major achievements of the CALS is the development of its strategy called P-PA-IA, which has become an important reference source for the NAPAD and the quality certification system 'Vážka' [8].

The CALS strategy: P-PA-IA

This strategy has been a result of many discussions ran by the CALS and through workshops and meetings. In 2006, the CALS developed (and repeatedly revised) a strategy of care for people with dementia. It was based on practical experience of care providers from the health and social care systems, discussions with dementia care experts, the experience of people with dementia and family caregivers, and consultations with important stakeholders (including the Public Defender of Rights, i.e. the ombudsman). This strategy, called P-PA-IA (acronym for support and care for the three phases of dementia), is compatible with the functional staging of the dementia syndrome, according to the Reisberg scale, and, in principle, it is based on the needs of people with dementia and the possible response to these needs by existing services in the Czech Republic.

Principles of the P-PA-IA strategy

This strategy enables dementia to be defined as three main phases, according to the severity of the disease and care needs. The aim is to improve or preserve the quality of life and comfort of people with dementia (and their family caregivers) through adequate support, therapy, and care. The strategy defines critical factors of quality care and needs of people with dementia and their caregivers along the course of the three phases of dementia. These key factors reflect the situation of health and social services. The strategy also defines the type of care that people with dementia need during the progression of the disease.

1. P: people are relatively independent and only need some assistance, support, and supervision, which should be provided regularly, but do not need permanent care and supervision.

2. PA: people with dementia gradually lose their functional ability, become disorientated, and need permanent supervision and assistance. However, it is important to keep in mind that people in this phase of dementia can still perform different activities (albeit under supervision and in a protected environment) and have a good quality of life—even very good in many aspects. Their behavioural problems are usually manageable using non-pharmacological and restraint-free methods. Therefore, the 'day care unit' and 'social type' of care would be appropriate for this group of patients.

3. IA: people in this phase of dementia need skilled nursing, social, and palliative care. This phase roughly corresponds to stages 6 and 7 of the Reisberg's scale. These patients might have neuropsychiatric and somatic complications. In institutional care, skilled nursing (and medical supervision) is necessary [9].

Quality certification system 'Vážka'

The quality of care provided in care homes has become a subject of concern and discussions. In the last decade, several systems of quality evaluation and monitoring in the Czech Republic have been developed. However, these systems are implemented separately in the health and social care systems, and not at the interface between these two care systems and with no coordination of services in line with patients' needs, which is a very important aspect of the quality of care for people with dementia.

'Vážka' ('dragonfly'), which was the original logo of the CALS, over time became a symbol of care for people with dementia. Thus, within the first decade of CALS' existence, services for people with dementia were denoted by CALS' dragonfly. With the rising awareness of AD and other causes of dementia in the Czech Republic and the recognition of CALS as an important and respected stakeholder in this field, it was an ideal opportunity for care providers to be a contact point of CALS. However, some care providers did not contribute to the good credit of CALS. Therefore, it was decided, after many discussions within the board, as well as with our members and dementia care specialists, to establish and define quality of care criteria, which would be relevant to the standard of care provision in the Czech Republic. The CALS evaluated these criteria in practice in a pilot evaluation and established standards that are achievable in the complex system of dementia care in the country. Thus, Vážka has been registered as a protected mark which can be used by care providers only after having successfully met these certification criteria. Quality Criteria Vážka˚ are complementary to other systems of quality evaluation of the care for older people, and they express the values and opinion of the CALS [10].

National Action Plan on Alzheimer's Disease and Similar Disorders

This Action Plan was prepared by the Ministry of Health and approved by the Government of the Czech Republic in February 2016. It includes the following chapters: diagnosis, care, and treatment guidelines; better diagnosis of dementia; better quality and accessibility of care; support of caregivers; destigmatization and communication; education of the public—ethics and attitudes towards the elderly and people with dementia; education of professional caregivers in health and social care; education of employees in the public sectors, as well as teachers; research; data collection and epidemiology of dementia; and European collaboration [11].

Psychiatric reform

This reform is currently being implemented with the financial support of the Ministry of Health [12]. The main aims of this reform is to transform institutional care into community-based care, to create psychiatric centres, and to promote multidisciplinary collaboration in the care of psychiatric patients.

The original aim of the reform (which was to focus on mental health) has been changed to focus on psychiatric care. Therefore, dementia has been, until now, marginalized in the reform developments.

Conclusion

The prevalence of dementia is increasing very rapidly in the Czech Republic. It represents a challenge not only for people with dementia and their families, but also for services and the public sector, and has become an important topic of public discussion. The NAPAD was approved by the Czech Government in 2016. The CALS has been playing an important role in the last two decades in raising awareness, promoting a better quality of care, introducing practical tools, and helping in case finding and organizing other activities. The Alzheimer Foundation has been supporting young scientists, as well as useful projects on improvement of care. Still, there is much to do for people with dementia and their family caregivers. The goals of the NAPAD set the trends in the right direction, but they need to be implemented with the official support of institutions at different levels and also through the allocation of adequate funding. It is necessary to better integrate services provided by both the health and social care systems, to incorporate dementia into educational curricula at all levels (from primary schools to postgraduate specialized courses), to effectively communicate with the public and promote destigmatization, to create a dementia-friendly environment, and to support research and international collaboration in dementia.

References

1. Mátl O, Mátlová M, Holmerová I. *Zpráva o stavu demence 2016* [Report on Dementia 2016]. Praha: Česká Alzheimerovská Společnost; 2017

2. Holmerová I. [Alois Alzheimer a Oskar Fischer—110 let od jejich průkopnických publikací] (AA and OF—110 years anniversary of their publications). *Geriatrie a Gerontologie.* 2017;**16**:141–3.

3. Zákon 108/2006 Sb. o sociálních službách (Act on Social Services). Sbírka zákonů. Praha; 2006.

4. Sanford A, Orrell M, Tolson D, *et al.* An International definition for 'nursing home'. *Journal of the American Medical Directors Association.* 2015;**2015**:181–4.

5. Vaňková H, Hradcová D, Jedlinska M, Holmerová I. [Prevalence kognitivních poruch v pobytových zařízeních pro seniory]. *Geriatrie a Gerontologie.* 2013;**2**:111–14.

6. Wija P. *Podkladový materiál k problematice dlouhodobé péče a zdravého stárnutí* (Discussion paper on long-term care and healthy ageing). Praha: UK FHS a MZ ČR; 2013.

7. Haškovcová H. *Fenomén stáří* (Phenomenon of aging). Praha: Havlíček Brain Team; 2010.

8. **Czech Alzheimer Society**. Available from: http://www.alzheimer.cz [accessed 15 August 2018].

9. **Holmerova I, Balackova N, Baumanova M, et al.** [Strategie České alzheimerovské společnosti P-PA-IA] (Czech Alzheimer Society Strategy P-PA-IA). *Geriatrie a Gerontologie.* 2013;2:158–64.

10. **Hradcová D, Hájková L, Mátlová M, Vaňková H, Holmerová I.** Quality of care for people with dementia in residential care settings and the 'Vážka' Quality Certification System of the Czech Alzheimer Society. *European Geriatric Medicine.* 2014;5:430–4.

11. **Ministry of Health.** *National Action Plan on Alzheimer's disease and similar disorders.* Praha: Ministry of Health; 2016. Available from: http://www.mzcr.cz/dokumenty/narodni-akcni-plan-pro-alzheimerovu-nemoc-a-dalsi-obdobna-onemocneni-na-leta-201_12997_3216_1.html [accessed 15 August 2018].

12. **Reform of Czech Psychiatry.** Available from: http://www.reformapsychiatrie.cz/ [accessed 15 August 2018].

Chapter 20

England

Alistair Burns

Summary

The National Dementia Strategy (published in 2009) set the
scene for a sea change in dementia care in England. Work was
commenced in a number of areas, including a service to recognize
the work of general practitioners in identifying and diagnosing
dementia in primary care, an initiative to reward hospitals for
the correct assessment of people with suspected dementia
admitted as emergencies to general hospitals, reducing the level
of prescriptions of antipsychotic medication, raising awareness
of dementia in care homes, and ameliorating the effects of
stigma. In 2012, there was the first Prime Minister's Challenge on
Dementia, which had three major areas of focus. First, based on
the fact that dementia is the most feared illness in people over
the age of 50, a programme to reduce stigma was developed;
this challenged the notion that dementia was considered part of
normal ageing. Second was to increase the diagnosis rate, but
also to eliminate variation across the country. Third was in terms
of dementia research and the aspiration to improve the amount of
resources going into research. More recently, a five-point plan of
looking at the care and support of people with dementia has been
developed, emphasizing the importance of care across the care
pathway—Preventing Well, Diagnosing Well, Supporting Well,
Living Well, and Dying Well.

Background

In England, two landmark reports were published in 2009 which helped change
the face of the profile of dementia. The first was The National Dementia Strategy
('Living Well with Dementia') [1] (see Fig. 20.1); the results of a large consultation exercise, including people with dementia and their families, about what

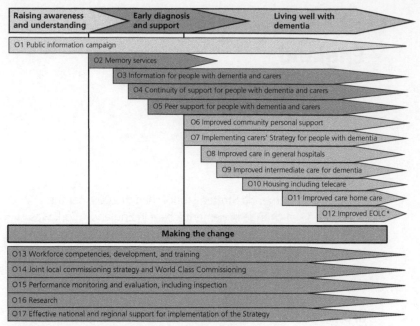

Fig. 20.1 The National Dementia Strategy (2009).
© Crown copyright 2009.

is important in terms of dementia care set the scene in determining the main aspects of better dementia care, including better public and professional understanding, earlier diagnosis, and improved quality of care. The second, called 'Time for Action' [2], highlighted the inappropriate use of antipsychotics in people with dementia, calling for a review of their prescription and estimating that there were 1800 excess deaths and 1600 excess strokes as a result of their use. At the same time, the National Audit Office (an independent group that considers any aspects of public life and have the ability to hold governments to account) chose to look at dementia care, including support for caregivers [3].

The Dementia UK report (2014) [4] highlighted the number of people with dementia in the United Kingdom (UK) (850,000), with the associated costs (£26 billion).

Prime Minister's Challenges

In 2012 (and further in 2015) [5, 6], there were two high-level initiatives on dementia by the then Prime Minister David Cameron. There were three areas of particular interest. First was the diagnosis rate. Figures from the Alzheimer's Society suggested that only 40% of people nationally were receiving a diagnosis, and surveys had confirmed that is what people with dementia and their care-givers wanted. Second was research. Alzheimer's Research UK (then the Alzheimer's Research Trust) cited powerful statistics looking at the comparison of dementia research and cancer research, the former being relatively under-funded, compared to the latter. Third was stigma. It was known that, for people over the age of 50, dementia is the most feared illness and there was a need to raise awareness. An initiative called 'Dementia Friends' was started—a social movement to make people more aware of the issues around dementia. Each of these strands was codified in a governance structure to deliver on the Prime Minister's Challenge on Dementia.

The 2015 Prime Minister's Challenge on Dementia was a re-articulation of the importance of the subject enshrined in the 2020 Prime Minister's Challenge on Dementia, to acknowledge the great advances that had been made in terms of the diagnosis rate—the rate had risen from around 40% to nearly 70% by the end of 2016, reflecting the fact that some 150,000 more people with dementia had been given their diagnosis and therefore had access to the bespoke post-diagnostic dementia services that are available. These developments are sum-marized in Fig. 20.2.

Dementia diagnosis rate

In 2011, the rate (i.e. the number of people with a formal diagnosis of dementia divided by the estimated number of people with dementia in the population, expressed as a percentage) was around 40%.

There was a specific ambition that two-thirds of the estimated number of people with dementia should have a diagnosis and have access to post-diagnostic support. A programme of work was created with colleagues in primary care to emphasize the needs for timely diagnosis and referral for investigations. There was debate as to whether GPs themselves could diagnose dementia; the National Institute for Health and Care Excellence (NICE) guidance [7] sug-gested that people with a suspected diagnosis of dementia should be seen and diagnosed in primary care or if everyone needed to be assessed in a specialist memory clinic. This mirrored a conversation which was had regarding the need for everyone with suspected dementia to have a brain scan—the guidance was adapted to reflect the fact that, in people with established disease, a brain scan was not always necessary.

Antipsychotics in dementia

The Time for Action Report [2] showed the potential dangers of prescribing antipsychotic drugs to people with dementia—an estimated 1800 excess deaths

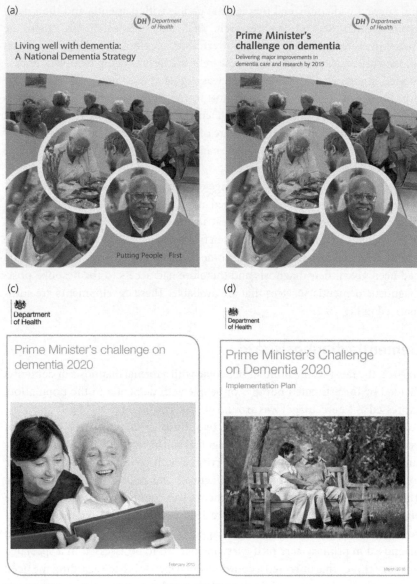

Fig. 20.2 Key milestones in dementia in England.
© Crown copyright.

and 1600 excess strokes a year. A campaign was launched to reduce their prescription, based on the idea that person-centred care, particularly in care homes, resulted in a better quality of care and less of a need for the drugs. A survey showed that a reduction of around 50% was achieved [8].

The 'I Statements'

Some other national initiatives have taken place, for example, the 'I Statements' were created (from work in cancer) which simply stated what a person with dementia and their caregivers could expect to see. Their genius was in their simplicity. They have gone through a number of iterations and are now being used as a measure of the effectiveness of care and services.

There have been a number of iterations, but the current 'I Statements' [9], due to be refreshed in May 2017), are:

- I have personal choice and control or influence over decisions about me.
- I know that services are designed around me and my needs.
- I have support that helps me live my life.
- I have the knowledge and know-how to get what I need.
- I live in an enabling and supportive environment where I feel valued and understood.
- I have a sense of belonging and of being a valued part of the family, the community, and civic life.
- I know there is research going on which delivers a better life for me now and hope for the future.

Dementia Friends

An initiative called Dementia Friends [10] was created, based on the Japanese model whereby a campaign was launched to bust some of the myths around dementia. The five key messages were:

- Dementia is not part of normal ageing.
- It is caused by brain diseases such as AD.
- There is more to dementia than memory loss.
- There is more to the person than dementia.
- It is possible to live well with dementia.

This has been a very successful campaign, with studies from the Alzheimer's Society showing that it has a positive impact in terms of people's understanding and awareness of dementia. The most recent figures (early 2017) suggest 1.8 million Dementia Friends, as well as dementia-friendly towns and cities, Dementia Friends' communities, and dementia-friendly businesses. Work in schools has highlighted the benefits of schoolchildren being aware of dementia, and a nationwide campaign to raise awareness of dementia and to encourage people to visit their doctor if they were worried that they had symptoms suggestive of dementia was launched.

Prevention of dementia

Prevention of dementia has recently become of interest in relation to the knowledge that a proportion of people with dementia have vascular disease and by paying attention to these risk factors, a proportion of diagnoses could be avoided. Information from Alzheimer's Research UK [11] showed that some 80% of the population do not know it is possible to reduce a person's individual risk of developing dementia, but that half of people would do something about it once they realized it. The Blackfriars consensus has emphasized the importance of prevention [12].

Dementia research

This has been a priority, and inevitably comparisons were made with cancer research which has been comparatively generously funded. In 2016, a National Dementia Research Institute was launched with £150 million of government money and £50 million each from Alzheimer's Research UK and the Alzheimer's Society charities.

The G8 summit was a key initiative [13] in raising the profile of dementia research and looking at the importance of a joined-up approach to dementia care across the world. From that, a dementia envoy was created, as well as work on a Global Dementia Observatory to bring together information. A Dementia Drug Discovery Fund was created, led by the UK, and made investments in more speculative new products more possible.

The dementia well-being pathway

More recently, based on the work of the National Dementia Strategy in 2009, a five-point way of looking at the care of people with dementia has been developed—Preventing Well, Diagnosing Well, Supporting Well, Living Well, and Dying Well (see Fig. 20.3).

Conclusion

There have been significant improvements in dementia care over the last decade, with increases in the diagnosis rate, more anti-dementia drugs being prescribed, and less antipsychotics being given [14]. Awareness is high, and political support is strong. There has been an emphasis on the earlier stages of dementia, but the experience across the pathway (from prevention to end of life) is now recognized as being important. Much has been done, but more needs to be done.

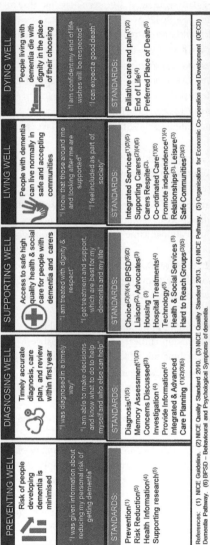

NHS ENGLAND TRANSFORMATION FRAMEWORK – THE WELL PATHWAY FOR DEMENTIA

PREVENTING WELL	DIAGNOSING WELL	SUPPORTING WELL	LIVING WELL	DYING WELL
Risk of people developing dementia is minimised	Timely accurate diagnosis, care plan, and review within first year	Access to safe high quality health & social care for people with dementia and carers	People with dementia can live normally in safe and accepting communities	People living with dementia die with dignity in the place of their choosing
"I was given information about reducing my personal risk of getting dementia"	"I was diagnosed in a timely way" "I am able to make decisions and know what to do to help myself and who else can help"	"I am treated with dignity & respect" "I get treatment and support, which are best for my dementia and my life"	"I know that those around me and looking after me are supported" "I feel included as part of society"	"I am confident my end of life wishes will be respected" "I can expect a good death"
STANDARDS: Prevention[1] Risk Reduction[5] Health Information[4] Supporting research[5]	**STANDARDS:** Diagnosis[1][5] Memory Assessment[1][2] Concerns Discussed[3] Investigation[4] Provide Information[4] Integrated & Advanced Care Planning[1][2][3][5]	**STANDARDS:** Choice[2][3][4], BPSD[6][2] Liaison[2], Advocates[3] Housing[3] Hospital Treatments[4] Technology[5] Health & Social Services[3] Hard to Reach Groups[3][5]	**STANDARDS:** Integrated Services[1][3][5] Supporting Carers[2][4][5] Carers Respite[2], Co-ordinated Care[1][6] Promote independence[1][4] Relationships[3], Leisure[3] Safe Communities[3][5]	**STANDARDS:** Palliative care and pain[1][2] End of Life[4] Preferred Place of Death[5]

References: (1) NICE Guideline. (2) NICE Quality Standard 2010. (3) NICE Quality Standard 2013. (4) NICE Pathway. (5) Organisation for Economic Co-operation and Development (OECD) Dementia Pathway. (6) BPSD – Behavioural and Psychological Symptoms of dementia.

RESEARCHING WELL
- Research and innovation through patient and carer involvement, monitoring best-practice and using new technologies to influence change.
- Building a co-ordinated research strategy, utilising Academic & Health Science Networks, the research and pharmaceutical industries.

INTEGRATING WELL
- Work with Association of Directors of Adult Social Services, Local Government Association, Alzheimer's Society, Department of Health and Public Health England on co-commissioning strategies to provide an integrated service ensuring a seamless and integrated approach to the provision of care.

COMMISSIONING WELL
- Develop person-centred commissioning guidance based on NICE guidelines, standards, and outcomes based evidence and best-practice.
- Agree minimum standard service specifications for agreed interventions, set business plans, mandate and map and allocate resources.

TRAINING WELL
- Develop a training programme for all staff that work with people with dementia, whether in hospital, General Practice, care home or in the community.
- Develop training and awareness across communities and the wider public using Dementia Friends, Dementia Friendly Hospitals/Communities/Homes.

MONITORING WELL
- Develop metrics to set & achieve a national standard for Dementia services, identifying data sources and set 'profiled' ambitions for each.
- Use the Intensive Support Team to provide 'deep-dive' support and assistance for Commissioners to reduce variance and improve transformation.

Fig. 20.3 The well-being pathway for dementia.

Contains public sector information licensed under the Open Government Licence v3.0.

References

1. Department of Health and Social Care. *Living well with dementia: a national dementia strategy.* 2009. Available from: https://www.gov.uk/government/publications/living-well-with-dementia-a-national-dementia-strategy [accessed 15 June 2018].

2. Medicines and Healthcare Products Regulatory Agency. *Antipsychotics: initiative to reduce prescribing to older people with dementia.* 2012. Available from: https://www.gov.uk/drug-safety-update/antipsychotics-initiative-to-reduce-prescribing-to-older-people-with-dementia [accessed 15 June 2018].

3. National Audit Office. *Improving services and support for people with dementia.* 2007. Available from: https://www.nao.org.uk/report/improving-services-and-support-for-people-with-dementia/ [accessed 15 June 2018].

4. Alzheimer's Society. *Dementia UK report.* 2014. Available from: https://www.alzheimers.org.uk/info/20025/policy_and_influencing/251/dementia_uk [accessed 15 June 2018].

5. Department of Health and Social Care. *Prime Minister's challenge on dementia.* 2012. Available from: https://www.gov.uk/government/publications/prime-ministers-challenge-on-dementia [accessed 15 June 2018].

6. Cabinet Office, Department of Health and Social Care, and Prime Minister's Office, 10 Downing Street. *Prime Minister's challenge on dementia 2020.* 2015. Available from:https://www.gov.uk/government/publications/prime-ministers-challenge-on-dementia-2020 [accessed 20 August 2018].

7. National Institute for Health and Care Excellence. *Dementia: supporting people with dementia and their carers in health and social care.* Clinical guideline [CG42]. 2006, updated 2016. Available from: https://www.nice.org.uk/guidance/cg42 [accessed 15 June 2018].

8. NHS Digital. *National dementia and antipsychotic prescribing audit.* Available from: https://digital.nhs.uk/data-and-information/clinical-audits-and-registries/national-dementia-and-antipsychotic-prescribing-audit [accessed 20 August 2018].

9. Dementia Action Alliance. *National Dementia Declaration.* 2010. Available from: http://www.dementiaaction.org.uk/nationaldementiadeclaration [accessed 15 June 2018].

10. Dementia Friends. Available from: https://www.dementiafriends.org.uk [accessed 15 June 2018].

11. Alzheimer's Research UK. *Dementia risk reduction and prevention policy statement.* 2017. Available from: http://www.alzheimersresearchuk.org/wp-content/uploads/2015/01/Dementia-Prevention-Policy-Statement-ARUK-April16.pdf [accessed 15 June 2018].

12. Lincoln P, Fenton K, Alessi C, *et al.* The Blackfriars Consensus on brain health and dementia. *The Lancet.* 2014;**383**:1805–6.

13. Department of Health and Social Care. *G8 dementia summit declaration.* 2013. Available from: https://www.gov.uk/government/publications/g8-dementia-summit-agreements/g8-dementia-summit-declaration [accessed 15 June 2018].

14. Donegan K, Fox N, Black N, Livingston G, Banerjee S, Burns A. Trends in diagnosis and treatment for people with dementia in the UK from 2005 to 2015: a longitudinal retrospective cohort study. *The Lancet Public Health.* 2017;**2**:e149–56.

Useful links

Alzheimer's Society. Available from: https://www.alzheimers.org.uk [accessed 15 June 2018].

Alzheimer's Society. *Dementia advisers*. Available from: https://www.alzheimers.org.uk/ [accessed 20 August 2018].

Dementia Academy. *New dementia toolkit is an Aladdin's cave of information*. 2017. Available from: https://dementiaacademy.co/2017/02/13/new-dementia-toolkit-is-an-aladdins-cave-of-information [accessed 20 August 2018].

Dementia United. Available from: http://dementiaunited.net/ [accessed 15 June 2018].

MODEM. *Modelling outcome and cost impacts of interventions for dementia*. Available from: http://www.modem-dementia.org.uk [accessed 15 June 2018].

NHS Benchmarking Network. Available from: https://www.nhsbenchmarking.nhs.uk/ [accessed 15 June 2018].

NHS England. *Clinical Commissioning Group improvement and assessment framework indicators*. Available from: https://www.england.nhs.uk/commissioning/ccg-assess/iaf/ [accessed 15 June 2018].

NHS England. *Integrated care: local partnerships to improve health and care*. Available from: https://www.england.nhs.uk/stps/ [accessed 15 June 2018].

NHS England. *NHS RightCare*. Available from: https://www.england.nhs.uk/rightcare/ [accessed 20 August 2018].

NHS England. *CCG data packs*. Available from: https://www.england.nhs.uk/rightcare/ intel/cfv/data-packs/ [accessed 15 June 2018].

NHS England. *Dementia: care planning in dementia*. Available from: https://www.england. nhs.uk/mental-health/resources/dementia/ [accessed 15 June 2018].

Public Health England. *Dementia profile*. Public Health England fingertips tool. Available from: https://fingertips.phe.org.uk/profile-group/mental-health/profile/dementia [accessed 15 June 2018].

Chapter 21

France

Philippe Robert, Renaud David,
and Valeria Manera

Summary

In 2011, France began the launch of its National Alzheimer Plans
to fund research on Alzheimer's disease (AD) and related disorders,
which resulted in a significant increase in French scientific research
output, particularly after implementation of the Third National
Alzheimer Plan (2008–2012). The 2014–2019 Neurodegenerative
Disease Plan and the new Action and Prevention of Loss of
Autonomy National Plan aim at extending the positive research
outcomes in AD to other neurodegenerative pathologies.
Interestingly, these plans also assign an important role to
Information and Communication Technologies in the assessment
and training of people with AD, frailty, and related disorders. This
may contribute to shaping the new Silver Economy by creating
new challenges and opportunities.

National Alzheimer, Neurodegenerative Diseases, and Loss of Autonomy Plans

AD has been recognized in France as a major public health problem and has
led to the development of three National Plans, the first of which was launched
in 2001.

The Third National Alzheimer Plan (2008–12) was a major public health
initiative in France that included €200 million of funding for research in AD
and related disorders, most particularly to strengthen research in AD, promote early diagnosis and improve management, and enhance support for caregivers. Haeffner-Cavaillon et al. [1] compared the impact of this plan over a
5-year period immediately before and after its initiation. The authors found
that worldwide publication of original scientific articles between the periods of

2004–2008 and 2009–2013 increased by 39%, and those specifically on AD by 46%. The absolute increase in French academic research output on AD (54.6%) was greater than that for stroke, Parkinson's disease, acquired immune deficiency syndrome (AIDS), or diabetes. Globally, France had the third largest relative increase in academic research output on AD (1.7-fold), behind only India (2.5-fold) and China (1.9-fold).

Based on these findings, one of the questions was whether the priority given to the mobilization against AD could be shared for the benefit of other diseases. Along this line, the report *'Evaluation of the Alzheimer's Plan 2008–12'* put forward recommendations that were useful for developing a new plan around two issues: continuation of measures taken from the previous plan, and 'expansion of the plan to also reach people affected by other diseases such as Parkinson's disease, multiple sclerosis (MS), and also punctually amyotrophic lateral sclerosis (ALS) and Huntington's disease'. After 2 years without a plan since 2012, France now has the 2014–2019 Neurodegenerative Diseases Plan.[1]

In parallel, frailty is another concept that has attracted the attention of clinicians and public authorities. Frailty is defined as a multidimensional geriatric syndrome, characterized by increased vulnerability to stressors as a result of a reduced capacity of different physiological systems. Traditionally, the concept of frailty has mainly focused on the physical domain. Recent work has begun to study in more detail cognitive impairment due to physical frailty, leading to the definition of cognitive frailty, which is defined as the simultaneous presence of both physical frailty and cognitive impairment without the presence of a concomitant neurological disease [2]. Cognitive frailty is viewed as a potential precursor of neurodegenerative processes, with good reversibility potential, and thus is the ideal target for early intervention. In addition, psychological aspects are an important factor of frailty, even if less explored today.

This led to the launch in September 2015 of another plan called the Action and Prevention of Loss of Autonomy National Plan.[2] This plan does not include measures described in the various previous plans and recommendations published to date but emphasizes the implementation of prioritized. It is designed specifically for conference funders in the prevention of the loss of 'autonomy of the elderly that will be implemented within the framework of the law on the adaptation of society to ageing'. The issues are summarized in Table 21.1.

---

[1] http://social-sante.gouv.fr/IMG/pdf/Plan_maladies_neuro_degeneratives_def.pdf

[2] http://social-sante.gouv.fr/IMG/pdf/plan_national_daction_de_prevention_de_la_perte_dautonomie.pdf

Table 21.1 Axes, issues, and measures comprised in the Action and Prevention of Loss of Autonomy National Plan

Axis	Issues	Measures
I—to improve the broad determinants of health and autonomy	1. To ensure the health of seniors	1. To promote a healthy diet 2. To encourage physical and sports activities 3 and 4. To keep older workers active in the context of longer careers and promote their entry into retirement without incapacity 5. To adopt measures for the health of caregivers
	2. To prepare the transition to retirement	6. In the preparation and transition to retirement: to promote the emergence of a new life project through retirement preparation sessions
	3. To fight against isolation and promote social links and intergenerational and cognitive activities	7. To prevent, detect, and manage failure risk factors of social ties and the effects of isolation on the health and social life of the elderly 8. To maintain social ties and prevention tips: develop testing services baskets, offer diverse home
	4. To provide foster home support in individual or collective housing and adapt the environment to the consequences of ageing	9. To promote the home's autonomy and preservation of autonomy of its residents and to adapt their environment
	5. To adapt the environment to the consequences of ageing	10. To promote a global approach to creating 'age-friendly cities' in France 11. To integrate ageing issues in planning documents 12. To ensure mobility and easy access in neighbourhoods
	6. To support the availability of assistance and coordinate the arrangement of courses and tracking the loss of autonomy and frailty	13. To ensure the elderly have access to information and guidance, as well as access to their rights and rapid, relevant support to aid, trade, services, and devices adapted to their situation 14. To ensure the identification and management of risk factors for frailty and fragility 14a. To ensure the identification and management of risk factors for frailty

(continued)

Table 21.1 Continued

Axis	Issues	Measures
II—to prevent loss of autonomy	7. To delay the onset of loss of autonomy through preventive and coordinated interventions	15. To improve and coordinate practices for granting technical aids, diagnostic services, and housing adaptation 16. To fight against physical inactivity, strengthen the maintenance of mobility balance, walking, and falls prevention 17. To prevent the risks for depression so to avoid its effects on autonomy 18. To prevent any associated sensory disturbances 19. To preserve maximum possible independence of residents living in nursing homes in terms of their activities of daily living
III—to avoid worsening situations already characterized by an inability	8. To prevent and limit worsening of loss of autonomy	20. To reduce malnutrition among the elderly and improve their nutritional management 21. To improve the health conditions of elderly people with loss of autonomy 22. To educate hospitals on the risk of loss of independence in elderly patients during hospitalization and to encourage hospitals to ensure their safe return home upon discharge 23. To inform, educate, and train all professionals working in nursing homes on the prevention of risks related to the health and vulnerability of their residents to optimize their health potential
IV—to reduce social health inequalities		
V—to train professionals in the prevention of loss of autonomy	9. To train professionals to facilitate implementation of other measures of the prevention plan	24, 25, and 26. To improve skills, update professional practices, and disseminate good practices and training experiments in various fields related to the prevention of loss of autonomy

VI—to develop research	10. To expand research in risk factors for frailty and dependence and to give new impetus to research in the prevention of dementia	27 and 28. To develop research in autonomy and frailty risk factors in order to determine appropriate action plans and organize optimal support, and to give new impetus to research in frailty and dementia
	12. To strengthen the role of interface and intermediation of longevity and ageing research group among researchers and between researchers and decision-makers	29. To promote the role of interface and intermediation of longevity and ageing French centre to strengthen human and social scientists on issues related to ageing

The plan is structured around six axes: (1) to improve the broad determinants of health and autonomy, (2) to prevent loss of autonomy, (3) to avoid worsening of situations already characterized by an inability, (4) to reduce social health inequality, (5) to train professionals in the prevention of loss of autonomy, and (6) to develop research.

The plan consists of 'action sheets' designed to be practical and operational. Each 'action sheet' specifies the context and issues, objectives, measurements, tools and best practices, involved specialists and required training, operators, and evaluation criteria (process and outcome indicators).

Role of Information and Communication Technologies

Some of the National Plan's issues emphasize the important role that technology holds and will hold in the future. In the last decades, there has been a growing interest in the use of Information and Communication Technologies (ICT) to help assess and evaluate patients' functional impairments, as well as to help and support patients in daily activities. ICT plays an important role in clinical assessment, allowing the development of new methods to evaluate more objectively behavioural and functional deficits [3]. This is important for clinical, as well as for research, purposes. Beyond its importance in clinical assessment, ICT can also play a key role in patient treatment, stimulation, and rehabilitation [4].

Focusing research on innovative technologies for ageing is also a vital part of the European Union's framework programmes for research (FP7 and H2020). Over the last few years, hundreds of millions of euros have been invested in research on health-related issues of ageing and neurodegenerative diseases, including projects focusing on the use of ICT in the prevention, assessment, and treatment of age-related disorders. The H2020 framework programme is currently under way and consists of research projects specifically aimed at employing ICT to facilitate better ageing.

The importance of technological innovations is also underlined in the concept of the Silver Economy defined as economy that serves the elderly. Its aims are to enable and encourage innovations that will support an ageing society and help reverse the loss of autonomy in old age. As indicated by the Ministry of Social Affairs and Health, the Silver Economy is a sector that must be organized and structured, so as to consolidate and federate all companies acting for, or working with, the elderly.

The targets are to create custom services and innovative technologies to maintain autonomy, including home automation and connected objects—in other words, to develop over the coming years as many products and services as possible that will soon prove essential to an ageing society.

The Silver Economy is a new and promising sector opening up areas for economic growth and employment in the years to come. It also stands as a new partner for the traditional health stakeholders including patients, caregivers, and healthcare professionals. Finally, it also represents a new ethical challenge. The times they are a changing.

References

1. Haeffner-Cavaillon N, Devos P, Ledoux S, Menard J. The Third French Alzheimer Plan: analysis of the influence of a national public health initiative on scientific research productivity and impact. *Alzheimer's Research and Therapy*. 2015;7:60.

2. Kelaiditi E, Cesari M, Canevelli M, *et al.* Cognitive frailty: rational and definition from an (I.A.N.A./I.A.G.G.) international consensus group. *Journal of Nutrition, Health and Aging*. 2013;**17**:726–34.

3. Konig A, Aalten P, Verhey F, *et al.* A review of current information and communication technologies: can they be used to assess apathy? *International Journal of Geriatric Psychiatry*. 2014;**29**:345–58.

4. Robert PH, Konig A, Amieva H, *et al.* Recommendations for the use of Serious Games in people with Alzheimer's Disease, related disorders and frailty. *Frontiers in Aging Neuroscience*. 2014;**6**:54.

Chapter 22

Germany

Jochen René Thyrian

Summary

In recent years, there have been considerable efforts and many comprehensive developments in Germany to address the challenge that demographic change poses on dementia care on both regional and federal levels. Consequently, dementia care has changed considerably in the last decades. These changes have been published by the Alliance for People with Dementia and will be available on databases in the near future. However, Germany has only just begun to integrate important stakeholders and players into this concerted process. The efficacy and efficiency of this action plan have not been evaluated or assessed systematically, and its impact on dementia care is not yet clear. This needs to be investigated in prospective long-term studies. A national plan is to be established in 2018 as the successor of the existing action plan. As such, it is not expected to differ much from the existing action plan and should also be comparable to current plans or strategies in place worldwide.

Background

In Germany, the number of people living with dementia has been increasing steadily over the last decades and is estimated to be currently 1.6 million. As a result of demographic changes and ageing being the main risk factor for dementia, it is expected that the number of people affected by dementia will reach 3 million in 2050 if no progress is made in dementia prevention, treatment, or care support.

The profound impact of an ageing German population on various aspects of society has been acknowledged by the Federal Government of Germany. In April 2012, the Federal Ministry of Internal Affairs (BMI) initiated a dialogue process called 'Every age counts' (*Jedes Alter zählt*). It convened delegates from the government, federal ministries, state institutions, municipalities, and social associations, stakeholders in economy, research, and healthcare, members of civil society institutions, and German citizens. Discussions were focused on various topics, including the impact of demographic change on families, youth, workforce, autonomy in old age, geographic regions, and dementia care [1]. One working group in this process has been designated to focus on dementia and has been named 'Alliance for People with Dementia' (*Allianz für Menschen mit Demenz*). It is jointly led by the German Alzheimer's Association, the Federal Ministry of Health (BMG), and the Federal Ministry of Families, Senior Citizens, Women, and Youth (BMFSFJ), and brings together public agencies and civil society organizations, including self-help groups, which work to support people with dementia at federal, state, and municipal levels, and pools forces from all responsible stakeholders. The Alliance was founded on 19 September 2012 upon a joint declaration of all partners, which provided the foundation for its future work.

Alliance for People with Dementia

The Alliance (https://www.allianz-fuer-demenz.de/startseite.html; in German) has agreed to work jointly on: (1) raising awareness, (2) enhancing sensibility towards, and improving understanding of, dementia, (3) influencing dementia care and preventing societal exclusion, (4) ensuring societal participation, (5) linking existing measures and initiatives, as well as complementing and developing them further, and (6) supporting local alliances for dementia on a regional level. On 15 September 2014, the Alliance published its detailed action plan (https://www.allianz-fuer-demenz.de/fileadmin/de.allianz-fuer-demenz/content.de/downloads/Alliance_for_people_with_dementia.pdf), in which four action fields are identified (science and research, social responsibility, support for people with dementia and their families, and structuring the support and healthcare system). For each action field, several focus areas are described, each with its own goal, as well as a resolution of commitment of the Alliance partners, including a description of the partners' contributions towards reaching these goals. A total of 155 measures were introduced, together with a monitoring process for their implementation. In September 2016, an interim report on the progress of the Alliance's action plan was published (http://www.allianz-fuer-demenz.de/service/meldungen/zwischenbericht-zur-umsetzung-der-agenda.html; in German). Based on the outcomes of its action plan, the Alliance is expected to initiate a National Dementia Plan in 2018. It is expected that a National Dementia Plan will be proposed in the following years.

Science and research

Scientific research and disseminating their findings are of central importance to providing quality treatment and healthcare services for people with dementia and ensuring their active integration in society. Special emphasis is placed on biomedical/clinical research, healthcare research, gerontology research in social and behavioural sciences, nursing research, and empirical principles and epidemiological research.

Furthermore, the different fields of research involved need interdisciplinary research structures designed for the long term. The goal of such structures is to efficiently link the individual phases of the research process, from biomedical basic research and clinical studies to population studies. New findings should be made useful to patients as quickly as possible in the fields of prevention, diagnostics, and treatment.

Social responsibility

People with dementia are dependent, above all, on competent contacts and a dementia-friendly environment. Only in this way can they participate, with self-determination, in life in society. Being able to treat people with dementia with respect and as equals in society requires knowledge of dementia and an understanding of the impact of the disease on their life. Consequently, social integration of all those involved continues to be a challenge. Local community support can help to alleviate the situation to some extent. In addition, new forms of cooperation must be developed and civic/volunteer participation should be encouraged.

Particular emphasis in this action field is placed on enabling people with dementia to be active participants in society by creating dementia-friendly communities, maintaining accessibility, networking between healthcare and support programmes, ensuring legal questions are addressed appropriately (legal capacity, traffic and administrative law, legal planning, compulsory measures), raising awareness, and promoting public relations.

Support for people with dementia and their families

At present, approximately two-thirds of people with dementia live in their accustomed social environment, with the majority at home with their families and others living in communities with mobile nursing care or inpatient care facilities. Supporting and caring for a dementia patient is a tremendous challenge for families, but also for friends and neighbours, particularly when caregiving extends over a long period of time. Ensuring healthcare and supporting patients in their home environment can completely overwhelm family members, putting the latter at risk of falling ill themselves. To avoid jeopardizing the quality of care provided to patients and the quality of life of both patients and their families, help and support should be provided to both patients and family caregivers.

In this action field, for people with dementia, there should be focus on providing them with counselling and support, ensuring their participation in society, structuring their home and living environment, ensuring their freedom of mobility and protection, and ensuring their protection against violence. For family caregivers, the focus should be on providing them with supportive counselling and promoting their competencies, volunteer work, and active citizenship.

Structuring the support and healthcare system

Dementia patients and their relatives need a holistic, cross-sectoral system of support and healthcare that takes into account not only the various clinical presentations and severity of the disease, but also patients' individual needs to allow their participation in community life. The healthcare system thus should be geared to the individual needs and circumstances of patients with dementia, ensuring a coordinated provision of support for all degrees of severity and forms of the illness, including the patient's age (young versus old), the patient's background (e.g. those with an immigrant background), and the patient's living situation (e.g. living alone or with good family networks). In rural areas, bottlenecks in medical and nursing care must be avoided, and access to benefits of the health system, including rehabilitation and prevention, must be guaranteed, as well as access to medical care at home. To be able to individualize existing support provision and to address the specific requirements of patients and their families in the respective phases of dementia, there is a need for: (1) the availability of different forms of accommodation and assistance tailored to their respective requirements, (2) effective networking between outpatient and inpatient healthcare service providers, (3) qualification of all professionals involved, and (4) quality assurance for both inpatient and home care sectors.

In this action field, healthcare structures focused on include: accommodation and living in neighbourhoods, rehabilitation, medical/nursing care, and healthcare in acute care hospitals, with particular emphasis on qualified personnel and quality of healthcare.

Results of the Alliance

An interim report, published in 2016, focused on developments in the action field of support for people with dementia and their families and on developments overarching the various action fields (http://www.allianz-fuer-demenz. de/service/meldungen/zwischenbericht-zur-umsetzung-der-agenda.html; in German). Furthermore, a joint database and information resource for all partners has been developed to improve information exchange and facilitate cooperation. As already evident, results of the Alliance include, for example, for the annual week of dementia in 2017, a joint logo, joint materials, and a joint press release were made available to all partners—all of which help to create synergies and places the work of each individual partner in a bigger frame, making it more recognizable. Another example is the introduction of the global initiative Dementia Friends (Demenz Partner; https://www.demenz-partner. de) into the Alliance, which has improved and facilitated the roll-out of this programme. In 2018, the Alliance is expected to publish its final evaluation of the action plan. As part of this evaluation, a National Dementia Strategy will also be planned and proposed.

Dementia plans in Germany

Besides the National Dementia Strategy, there have been several dementia plans in Germany generated by the federal system of the country. The federal states of Bavaria, Saarland, and Schleswig-Holstein (in alphabetical order) have dementia plans in place that give recommendations at a state level. These plans differed in their development process, e.g. in Saarland, it was a top-down process, but a bottom-up process in Schleswig-Holstein. Furthermore, the plans are regionally tailored, putting emphasis on resources and challenges specific to each federal state. A scientific evaluation or reports of their impact on dementia care have not been published so far.

Reference

1. **Federal Ministry for Family Affairs, Senior Citizens, Women and Youth and Federal Ministry of Health.** *Alliance for people with dementia. The fields of action.* 2014. Available from: https://www.allianz-fuer-demenz.de/fileadmin/de.allianz-fuer-demenz/ content.de/downloads/Alliance_for_people_with_dementia.pdf [accessed 31 July 2018].

Chapter 23

Greece

Stelios Zygouris and Magda Tsolaki

Summary

In Greece, there is an ongoing effort for the implementation of a
national dementia plan. In 2014, a national dementia observatory
was established after appropriate legislation was implemented.
National and local Alzheimer's associations have developed
an ongoing collaboration with the health ministry and other
regulatory authorities in order to draft a national dementia plan
and promote the necessary changes that will lead to improved
services for dementia patients and caregivers. This chapter
provides an outlook on dementia care in Greece. It outlines the
diagnostic process and issues related to disclosure of the diagnosis
and various aspects of competence assessment, including mental,
functional, financial, driving, and personality competences, as well
as issues related to advance directives and end-of-life decisions.
Management and treatment of dementia in Greece is also
outlined. An overview of available pharmacological treatments is
presented. At the same time issues concerning reimbursement,
initiation and discontinuation of treatment and new therapies are
discussed. Non-pharmacological treatments for all stages of preclinical and clinical dementia, as well as their availability, are also
discussed. The chapter also includes a section dedicated to family
and caregiver support programs and services in Greece

Current dementia care in Greece

In Greece, dementia care is provided by the public healthcare system in collaboration with Alzheimer's associations under the umbrella of the Panhellenic
Federation of Alzheimer's Disease and Related Disorders (PFADRD). Older
adults can access diagnostic and support services through the public healthcare
system, Alzheimer's associations, or doctors in private practice. All currently

existing pharmacological therapies are available in Greece, with reimbursement covering 75–90% of medication costs through the public healthcare system [1, 2]. In addition, support services and cognitive rehabilitation programmes are offered by Alzheimer's associations, while a public-funded programme offers home assistance.

The legal framework concerning dementia remains fragmented and inadequate. Some areas such as driving competence are covered by legislation; however, implementation of the necessary screening procedures is often flawed. Moreover, there is no legal framework concerning financial competence of older adults, leaving them vulnerable to fraud and putting strain on caregivers. There is also no legal framework for the implementation of advance directives, end-of-life decisions, and euthanasia in Greece, which often leads to patients' wishes being overruled by doctors or relatives.

A huge effort is being made to improve dementia care and dementia-related legislation in Greece. A plethora of services related to dementia diagnosis, treatment, and support are currently available. However, organizational changes and updated legislation are necessary.

Diagnosis and assessment of competence

In Greece, dementia diagnosis is a medical diagnostic procedure that is usually carried out by neurologists or one of the 22 specialized memory clinics throughout Greece. GPs are also allowed to diagnose dementia [1], despite not receiving specialist training in dementia [2]. The usual diagnostic procedure includes a medical examination and cognitive assessment using brief neuropsychological tests such as the MMSE [3] and the Montreal Cognitive Assessment (MoCA) [4], although there are no set guidelines on the tests that should be used [2]. Often depression screening is conducted either informally during clinical assessment or using standardized questionnaires such as the Geriatric Depression Scale (GDS) [5]. The main barriers to effective diagnosis are related to personal factors such as fear of stigmatization, denial of memory problems, etc. [1]. There is no set framework for the disclosure of diagnosis, and thus patients are not routinely informed about their diagnosis. The wishes of the patient's family also affect disclosure [1]. Lately, there has been some effort, mainly by the Greek Association of Alzheimer's Disease and Related Disorders (GAADRD), to utilize computerized instruments in the diagnostic procedure and create novel computerized instruments tailored to the needs of Greek older adults [6–8].

A more comprehensive diagnostic protocol has been implemented in the day centres of the GAADRD [9]. Unfortunately, due to time and budget constraints, this protocol has not been adopted by other healthcare services. The protocol consists of the following steps:

◆ The patient is first examined by a neurologist who refers the patient for laboratory investigations.

◆ The patient is examined by a neuropsychologist using a comprehensive battery of neuropsychological tests to evaluate global cognition, specific cognitive domains, and everyday functionality, and also to assess for the presence of anxiety or depression.

◆ All clinical, laboratory investigation, and neuropsychological findings are assessed by a neurologist who makes the final diagnosis, after consulting the head psychologist of the day centre.

◆ Additional investigations, such as MRI, electroencephalography (EEG), or measurement of event-related potentials (ERP), may be conducted in order to provide a clearer clinical picture and allow for more effective interventions.

Competence assessment

In the Greek legal framework, competence is defined as a person's ability to live autonomously without the need for a caregiver. Assessment of competence in dementia patients is based both on objective criteria, such as use of standardized neuropsychological tests, and on each patient's own personal circumstances such as family structure, socio-economic status, etc. [10].

Mental and functional competence

Assessment of mental competence is carried out during the diagnostic procedure and in follow-up examinations. At the same time, functional assessment is performed either informally during the diagnostic interview or using standardized tests such as the Functional Rating Scale for Symptoms of Dementia (FRSSD) or the Functional Cognitive Assessment Scale (FUCAS) [11].

Often dementia remains undiagnosed until the onset of mental and functional decline which prompts the individual or their family to seek treatment. Assessment of competence is also offered through the European 'Help at Home' programme for older adults who are unable to visit appropriate health services [10].

Financial competence

Financial competence refers to the ability of an individual to participate in financial transactions, knowledge of basic financial concepts, and financial judgement [12]. In Greece, there is no legal framework concerning the financial competence of people with dementia, who are covered under the same framework as people with mental health issues. People with dementia can often fall victim to fraud, usually by individuals pretending to be relatives or utility company employees [10]. According to Greek law, a person's will is valid if it was drawn up before the onset of dementia. Wills written after the onset of dementia can be disputed in court by the patient's relatives.

Driving competence

Driving competence is impaired in people with dementia. Impairment begins at the preclinical or mild cognitive impairment (MCI) stage and increases in severity as the disease progresses. A research study demonstrated that Greek older drivers experience similar difficulties, compared to drivers in other countries, and employ similar mechanisms to compensate for their difficulties, namely driving less or driving in less challenging conditions [13]. There is no legal framework concerning discontinuation of driving. People aged over 65 years are obliged to undergo an ophthalmological and clinical examination. However, as the examination is carried out by private doctors and driving schools, its reliability is often questionable and bribery remains an issue. Usually the decision to discontinue driving is based on a consensus reached between the patient's family and the clinician, which often leads to disputes between the patient and their family [10].

Personality competence and nursing homes

Loss of language and communication skills, functional decline, and emergence of behavioural/neuropsychiatric problems, in combination with limited free time on the part of the caregivers, are the main reasons for placement of patients in nursing homes and similar institutions. Of note, 25% of institutionalized patients have no children or close (second-degree or closer) relatives. Of those who have a family or close relatives, 62% are placed in nursing homes by their children and 35% by their spouse [9].

Advance directives and end of life

In Greece, there is no legal framework concerning advance directives, end-of-life decisions, and euthanasia. Since patients with severe dementia have impaired decision-making capacity, decisions concerning treatment withdrawal are made by the patient's family in consultation with healthcare specialists. Caregivers can receive support and counselling on these subjects from nonprofit organizations [10].

Management of dementia

In Greece, a variety of pharmacological and non-pharmacological treatments are available for patients with dementia. Whenever possible, combined pharmacological and non-pharmacological treatment is provided for improved outcomes [14, 15].

Pharmacological treatments

All three second-generation cholinesterase inhibitors donepezil, rivastigmine, and galantamine, as well as the *N*-methyl-*D*-aspartate (NDMA) receptor antagonist memantine, are available in Greece [1], with reimbursement covering 75–90% of their costs through the public healthcare system [2]. The initial treatment decision should be taken by a neurologist or psychiatrist [1, 2]. However, in practice, GPs sometimes initiate pharmacological treatment, due to lax controls by the state [2]. Ongoing evaluation of dementia severity and adjustment of pharmacological treatment can be conducted by any doctor, including GPs [1, 2]. Patients usually visit a doctor 1–3 times each year [1]. There is no framework or specific MMSE cut-off score for discontinuation of treatment and thus, this decision is taken by the clinician treating the patient [1, 2].

There has been an effort to introduce pharmacological treatments based on natural Mediterranean products such as olive oil [16] and *Crocus sativus* (saffron) [17]. These treatments are aimed mostly at patients with MCI (preclinical dementia) for whom conventional drug treatments are unavailable. Initial results are promising, and an effort is being made to introduce these treatments to public health services.

Non-pharmacological treatments

Various non-profit organizations under the umbrella of the PFADRD offer non-pharmacological interventions for people with dementia or MCI. These interventions are based on the work carried out by the GAADRD, which was the first organization to provide such services. A variety of complex cognitive exercises, including computerized cognitive training, are available to patients with preclinical dementia/MCI [9, 18]. Patients with mild dementia can participate in cognitive neurorehabilitation programmes focusing mainly on attention and executive function [19]. Patients with moderate dementia can participate in art therapy programmes which focus on emotional expression, as emotional capacity is retained at this stage [20, 21]. Reminiscence therapy, offered in a group setting, is available to people with moderate and severe dementia, with the aim of improving emotional well-being and social interaction [9]. Physical exercise and physiotherapy programmes are available to all dementia patients, aimed at improving physical fitness and reducing the risk of falls.

Family and caregiver support

Weekly caregiver support groups are available across Greece. The GAADRD also provides a Skype-based evening support group for caregivers who are unable to participate in face-to-face meetings. Once-monthly 'Alzheimer Café' gatherings, open to patients, caregivers, and the general public, are organized in various cities. These events begin with an informal discussion, followed by a presentation given by a dementia specialist who has hands-on experience in the topic of discussion [9].

Conclusion

There are some issues concerning the legal framework for competence assessment in Greece. At the same time, all available therapies for dementia are fully accessible to dementia patients, and 75–90% of medication costs are covered by reimbursement. There is considerable effort by the PFADRD to improve the diagnostic procedure, treatment, and available services for patients with dementia and caregivers.

References

1. **Alzheimer Europe**. *Dementia in Europe Yearbook 2014*. Luxembourg: Alzheimer Europe; 2014.
2. **Alzheimer Europe**. *Dementia in Europe Yearbook 2012*. Luxembourg: Alzheimer Europe; 2012.
3. **Fountoulakis KN, Tsolaki M, Chantzi H, Kazis A**. Mini Mental State Examination (MMSE): a validation study in Greece. *American Journal of Alzheimer's Disease and Other Dementias*. 2000;**15**:342–5.
4. **Nasreddine ZS, Phillips NA, Bedirian V**, *et al*. The Montreal Cognitive Assessment, MoCA: a brief screening tool for mild cognitive impairment. *Journal of the American Geriatrics Society*. 2005;**53**:695–9.
5. **Fountoulakis KN, Tsolaki M, Iacovides A**, *et al*. The validation of the short form of the Geriatric Depression Scale (GDS) in Greece. *Aging Clinical and Experimental Research*. 1999;**11**:367–72.
6. **Tsolaki M, Zygouris S, Lazarou I**, *et al*. Our experience with informative and communication technologies (ICT) in dementia. *Hellenic Journal of Nuclear Medicine*. 2015;**18**(Suppl 1):131–9.
7. **Zygouris S, Giakoumis D, Votis K**, *et al*. Can a virtual reality cognitive training application fulfill a dual role? Using the Virtual Super Market cognitive training application as a screening tool for mild cognitive impairment. *Journal of Alzheimer's Disease*. 2015;**44**:1333–47.

8. **Zygouris S, Tsolaki M.** Computerized cognitive testing for older adults: a review. *American Journal of Alzheimer's Disease and Other Dementias.* 2015;**30**:13–28.

9. **Tsolaki M.** The practice of dementia care: Greece. In: **Burns A** (ed). *Standards in Dementia Care.* Boca Raton, FL: CRC Press; 2005. pp. 55–63.

10. **Tsolaki M, Tsantali E.** Practice of competence assessment in dementia: Greece. In: **Stoppe G** (ed). *Competence Assessment in Dementia.* Vienna: Springer Vienna; 2008. pp. 121–4.

11. **Kounti F, Tsolaki M, Kiosseoglou G.** Functional cognitive assessment scale (FUCAS): a new scale to assess executive cognitive function in daily life activities in patients with dementia and mild cognitive impairment. *Human Psychopharmacology.* 2006;**21**:305–11.

12. **Marson DC.** Clinical and ethical aspects of financial capacity in dementia: a commentary. *American Journal of Geriatric Psychiatry.* 2013;**21**:392–400.

13. **Katsouri I, Athanasiadis L, Bekiaris E, Touliou K, Tsolaki M.** Mild cognitive impairment and driving habits. *International Journal of Prevention and Treatment.* 2015;**4**(2A):1–10.

14. **Buschert V, Bokde ALW, Hampel H.** Cognitive intervention in Alzheimer disease. *Nature Reviews Neurology.* 2010;**6**:508–17.

15. **Matsuzono K, Hishikawa N, Takao Y,** *et al.* Combination benefit of cognitive rehabilitation plus donepezil for Alzheimer's disease patients. *Geriatrics and Gerontology International.* 2016;**16**:200–4.

16. **Martinez-Lapiscina EH, Clavero P, Toledo E,** *et al.* Virgin olive oil supplementation and long-term cognition: the PREDIMED-NAVARRA randomized trial. *Journal of Nutrition, Health and Aging.* 2013;**17**:544–52.

17. **Tsolaki M, Karathanasi E, Lazarou I,** *et al.* Efficacy and safety of *Crocus sativus L.* in patients with mild cognitive impairment: one year single-blind randomized, with parallel groups, clinical trial. *Journal of Alzheimer's Disease.* 2016;**54**:129–33.

18. **Tsolaki M, Kounti F, Agogiatou C,** *et al.* Effectiveness of nonpharmacological approaches in patients with mild cognitive impairment. *Neurodegenerative Diseases.* 2011;**8**:138–45.

19. **Aguirre E, Woods RT, Spector A, Orrell M.** Cognitive stimulation for dementia: a systematic review of the evidence of effectiveness from randomised controlled trials. *Ageing Research Reviews.* 2013;**12**:253–62.

20. **Elferink Maaike W-O, van Tilborg I, Kessels Roy PC.** Perception of emotions in mild cognitive impairment and Alzheimer's dementia: does intensity matter? *Translational Neuroscience.* 2015;**6**:139–49.

21. **Lee KH, Algase DL, McConnell ES.** Daytime observed emotional expressions of people with dementia. *Nursing Research.* 2013;**62**:218–25.

Chapter 24

Ireland

Catherine Dolan and Brian Lawlor

Summary

This chapter examines the prevalence and pathways to the diagnosis of dementia, as well as dementia care infrastructure, in the Republic of Ireland. The economic burden of dementia in Ireland is explored, including both formal and informal costs. Dementia care in the community, residential, and acute hospital settings is described. Associated policy, legislation, standards, and guidelines relevant to dementia care in Ireland are addressed. Current funding structures are examined. The contributions of dementia-specific educational efforts and relevant research in Ireland are highlighted. Challenges encountered in moving from a more traditional medical model of dementia care to a psycho-social, person-centred care model in Ireland, including inequitable funding allocation, are outlined.

Introduction

In 2014, an estimated 48,000 people with dementia lived in the Republic of Ireland (ROI), with a projected rise to 55,000 for the year 2016 [1]. Of the people with dementia in the ROI, in 2011, an estimated two-thirds were female and 4000 were aged under 65 years [1], with 700 people with Down syndrome and dementia [2]. By 2046, a rise to over 152,000 people with dementia in the ROI [1] is projected, consistent with global trends in population ageing.

The government annual spend on dementia is unclear, but as per estimates in a 2014 report [3], the baseline economic and social cost of dementia in the ROI in 2010 was €1.69 billion.

Dementia assessment and diagnosis

As no national dementia register exists, the ROI lacks reliable data on how many people with dementia receive a diagnosis or where dementia diagnosis occurs. In the main, GPs, geriatricians, neurologists, and old age psychiatrists undertake dementia assessment and diagnosis, in addition to dedicated memory clinics. Difficulties experienced by Irish GPs in dementia assessment include problems differentiating dementia from normal ageing [4]. Where expertise is required in dementia diagnosis, GPs are advised to refer patients to a specialized multidisciplinary team for further assessment [5].

There are 17 memory clinics in the ROI [6]. In a 2011 profile of 14 Irish memory clinics [7], mainly led by old age psychiatrists or geriatricians, less than half had input from allied health professionals, including neuropsychologists. Some memory clinics focused on diagnostic assessment only, with other services also focusing on aftercare and follow-up of people with dementia. There is no dedicated service for assessment, diagnosis, and management of early-onset dementia in the ROI.

Models of care

The Irish National Dementia Strategy [8], launched in 2014, reinforces the aim of the Irish government policy since 1988 [9], which is to facilitate continued community living of people with dementia where practicable.

However, current funding structures to support the move from a traditional medical model of dementia care to a health and social care approach are inadequate. In the ROI, access to community care—unlike access to long-term residential care—is not underpinned by legislation. In addition, specialized dementia services in the ROI lack integration and are set up and funded through separate clinical programmes, generally within the specialties of geriatrics, psychiatry, and neurology. This service approach leads to fragmented cross-disciplinary care of people with dementia.

Community care

In 2011, an estimated 30,000 people with dementia lived in the community in the ROI, with a doubling in this number projected over the next 20 years [1]. Despite these projections, there has been a decrease in the provision of home help hours by the State, from 12.6 million hours in 2008 to 10.3 million hours in 2014 [10, 11]. Ireland's healthcare provider—the Health Service Executive (HSE)—provides a number of community supports for people with dementia through its own staff or through private agencies. The Alzheimer Society of Ireland, a voluntary organization, also provides a range of specialist dementia services, including day care, respite care, and a support telephone service—the Alzheimer National Helpline.

Private home care (for people with dementia) in the ROI is not regulated, despite a rise in private home care service providers in recent years. Many families in the ROI also make arrangements privately with individuals to provide home care.

Prioritized in the National Dementia Strategy is the implementation of intensive home care packages (HCPs) for people with dementia, with €22 million in funding allocated over the period of 2015–18. However, recent criticism relates to the low number of beneficiaries of HCPs among people with dementia and strong links between delayed hospital discharge and granting of HCPs [12].

Scarcity of day services and respite beds country-wide increases stress on caregivers of people with dementia, with just 66 respite beds available across 54 dementia-specific care units (SCUs) in the ROI [13].

Residential care

A 2015 survey [13] of 469 Irish nursing homes highlighted the division of residential care provision for people with dementia, with two-thirds privately operated, approximately 20% provided by the HSE, and approximately 13% delivered by voluntary and not-for-profit organizations.

Of residential facilities surveyed, only 11% had SCUs, with wide variations in location, physical environment, and availability of appropriately stimulating activities [13], indicating an inconsistency with the National Quality Standards [14]. Furthermore, approximately 60% of privately employed care staff had undergone specialist dementia training, compared with only 30% of staff in publicly run facilities [13].

The Nursing Homes Support Scheme (NHSS) [15], underpinned by legislation, funds the cost of long-term nursing home care for the majority of nursing home residents within a capped budget of approximately €900 million to €1 billion per annum since 2009 [16].

An individual's contribution is based on their means, and the State pays the balance of the costs in approved nursing homes.

Policy reform [17] and the establishment of a statutory agency—the Health Information and Quality Authority (HIQA)—in 2007 resulted in the development of a set of national care standards for older people in residential care in the ROI [14], which have been recently revised [18]. Accordingly, all registered Irish nursing homes are subject to regular inspections since 2009.

Acute hospital setting

The first Irish National Audit of Dementia Care [19] in acute hospitals was undertaken in 2013. It found that less than one-third of hospitals had a policy for management of challenging behaviour and 33 of 35 acute hospitals had no dementia care pathway in place.

Current policy and legislation

The 2014 publication of the National Dementia Strategy builds on a number of earlier reports, including *An Action Plan for Dementia* (APD) [20]. Priority action areas include better dementia awareness, timely diagnosis and intervention, integrated dementia services, training and education, research, and leadership. Funding of €27.5 million to cover implementation of the Strategy over the period of 2014–17 was contributed by The Atlantic Philanthropies and the Department of Health, through the HSE.

The Assisted Decision Making (Capacity) Act 2015 [21], due for commencement during 2016, is relevant to people with dementia. It reforms Ireland's capacity legislation, establishing a statutory framework to support and assist decision-making among individuals who lack or who may lack capacity to make legally binding agreements or decisions about their welfare, property, or affairs unaided.

Primary prevention, education, and research

Current government strategy promotes healthy lifestyle behaviours [22, 23]. As part of the National Dementia Strategy, an awareness campaign, launched in 2015, aims to make Ireland more dementia-friendly, reduce stigma, and raise awareness of modifiable risk factors for dementia.

The Dementia Services Information and Development Centre (DSIDC) is a national research and education resource for healthcare professionals. The Alzheimer Society of Ireland and the HSE also provide dementia education programmes for healthcare providers and caregivers of people with dementia.

The HSE in their 2016 Service Plan commits to continued dementia-specific education for GPs [24].

A 2011 report [25] by the European Union Joint Programme–Neurodegenerative Disease Research (JPND) estimated the annual investment in research related to neurodegenerative disorders in Ireland to be €5.88 million. The investment breakdown across basic, clinical, and service areas is shown in Fig. 24.1. Since the publication of this report, there have been a number of service and research developments in the ROI. The HSE & Genio Dementia Programme, with support from The Atlantic Philanthropies, funded the piloting of a number of innovative service models aligned with government policy. These include the development of integrated dementia care pathways in three acute hospitals in the ROI and community care innovations for people with dementia at four sites around Ireland. Dementia and Neurodegeneration Network Ireland (DNNI) (http://www.dementia-neurodegeneration.ie), an interdisciplinary research network which aims to promote multisectoral

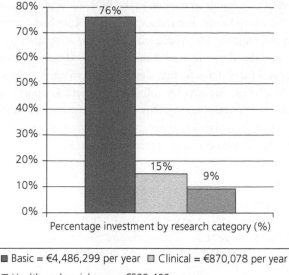

Fig. 24.1 Breakdown of investment in neurodegenerative disease-related research in Ireland.
Source data from EU Joint Programme–Neurodegenerative Disease Research. *JPND Mapping Exercise Report*, 2011.

research in dementia, was established in 2015 with the support of the Health Research Board (HRB), the lead agency involved in funding health research in the ROI.

Additional research funding of €4.5 million was provided by the HRB and The Atlantic Philanthropies in 2016, as part of the research arm of the National Dementia Strategy. Despite recent funding injections and considering the societal challenge posed by dementia, research in dementia, particularly that related to health and social care, remains relatively underfunded in the ROI.

Conclusion

Despite major progress in dementia care in the ROI in the last decade, a number of challenges remain. Promotion of timely diagnosis of dementia requires awareness and education at the general public and primary care level and the implementation of integrated care pathways between primary care and specialist and hospital services. Memory clinics are poorly developed and resourced, and there are no dedicated services for people with early-onset dementia.

Prioritization of investment in community supports for people with dementia and their caregivers, including equitable access to home care, day, and respite services, will decrease caregiver burden in the ROI, allow people with dementia to remain in their own home, and reduce long-term care bed occupancy.

Residential care funding for people with dementia should recognize the importance of specialized services with appropriately designed long-term care environments and incentivize further development of such units with suitably trained staff and infrastructure. Ongoing government support for dementia-specific education and training, together with investment in research to create evidence that can be translated into policy and practice, is key to the continued enhancement of dementia care and services in the ROI.

References

1. Pierce M, Cahill S, O'Shea E. *Prevalence and projections of dementia in Ireland, 2011–2046*. Trinity College Dublin, National University Of Ireland Galway, and Genio; 2014.

2. Cahill S, O'Shea E, Pierce M. *Future dementia care in Ireland, sharing the evidence to mobilise action*. Trinity College Dublin and National University Of Ireland Galway; 2012.

3. Connolly S, Gillespie P, O'Shea E, Cahill S, Pierce M. Estimating the economic and social costs of dementia in Ireland. *Dementia (London)*. 2014;13:5–22.

4. Cahill S, Clark M, Walsh C, O'Connell H, Lawlor B. Dementia in primary care: the first survey of Irish general practitioners. *International Journal of Geriatric Psychiatry*. 2006;21:319–24.

5. Foley T, Swanwick G. *Dementia: diagnosis and management in general practice*. Dublin: Irish College of General Practitioners; 2014.

6. Gibb M, Cahill S, Moore V, Pierce M. *Memory clinics in Ireland: a guide for family caregivers and health service*, 3rd ed. Dublin: Dementia Services Information and Development Centre; 2014.

7. Cahill S, Pierce M, Moore V. A national survey of memory clinics in the Republic of Ireland. *International Psychogeriatrics*. 2014;26:605–13.

8. Department of Health. *The Irish national dementia strategy*. Dublin: Department of Health; 2014.

9. National Council on Ageing and Older People. *The years ahead report: a review of the implementation of its recommendations*. Report No. 48. Dublin: Stationery Office; 1988.

10. Health Service Executive. *Annual report and financial statements 2008*. Dublin: Health Service Executive; 2008.

11. Health Service Executive. *Annual report and financial statements 2008*. Dublin: Health Service Executive; 2014.

12. Alzheimer Society of Ireland. *The Alzheimer Society of Ireland pre-budget submission 2017*. Dublin: Alzheimer Society of Ireland; 2016.

13. Cahill S, O'Nolan C, O'Caheny, Bobersky A. *An Irish national survey of dementia in long-term residential care*. Dublin: Dementia Services Information and Development Centre; 2014.

14. Health Information and Quality Authority. *National quality standards for residential care settings for older people in Ireland*. Dublin: Health Information and Quality Authority; 2009.

15. **Nursing Home Support Scheme Act 2009**. Act Number 15 of 2009. Available from: http://www.irishstatutebook.ie/eli/2009/act/15/enacted/en/pdf [accessed 1 September 2016].

16. **Department of Health**. *Review of the nursing homes support scheme, A fair deal*. Available from: http://health.gov.ie/wp-content/uploads/2015/07/Review-of-Nursing-Homes-Support-Scheme.pdf [accessed 1 September 2016].

17. Health Act 2007. Act Number 23 of 2007. Available from: http://www.irishstatutebook. ie/eli/2007/act/23/enacted/en/pdf [accessed 1 September 2016].

18. **Health Information and Quality Authority**. *National standards for residential care settings for older people in Ireland, 2016*. Dublin: Health Information and Quality Authority; 2016.

19. **De Siún A, O'Shea E, Timmons S**. *Report of the Irish national audit on dementia care in acute hospital*. Cork: National Audit of Dementia; 2014.

20. **O'Shea E, O' Reilly S**. *An action plan for dementia*. National Council on Ageing and Older People. Report No. 54. Dublin: National Council on Ageing and Older People; 1999.

21. **Assisted Decision-Making (Capacity) Act 2015**. Act Number 64 of 2015. Available from: https://www.oireachtas.ie/documents/bills28/acts/2015/a6415.pdf [accessed 1 September 2016].

22. **Department of Health**. *The national positive ageing strategy*. Dublin: Department of Health; 2013.

23. **Department of Health, Healthy Ireland**. *A framework for improved health and wellbeing 2013–2025*. Dublin: Department of Health; 2013.

24. **Health Service Executive**. *National service plan 2016*. Dublin: Health Service Executive; 2016.

25. **EU Joint Programme–Neurodegenerative Disease Research**. *JPND mapping exercise report*. 2011. Available from: http://www.neurodegenerationresearch.eu/fileadmin/Documents/2012/SRA-related/JPND_Mapping_Report__Final__01.pdf [accessed 1 September 2016].

Chapter 25

Italy

Claudia Palumbo and Umberto Volpe

Summary

Italy is among countries in the world with the highest population of older people, with Italian elderly people accounting for over 20% of the total population of the country, and ranks second in Europe in terms of the 'ageing index' (i.e. the number of people aged 65 and above per 100 youths under the age of 15). In Italy, over 1 million people suffer from dementia, including approximately 600,000 cases of Alzheimer's disease. Since 2000, a specific National Dementia Plan was initiated and Alzheimer's Evaluation Units (UVAs) were introduced in all Italian regions to coordinate systematically the complex care process for dementia. Some Italian regions have recently deemed appropriate to change the denomination of UVAs to 'Evaluation Units of Dementia' (UVDs) and/or 'Centres for Cognitive Impairment'. More recently, the Italian Ministry of Health launched an initiative aimed at improving the essential levels of assistance/care (LEA). The LEA represent all activities and services deemed essential to all Italian citizens and that the Italian national health system has to ensure are available, either on a free basis or by paying a participation fee, depending on patients' situations. To provide directive indications for promoting and improving interventions in the dementia field, particularly focusing on the support of patients and families throughout specific pathways of care, the Italian Ministry of Health licensed an official update of the "Dementia National Plan" in October 2014. Within this initiative, a specific attention was given to ethical issues in dementia management and early onset dementias. Also, a crucial focus of the plan is to ensure timely diagnosis of dementia, as it is considered one of the main aspects which will be evaluated in order to apply further changes to the Italian dementia care strategy in the future.

Introduction

Italy is among countries in the world with the highest population of older people, with the proportion of people aged 65 years and above accounting for over 20% of the total Italian population. Italy ranks second in Europe, after Germany, in terms of the 'ageing index' (i.e. the number of people aged 65 years and above per 100 youths under the age of 15) [1]. Given the global trends in population ageing, along with the rising prevalence of chronic diseases, and dementia in particular, it is not surprising that in Italy, there are more than 1 million people suffering from dementia, which includes approximately 600,000 cases of AD, with more than 3 million people involved, either directly or indirectly, in dementia care [2]. Furthermore, demographic projections show an arithmetic progression of such indicators, with a projected ratio of 280 seniors to 100 young people in Italy by 2051 [3]. The progressive growth of the elderly population will result in a substantial increase in the prevalence of dementia. Therefore, significant changes in care needs for people with dementia are easily foreseeable in Italy in the coming years.

The Italian National Dementia Strategy

Since 2000, Alzheimer's Evaluation Units [*Unità di Valutazione per l'Alzheimer* (UVA)] were introduced in all Italian regions to coordinate systematically the complex care process for dementia. UVAs represent local health units specifically dedicated to the care of people with dementia by coordinating healthcare and social care services for dementia. Currently, more than 2000 health professionals (including GPs, neurologists, geriatricians, psychiatrists, rehabilitation staff, nurses, psychologists, and social workers) are involved in UVA activities [3]. Some Italian regions have recently deemed appropriate to change the denomination of UVAs to 'Evaluation Units of Dementia' (UVDs) and/or 'Centres for Cognitive Impairment', thus emphasizing the shift in focus from AD to a wider spectrum of dementia-related problems, including all types of dementia. However, the designation that appears more appropriate is probably 'Centres for Cognitive Diseases and Dementia' [*Centri per Disturbi Cognitivi e Demenze* (CDCD)].

Furthermore, at around the same time, the Italian Ministry of Health also launched another initiative aimed at improving the essential levels of care [*livelli essenziali di assistenza* (LEA)] [4]. The LEA represent all activities and services that are deemed essential to all Italian citizens and that the Italian national health system has to ensure are available and accessible, either on a free basis or by paying a participation fee. The LEA have also been defined specifically for geriatric medicine to ensure the most appropriate care for dementia

Table 25.1 Major objectives of the Italian National Dementia Plan

Objective 1	To promote health and social care interventions and policies
Objective 2	To create/strengthen the integrated network of services for dementia, based on an integrated approach
Objective 3	To implement strategies for promoting appropriateness and quality of care
Objective 4	To improve the quality of life of people with dementia and their families by supporting empowerment and destigmatization

Source data from *Annali dell'Istituto Superiore di Sanità*, **51**, 4, Di Fiandra T., Canevelli M., Di Pucchio A., Vanacore V., and the Italian Dementia National Plan Working Group, The Italian Dementia National Plan, pp. 261–264, 2015.

patients and also to effectively identify, in specific care contexts, critical areas in which it is likely or believed that the provision of basic levels of care might be suboptimal. The LEA system in geriatric medicine is also specifically aimed at ensuring a standardized, multidimensional evaluation of patients with dementia and a continuous flow of information between UVAs and the Ministry of Health concerning the planning and delivery of dementia care [4]. The LEA also address issues of dementia care at the three basic levels of Italian healthcare, namely residential/hospice care, UVA/district care, and maintenance care [4].

Finally, the first proper 'National Dementia Plan' was launched in October 2014 [3] by the Italian Ministry of Health, in close collaboration with the regional (political, health, and social) governing bodies, the National Institute of Health, and the major national associations of patients and caregivers. The overarching goal of this strategy is to provide guidance and recommendations on promoting and improving interventions in dementia care, not only limited to specialist and therapeutic measures, but also focusing particularly on support provision for patients and their families as part of care pathways. The four main objectives, which are shown in detail in Table 25.1, include promotion of healthcare policies, creation of service networks, implementation of specific care strategies, and improvement of the quality of life of people with dementia; each general objective is defined in terms of specific 'purposes' for each area, and 'actions' to be taken are also identified [3].

Strengths of the Italian National Dementia Strategy

Italy was probably the first country in the world to systematically introduce 'memory clinics' in its national healthcare system. The criteria set for the establishment of UVAs were centred on the identification of functional units based on the coordination of neurological, psychiatric, internal medical, and geriatric expertise (from hospital departments, specialist community services, home care, and general practice). Italy was indeed the first country that focused on the creation of specialist centres for dementia screening, assessment, and diagnosis and for coordinating treatment. Subsequently, France, Germany, the UK, Austria, and Ireland followed suit by promoting the establishment of 'memory clinics', based on the same principles. The 'CRONOS Project', launched in 2000 by the Italian Ministry of Health, has provided all Italian regions with more than 500 specific UVAs, thus encompassing all local health districts in the country. This initiative was one of the first in the field of dementia care aimed at standardizing, at a national level, prescriptions of acetylcholinesterase inhibitors, to assess their effects on defined outcomes (cognition, functional status, behaviour), and thus to help adopt a definite attitude towards the reimbursement of the costs of drug treatment, which had some detractors in Italy at the time [5].

Further to this, the long-standing Italian 'integrated management' model of care [6] has been fully incorporated into the current national plan for dementia care. The 1978 reform (Law No. 833/1978) created the national health system in Italy and introduced universal healthcare coverage for Italian citizens and those legally residing in Italy, establishing human dignity, health needs, and solidarity as the guiding principles of the health system. The new healthcare system was partly decentralized, to include national, regional, and local administration levels. Since then, the central government has been responsible for financing, as well as defining the criteria for the distribution of funds to, the regions of the country. The main aims and values of the 1978 reform have been retained in subsequent healthcare plans to guarantee everyone equal access to uniform levels of care, irrespective of income or location, to develop disease prevention schemes, to control health spending, and to guarantee public democratic control with a mixed financing model. In Italy, this model is still considered the best approach to improve care for people with chronic diseases, as this specific segment of the population needs effective treatments, modulated according to disease severity, without loss of continuity of care, information, and support, with the ultimate aim of achieving the highest possible level of self-management [6].

Current challenges in dementia care in Italy

Despite the valid initiatives for dementia care in Italy described in the previous section, several challenges still remain in this health sector. First, the traditional local socio-economic differences among the different regions of Italy are still present in the country, and they exert some relevant influence over the provision of dementia care. The management of dementia in Italy is still affected by a profound disparity among Italian regions in terms of available resources and services, with possible significant differences in care delivery from one region to another and a substantial lack of a national standard [3]. As a result, in Italy, it is highly likely that different aspects of dementia care are addressed in a fragmented manner—at different times and through different care processes. Thus, besides the declared aim of the 2014 National Dementia Care Plan to provide guidance on promoting and improving interventions in dementia care, the real possibility to achieve a uniform and fully integrated model of dementia care still remains an objective to be pursued in Italy. A critical element of the Italian healthcare system is the lack of integration between health and social services; it would be highly essential to establish a strategic process aimed at identifying pathways and structures that would help efficiently coordinate services provided by these two sectors. At the same time, it is also important to build on the positive experience gained from the UVA initiative over the last 15 years. Finally, the lack of full integration and collaboration between hospital care, primary care, home care, and community service providers in some Italian regions has to be acknowledged and the potential negative impact of non-continuity of care for dementia patients still remains to be addressed in Italy.

The future of dementia care in Italy

The Italian National Dementia Plan was launched in 2015, and full evaluation of its impact on dementia care will be known in the near future. The Plan aims to address the current challenges of dementia care in Italy by identifying precise quality standards for dementia care, by continuously monitoring the identified quality standards, by producing guidelines on crucial aspects of dementia management (including diagnosis disclosure, informed consent, and use of legal options). Particular attention should be given to ethical issues in dementia management (e.g. advance directives and accessibility of palliative care) and early-onset dementia. Moreover, the Italian Ministry of Health has provided some recommendations on optimization of the diagnostic process and strengthening of the social welfare process. Timely diagnosis, in fact, is one of the key points to consider in the future development of the National Dementia Strategy.

References

1. **National Institute of Statistics (Istituto Nazionale di Statistica).** *Annual report/ Rapporto annuale.* Rome: Istituto Nazionale di Statistica; 2014. Available from: https://www.istat.it/it/files/2014/05/Rapporto-annuale-2014.pdf [accessed 22 August 2018].

2. **ALCOVE Project. Alzheimer Cooperative Valuation in Europe.** 2016. Available from: https://www.alzheimer-europe.org/ [accessed 22 August 2018].

3. **Di Fiandra T, Canevelli M, Di Pucchio A, Vanacore V; the Italian Dementia National Plan Working Group.** The Italian Dementia National Plan. Commentary. *Annali dell'Istituto Superiore di Sanità.* 2015 **51**:261–4.

4. **Degani LE, Mozzanica R.** Integrazione socio-sanitaria. In: **Degani LE, Mozzanica R** (eds). *L'integrazione socio-sanitaria.* Torino: Giappichelli Editore; 2011. pp. 49–57.

5. **Bianchetti A, Padovani A, Trabucchi M.** Outcomes of Alzheimer's disease treatment: the Italian CRONOS project. *International Journal of Geriatric Psychiatry.* 2002;**18**:86–90.

6. **Ferré F, de Belvis AG, Valerio L,** *et al.* Italy: health system review. *Health Systems in Transition.* 2014;**16**:1–168.

Chapter 26

The Netherlands

Marcel Olde Rikkert

Summary

In the Netherlands, there is currently an ongoing transition whereby a relevant part of long-term institutionalized care for dementia patients is being shifted to care at home. Legislation was changed in 2015 to achieve this goal. However, primary and nursing home care still needs to be redesigned to meet the needs of dementia patients and society. Improving network care holds great promise for this transition, as current dementia care in the Netherlands still falls short in terms of fragmentation of care, ad hoc collaboration, lack of feedback on quality and efficiency of care to healthcare professionals involved, and inadequate implementation of established multidisciplinary guidelines.

Current Dutch dementia care

In the Netherlands, there is currently an ongoing transition whereby a relevant part of long-term institutionalized care for dementia patients is being shifted towards care at home. To date, DementiaNet—a collaborative care approach—and other network proposals have been embraced by the national Deltaplan for Dementia to achieve this transition. Networking among professionals, services, and institutions for dementia care has the potential to reduce disease burden on individuals, healthcare services, and society—the triple-aim improvement. Two crucial elements in improving and changing the highly complex dementia care include short-term quality improvement cycles and value-based care evaluations.

So far, approximately 80 dementia networks have been established, of which 20 are based on the DementiaNet model, mostly including, among various arrangements, individual case managers. These networks vary in quality of care and strength of collaboration, depending on local circumstances. Initial results show considerable variability in clinical practice, and DementiaNet and other network approaches can lead to triple-aim improvement in care quality. Ongoing research will identify barriers, facilitators, and merits of the network approach to increasing the quality of care and ultimately improving outcomes for patients, caregivers, health services, and society.

The complexity and variability of local care across the Netherlands mean that network-based interventions and complexity-proof evaluation methods are required to achieve sustainable, high-quality value-based dementia care for the next, still larger, generation of dementia patients in our ageing society.

Introduction

The number of Dutch patients diagnosed with dementia in primary care is currently 80,000 and this will rise to 140,000 by 2030, which is an increase of 70%. It is not exactly clear how many patients have not been diagnosed at the moment and what will happen exactly in the near future, given recent evidence of decreased incidence of dementia in high-income countries, including the Netherlands (see, for example, the Rotterdam Study for epidemiological results) [1]. According to the Dutch Alzheimer Society, the number of people with dementia is estimated to grow from 243,000 to 400,000 by 2030. Currently, 12,000 people younger than 65 years suffer from dementia and 70,000 people with dementia live in nursing homes, though the majority (50–70%) live at home. Also it is estimated that a substantial number of patients have not been given a diagnosis of dementia, which is likely due to the presence of multimorbidity and advanced age where the value of an additional diagnosis of dementia is less clear to primary care physicians who care for the majority of dementia patients. Nevertheless, in the Netherlands, dementia care is a health sector with the highest costs, now reaching approximately €5 billion yearly, which represents 5% of the country's net healthcare costs and nearly 1% of the total government expenditures per year. These dementia care costs are expected to rise by 2–2.5% yearly with unchanged policy. Therefore, in order to ensure sustainability of healthcare provision for dementia in this era of an ageing population, both the national government and health insurers have established plans to reduce the burden of dementia on society, as well as on the national economy.

Current challenges

As a result of the changed policy, the number of elderly people with cognitive impairment who are still living at home is likely to increase. Consequently, primary care physicians will be increasingly required to manage and optimize treatment for dementia patients, which underlines the need to improve dementia care within primary care. Although many initiatives have been set up recently, collaborative dementia care is still fragmented and far from optimal, due to lack of disease-specific expertise and training and limited communication among healthcare professionals [2]. A collaborative approach would be particularly important for dementia patients to determine their care needs, as disease manifestation is often complex and complicated by comorbidities, while loss of mental autonomy and disease awareness are specific to dementia. Dementia patients have to cope not only with dementia, but also with other chronic health and welfare issues. This is not a feature unique to Dutch healthcare, but a global issue, as shown in a large Scottish study in which 95% of dementia patients also had relevant comorbidities [3]. Yet, collaboration among Dutch healthcare professionals is mainly ad hoc, rather than structured. This was demonstrated in a Dutch study on the effectiveness of post-diagnosis dementia care provided by nine memory clinics compared with GPs [4]. In both study arms, the care process proved to be fairly unstructured. Furthermore, care was inadequately personalized, without formal assessment of individual problems and priorities and without sufficiently taking into account patients' individual context [5–7]. In order to tackle these shortcomings and meet future challenges, a number of dementia policy plans have been initiated recently.

Dementia care transition policy

The biggest transition took place in 2015 when the national law on long-term care reimbursement [*Algemene Wet Bijzondere Ziektekosten* (AWBZ)] was substantially changed and nursing homes and care facilities had to cut down on their bed capacity and improve efficiency, while case management was transferred to private health insurers. This change was fuelled by the fact that the national healthcare system is currently the most expensive in Europe, though it is also rated as delivering the best quality of care by European health consumer groups (https://healthpowerhouse.com). After adjusting for the country's population size and economy, the Dutch healthcare costs (17% of the national product) are higher than those in other European countries and follow behind American healthcare expenditures (25%), with Dutch long-term dementia care requiring a substantial part of the national budget. Overall, the planned transition over time should alleviate the national expenditure on dementia care, despite the growing number of people with dementia. However, it is not clear whether these changes in legislation will actually meet the goals of improving efficiency and lowering care costs while maintaining, or even improving, care quality. The government and various organizations have come together in the national Deltaplan for Dementia. The Deltaplan, named after the famous countrywide waterworks in the twentieth century, has several prioritized themes to achieve its goals: (1) safeguarding case management, (2) improving networking in dementia care, (3) promoting a dementia-friendly society, and (4) developing relevant innovation programmes and research. Dementia research is supported as part of the nationwide Memorabel research programme, as well as in European studies as part of the JPND.

Case management

Nationally and internationally, case management for dementia is regarded as one of the most important interventions to keep patients with dementia as independent as possible (see David Cameron's statement at the G8 meeting in London, 2014; https://www.gov.uk/government/speeches/global-dementia-legacy-event-david-camerons-speech). Case management is also listed as a top priority in the Dutch Care Standard, which was set in a consensus statement in 2013. The challenge now is to integrate case management into the local and regional settings and safeguard access for all within the private insurance regulations. Case management should also be adaptable to different phases over the long-term course of the disease; thus, intensive input is required in the status transition from health to disease, e.g. with changes in living arrangements and the occurrence of crisis situations, whereas case management can be light, or even dormant, in stable disease phases. Case management with such a flexible and tailor-made approach has not been achieved on a wide scale yet but has been included as part of innovative projects.

Dementia networks

The Nijmegen-based DementiaNet initiative represents an innovative example of network approach to care, which is prioritized in the Deltaplan for future dementia care. The DementiaNet central facility forms an overarching umbrella that facilitates effective and efficient organization, implementation, and maintenance of local primary care networks, which are in direct connection with secondary care facilities for dementia. DementiaNet was designed to support these networks towards becoming an independent, sustainable, and inter-professional collaborative care system, in which professionals can deliver better quality of care with improved effectiveness. Primary care for dementia patients in the Netherlands is characterized by complex social and financial developments, with overlapping interventions and inadequate coordination between health professionals. Due to the significant societal and economic impact of dementia, the Dutch government, in line with international policymaking, aims for high-quality and affordable dementia care, partly by cutting services that offer similar assistance and by supporting patient and family participation in care. Between 2005 and 2016, change was instigated through the financing of four successive national dementia and elderly care network improvement programmes. This has already created a nationwide regional network structure with dementia case managers and dissemination of multidisciplinary guidelines. However, inadequate implementation and lack of structured finance resulted in large variability in the uptake of, and adherence to, the new guidelines and regulations in clinical practice. Additionally, in 2015, the Dutch government introduced the above-mentioned radical reforms in the financial structure of primary healthcare, resulting in a shift of welfare and care responsibilities from national and regional levels to local governments at the municipality level. Thus, responsibility for welfare was transferred to local authorities. GPs in the Netherlands have long acted as 'gatekeepers' in medical care, including dementia care, and community nurses now determine the extent of nursing care required. Case management is not yet structurally financed, and therefore, funding varies between regions, and case managers are not available to all dementia patients.

This new financial arrangement has created much insecurity for healthcare professionals and institutions, as well as for patients and their caregivers, in primary care. The DementiaNet approach was designed to take into account this healthcare complexity by shifting responsibilities and great variability in clinical practice. Thus, preliminary results for the first 20 local networks indicate that this investment and support via short-term cycles of quality improvement may pay off in terms of triple aim outcomes for patients, caregivers, professionals, and society [8].

Dementia research

Memorabel is the research and innovation part of the Deltaplan for Dementia. Memorabel is an 8-year research and innovation programme, which was launched in 2013 on behalf of the Ministry of Health, Welfare, and Sport. Phase 1 ran from 2013 to 2016, and phase 2 is currently under way. In this second phase, research will continue on the same path, consolidating the benefits already gained by facilitating the most relevant and best-quality studies, spread across basic and translational research themes, but with greater focus on the use of knowledge. More efforts will be directed towards the government policy to foster participation of patients and caregivers. The goal of the second phase of 'Memorabel' is to gather knowledge that could help, in the long term, to adequately and sustainably serve the growing number of patients (caring for tomorrow's patients), improve the quality of life of people with dementia, and improve the care and support they receive (caring for today's patients). The programme prioritizes four themes: (1) cause and mechanism of the disease, (2) improvement in diagnostics, (3) innovations in treatment and prevention, and (4) last, but not least, improvements towards efficient patient- and caregiver-directed care and support.

Conclusion

The Dutch healthcare system has to address important challenges to achieve sustainable and high-quality healthcare for the increasing number of dementia patients. In particular, the expensive long-term care services are being redesigned, and patient and families are encouraged towards more participation and self-management. Improved and innovative case management and dementia networks are prioritized as the instruments to help achieve these goals and, as such, form pivotal parts of the nationwide Deltaplan for Dementia, which also promotes dementia research.

Initial results of the Deltaplan for Dementia show that clinical practice highly varies and that the DementiaNet and other network approaches may indeed lead to triple-aim quality improvement. The high level of complexity of, and variability in, local care means that complex interventions and innovative research and evaluation methods are required to realize value-based care in dementia practice. The effectiveness of network innovations probably cannot be proven in randomized controlled trials, because the networks adapt themselves to local contexts and thus cannot be strictly standardized. Therefore, both in terms of innovation, reimbursement, and research methods, the challenges posed by dementia care give fresh impetus to innovations, in which all stakeholders should be involved to maintain the Netherlands as a leader in the provision of high-quality dementia care.

References

1. Schrijvers EMC, Verhaaren BFJ, Koudstaal PJ, Hofman A, Ikram MA, Breteler MMB. Is dementia incidence declining? Trends in dementia incidence since 1990 in the Rotterdam Study. *Neurology.* 2012;**78**:1456–63.
2. Perry M, Drašković I, van Achterberg T, *et al.* Development and validation of quality indicators for dementia diagnosis and management in a primary care setting. *Journal of the American Geriatrics Society.* 2010;**58**:557–63.
3. Barnett K, Mercer SW, Norbury M, Watt G, Wyke S, Guthrie B. Epidemiology of multimorbidity and implications for health care, research, and medical education: a cross-sectional study. *The Lancet.* 2012;**380**:37–43.
4. Meeuwsen EJ, Melis RJ, Van Der Aa GC, *et al.* Effectiveness of dementia follow-up care by memory clinics or general practitioners: randomised controlled trial. *BMJ.* 2012;**344**:e3086.

5. van Dongen JJJ, Lenzen SA, van Bokhoven MA, Daniëls R, van der Weijden T, Beurskens A. Interprofessional collaboration regarding patients' care plans in primary care: a focus group study into influential factors. *BMC Family Practice.* 2016;**17**:1–10.

6. Schölzel-Dorenbos CJ, Meeuwsen EJ, Olde Rikkert MG. Integrating unmet needs into dementia health-related quality of life research and care: introduction of the hierarchy model of needs in dementia. *Aging and Mental Health.* 2010;**14**:113–19.

7. Bell J, Kaats E, Opheij W. Bridging disciplines in alliances and networks: in search for solutions for the managerial relevance gap. *International Journal of Strategic Business Alliances.* 2013;**3**:50–68.

8. Nieuwboer M, Richters A, van der Marck MA. Triple aim improvement for individuals, services and society in dementia care: The DementiaNet collaborative care approach. *Zeitschrift fur Gerontologie und Geriatrie.* 2017;**50**(Suppl 2):78–83.

Chapter 27

Northern Ireland

Emma Louise Cunningham, Stephen Todd,
Conor Barton, and Peter Passmore

Summary

The Northern Ireland (NI) Dementia Strategy was launched in
November 2011, with similar strategic issues and priorities to
those identified in the English, Welsh, and Scottish documents.
There are a number of aspects of dementia care in NI of which
the province can be proud, several of which are outlined. One
of the major achievements has been the successful production
of the Mental Capacity Act, which awaits implementation and
publication of a code of practice for clinicians. Other challenges
include the coordination of care for people with dementia across
the healthcare spectrum and the anticipation and incorporation
into practice of evolving diagnostic and therapeutic interventions.
There are three things which we feel NI does particularly well
in dementia care: we consistently outperforms other nations
and regions within the UK in dementia diagnosis rates; NI
is in the vanguard of provision of occupational therapy-led
memory rehabilitation programmes to maintain and support
functional performance and safety in daily activities and there
is an active cross-disciplinary dementia research programme at
Queen's University Belfast and Ulster University also participates
in dementia research. For the future, we would like to see
maintenance of, and improvement upon, our current high
diagnostic rates through further public awareness raising and
increased provision of specialist memory assessment services
which straddle primary and secondary care sectors; increased
access to and availability of novel diagnostic modalities to
augment the memory assessment process in specialist services
and further enhancement and expansion of our dementia friendly
communities and society to improve the lived experience of people
with dementia and their caregivers.

The Northern Ireland National Dementia Strategy

The Northern Ireland (NI) Dementia Strategy was launched in November 2011 [1]. The strategy recognizes the need to support the person with dementia and their caregivers, so that, in as far as possible, the person can remain in their own home environment and maintain their independence. There are several essential underlying principles: general awareness of dementia, reduction in risk factors that could contribute to dementia, enablement of people with dementia to live with dignity and without stigma, and recognition of the knowledge and skill requirements of any staff dealing with people with dementia. There is consistent emphasis throughout the document on the crucial role of caregivers and the imperative for early diagnosis. There is recognition of the significant role played by hospitals and private nursing homes in the provision of care for people with dementia, and the importance of research is emphasized. The strategy is the only one in the UK to refer to risk reduction. Many other strategic issues and priorities are similar to those identified in the English, Welsh, and Scottish strategies.

The strategy lists 44 points in the action plan and is associated with new monies to facilitate the development of these action points, overseen by a specifically convened strategy group. The major achievements have been the successful production of the mental capacity legislation (2016; see later in this chapter), the development of better signposting services and key workers in Health and Social Care (HSC) Trusts, and the growing role of occupational therapy in cognitive rehabilitation programmes. Many of the action plans have not been implemented within the intended timelines, however.

What can Northern Ireland be particularly proud of in dementia care?

There are a number of aspects of dementia care in NI of which the province can be proud:

1. NI consistently outperforms other nations and regions within the UK in dementia diagnosis rates. In NI, 64.8% of people with dementia had a recorded diagnosis, compared to 48% in England and 43.4% in Wales, in each nation's last reported figures. All five HSC Trusts in NI have dementia diagnosis rates well above the UK average year-on-year, based on the General Practitioner (GP) Quality Outcomes Framework data, with two of the five consistently within the top ten of all UK Trusts. Making the diagnosis of dementia is the first step to providing appropriate treatment, both pharmacological and non-pharmacological, information, and support to people with dementia and their caregivers.

2. NI is in the vanguard of provision of occupational therapy-led memory re-habilitation programmes to maintain and support functional performance and safety in daily activities. Important work from Belfast confirms the benefits of a customized programme delivered in patients' own homes over several weeks and that these gains are maintained over several months [2]. This programme has been rolled out to the other HSC Trusts in NI, as part of delivering on the regional dementia strategy. In Scotland, there has been an independent validation of the programme and there is now a national implementation plan.

3. Dementia Together NI, part of the 'Delivering Social Change' programme jointly funded by the NI Executive and The Atlantic Philanthropies, is currently working to build on the work of the regional dementia strategy and improve the quality of dementia care through raising awareness and providing information and support for people living with dementia; delivering training and development for those in the caring professions, both formally and informally; and providing respite, short breaks, and support for caregivers.

4. In order to achieve high diagnostic rates, good levels of public awareness and interest in referral from primary care are required. These are evident in NI. In addition, dementia remains a political priority. This has been reflected in a recent Dementia Innovation laboratory project driven by Assembly ministers.

5. In NI, all medications licensed for treatment of dementia have always been available, reflecting the priorities of local politicians since 1997. There are concerns about access to medications for dementia where those who are most deprived have lower rates of prescription. A recent publication [3] shows that, compared to English practices, medications for dementia were prescribed more often in NI and that NI prescribing had no relation to deprivation quintiles.

6. In NI, there are memory clinics/services in all areas. It is notable that there are a number of geriatricians involved in memory clinics in most Trusts, which, in addition to old age psychiatry services, allows more people to be assessed and treated.

7. NI has good availability of neuroimaging, including general access to CT, MRI, DaTscan, and also 18-fluoro-deoxyglucose positron emission tomography-CT (FDG-PET-CT). The latter is formally commissioned and allows evaluation of its role in terms of the proposed new diagnostic criteria [4].

8. There is an active cross-disciplinary dementia research programme at Queen's University Belfast, and Ulster University also participates in

dementia research. This has resulted in high-quality outputs in international journals and international recognition.

Current challenges in dementia

Political and financial challenges

The political settlement of the period of civil disorder known locally as 'The Troubles' has given NI a system of government substantially different to that in other areas of the UK.

Healthcare ties with the Republic of Ireland have been generally increasing. The economic effects of the UK's 2016 referendum decision to leave the European Union remain to be seen. Dementia services may be impacted if healthcare funding decreases. There may also be direct effects on cross-border cooperation in healthcare provision and research into dementia.

New mental capacity legislation

In 2016, NI's Assembly adopted new legislation combining mental capacity and mental health law in a single parliamentary Mental Capacity Act (Northern Ireland). This should bring NI's law broadly in line with that in the rest of the UK.

The new Mental Capacity Act awaits implementation and publication of a code of practice for clinicians. It is currently unclear how the new Act will affect healthcare resources, but all clinical staff will have a greater role to play in determining and interpreting capacity in all areas of care, and some effect on financial and time resources can be anticipated.

It is unclear if the new legislation will adequately address issues such as deprivation of liberty safeguards until more case law accumulates. This has been an area of protracted legal development in the UK, and amendments to the new legislation and its code of practice may be required in the immediate future.

Challenges in service provision

Dementia diagnosis is largely provided through secondary care by local care of the elderly, old age psychiatry, and neurology services. Most day-to-day management lies with primary care. Health and Social Services are integrated in a single body, substantially reducing transitions and barriers to care.

National demographic trends indicate that an increased number of older and younger people with dementia will need adequately resourced care [5]. Closer coordination between diagnostic services is being planned by the Department of Health to improve efficiency. Broader healthcare strategy currently calls for a shift to primary care. In dementia care, this may present challenges in expertise and resources to GPs and may affect diagnostic rates, particularly in atypical and young-onset forms of the disease.

Increased public awareness of memory problems and dementia has led to an increased number of referrals. The National Institute for Health and Care Excellence (NICE) guidance suggests regular review of people with dementia who are on medication. This contributes to a significant workload in clinics and services, and it is very difficult to avoid increased waiting times for initial assessment. This is a very delicate issue and will require creative solutions.

As highlighted in the previous section, while there is much to be proud of in terms of the high rates of diagnosis, there is scope for improvement, although the projected figures for the prevalence of dementia in NI may be inaccurate, given recent findings [6].

A final challenge will be incorporation of the increasingly specialized diagnostic biomarker modalities recommended in updated diagnostic criteria [4], such as analysis of amyloid and tau levels in the cerebrospinal fluid (CSF) and functional brain imaging, into routine clinical practice which is shifting more towards primary care.

How might these challenges be addressed and how will success be measured?

The key to addressing the numerous challenges faced is to ensure that dementia remains at the forefront of government priorities. Dementia necessitates structural reassessment of the lives of patients and caregivers and of health and care provision, both public and private. In addition, the critically important economic burden of dementia requires carefully considered future projections, so that the correct strategies can be developed well in advance. There is accumulating evidence of reductions in incidence and prevalence of dementia, but whether this will continue, as we see the emergence of risk factors such as obesity, remains to be seen. Much of this forward planning will relate to funding, e.g. new diagnostics, provision of new medications as they are licensed, and provision of monitoring (biomarkers, including neuroimaging), clinical services, and appropriate care.

The interface with primary care will become increasingly important, as the diagnosis and management of dementia evolve, and is fundamental in the management of referrals and reviews, waiting times, new diagnostics, and chronic disease. Education and upskilling in primary care, with good mentorship from secondary care, will be required. Project ECHO (Extension for Community Healthcare Outcomes) is one possible solution currently being trialled. This should facilitate a number of the challenges mentioned, including those related to implementation of the Mental Capacity Act. The need for better access to novel functional neuroimaging and the facilities required for CSF analysis must be factored into hospital business cases.

It is important we assume that the likely changes predicted in diagnostics, dementia prevalence, and appearance of new medications are inevitable, so that our practice is evolving in relation to dementia. It is crucial that the clinical dementia fraternity does not 'stand still' and we immediately seek to improve our systems and operational activities in order to be prepared for the eventualities, so that when a novel diagnostic or therapeutic intervention appears, there can be proportional and timely responses.

The future of dementia care, in particular treatment care and prevention, in Northern Ireland

Building on those plans outlined previously, the future of dementia care will rely on coordination across medical, nursing, and social disciplines, in primary and secondary care, and on improved communication with people with dementia and their families and caregivers.

Existing multidisciplinary meetings, including geriatricians, psychiatrists, neurologists, and radiologists, will need to be extended. Joint memory clinics, already in place in some HSC Trusts, will be set up across the province, with follow-up care shared between the appropriate specialist nursing and professions allied to medical teams.

Adequate post-diagnosis services are necessary if the push for improved early diagnosis is to see sustained success. Current studies of new, and the repositioning of existing, drugs will inform pharmacological treatment strategies. Acetylcholinesterase inhibitors and memantine are likely to remain integral to expanding drug regimens, as seen in other chronic diseases, necessitating better communication between healthcare professionals and patients and caregivers. Coordination between the relevant charities, patient groups, and community services is also improving. As the population ages and smaller families become more geographically spread out, communities and society are adapting to care for the many cognitively impaired elderly patients living alone who are often socially isolated, examples being the RECALL Good Morning Call and the Alzheimer's Society befriending services offered via charities here.

Community, residential, outpatient, and inpatient care settings must be cognizant of users with cognitive impairment. The appropriate care of people with dementia in acute hospital settings is gaining more attention. Explicit conversations are required, at healthcare and societal levels, regarding the palliative care of patients dying with dementia, especially relating to ceilings of care and feeding, so that the most appropriate care is delivered in the most appropriate settings.

People with dementia and caregivers in NI have traditionally embraced medical research, and ongoing, well-planned collaborative projects will improve early diagnosis, prognosis, drug and multidisciplinary treatments, and preventative strategies, including possible early interventions prior to the clinical manifestations of dementia. Public health initiatives focusing on physical activity, healthy diet, smoking cessation, and better control of other vascular risk factors at a population level are already felt to be reducing the age-related incidence of dementia [6].

References

1. **Department of Health, Social Services, and Public Safety Northern Ireland.** *Improving dementia services in Northern Ireland: a regional strategy.* 2011. Available from: https://www.health-ni.gov.uk/sites/default/files/publications/dhssps/improving-dementia-services-2011.pdf [accessed 3 August 2018].

2. **McGrath MP; The Health Foundation.** *Promoting safety in the home: the home-based Memory Rehabilitation Programme for persons with mild Alzheimer's disease and other dementias.* 2013. Available from: http://patientsafety.health.org.uk/sites/default/files/resources/promoting_safety_in_the_home.pdf [accessed 3 August 2018].

3. **Cooper C, Lodwick R, Walters K,** *et al.* Observational cohort study: deprivation and access to anti-dementia drugs in the UK. *Age Ageing.* 2016;**45**:148–54.

4. **Dubois B, Feldman HH, Jacova C,** *et al.* Advancing research diagnostic criteria for Alzheimer's disease: the IWG-2 criteria. *The Lancet Neurology.* 2014;**13**:614–29. Erratum in: *The Lancet Neurology.* 2014;13:757.

5. **Northern Ireland Statistics and Research Agency.** *Northern Ireland census data 2011.* Available from: https://www.nisra.gov.uk/statistics/census [accessed 20 August 2018].

6. **Matthews FE, Stephan BCM, Robinson L,** *et al.* A two decade dementia incidence comparison from the Cognitive Function and Ageing Studies I and II. *Nature Communications.* 2016;**7**:11398.

Chapter 28

Norway

Knut Engedal

Summary

Norway has 5 million inhabitants, of whom 200,000 are aged above 80 years. The country is a welfare state, with a tax system covering most health services for its citizens. It is estimated that 78,000 people in Norway suffer from dementia, of whom 60% live at home and the remainder in residential care. In 2007, the first National Dementia Plan was launched (2007–2015), and the second in 2016 (2016–2020). The main goals of the two Plans are to develop services across the country to improve the care and quality of life for all people with dementia and their family caregivers, as well as increase the knowledge of dementia among healthcare professionals. In addition, the Plans also aim to improve awareness of dementia in society as a whole and to develop and implement measures to help create a more dementia-friendly society.

Current services

In Norway, a variety of services are currently available such as memory clinics in specialist healthcare, dementia teams and dementia coordinators in municipalities, day care activities, and special care units (SCUs) in nursing homes. A helpline has been set up for family caregivers, and both family caregivers and health professionals are offered educational programmes across the country. More recently, new programmes have been set up, such as post-diagnosis 'follow-up', and there is also focus on user involvement (i.e. people with dementia and family caregivers) in service provision.

Norway has had two Dementia Plans, both of which have been successful. Efforts have focused on raising awareness and increasing knowledge of dementia in the general population and among families and health professionals.

New services have been implemented, to help improve the quality of life of people with dementia and their families.

What works well in Norway

A nationwide, comprehensive educational programme on dementia offered to all health professionals in primary care has proven very effective. Community dementia teams including a coordinator are also a valuable measure to improve the quality of care for, and quality of life of, people with dementia. In addition, SCUs in nursing homes with well-trained personnel have been established across Norway.

What we look forward to in Norway

A post-diagnosis follow-up programme should be offered to all people with dementia, as well as their families. Day care activities, tailored to patients' needs and wishes, should be made more accessible to people with dementia. More user (i.e. people with dementia and their families) involvement in care planning should also be encouraged.

The Norwegian health and social care system

Norway has 5 million inhabitants, including 1.3 million aged 65 years and above and 200,000 aged 80 years and above. The public sector plays a major role in providing health and social care and has its foundation in the socio-democratic welfare state. Until recently, the public healthcare system has been the only option for healthcare service provision, ideally according to citizens' needs and independently of age, gender, economic status, and place of residence. The private market is growing but so far plays only a modest role.

The country has a three-tier system for the provision of public health and social care, based on: (1) the Municipal Health Care and Social Health Care Act, (2) the Hospital Act, and (3) the National Insurance Act. The state is responsible for specialist healthcare services provided in hospitals. Hospital admissions and treatment, including medicines, are provided free of charge. Municipalities, currently a total of 428, are responsible for primary healthcare services that include care for the elderly at home (home help and 24-hour in-home nursing) and residential care, mainly in nursing homes. The national insurance scheme covers most of the costs of services provided in primary care, although patients have to pay a small contribution (out-of-pocket payments) towards the costs of medical examinations and treatment. The costs incurred for long-term care in nursing homes are calculated on a rising scale, depending on patients' annual income, but will never exceed their income.

According to epidemiological studies, it is estimated that there are 78,000 people with dementia in Norway, and the costs associated with formal care of people with dementia is calculated to be 28 billion Norwegian krones (about €4 billion) a year.

The Norwegian Dementia Plans 2007–2015 and 2016–2020

The first Norwegian Dementia Plan 2007–2015—'Making the most of the good days'—was launched by the Norwegian government and approved by the parliament in 2007 [1, 2]. It was an action plan aimed at improving the quality of care for, and the quality of life of, people with dementia and family caregivers. It did not include care for people with dementia in hospitals, e.g. at a specialist care level. The second Dementia Plan covers the period of 2016 to 2020 and is an extension of the first Plan—implementation of services takes time! The most interesting part of the second plan is emphasis on user involvement; thus, seven large open meetings across the country have been organized, involving the participation of people with dementia, family caregivers, volunteers, health professionals, and the Ministry of Health. Both Plans are based on the recognition that the services provided to people with dementia are not tailored to the patients' needs. Furthermore, the Plans aim to concretize important ethical principles, such as respect for individual autonomy and dignity, and therefore to educate health professionals in person-centred care.

Aims and principles of the Norwegian Dementia Plans

The overall aim of the Dementia Plans is to implement services in all municipalities, to improve the quality of care and life for all Norwegian citizens with dementia. The specific aims are to: (1) increase knowledge of dementia in society and among family caregivers and health professionals, thereby improving care provision, (2) develop and offer a range of day care programmes, and (3) adapt living facilities to patients' needs under the slogan 'small is beautiful'.

People with dementia are a heterogeneous group and have different interests, like everyone else. Therefore, care services provided to people with dementia should be individualized and based on the individual's background and special interests. Dementia care is therefore about providing personalized care for everyone, and the services should be tailored so that people with dementia feel secure and have a meaningful day-to-day life. Another principle is that the quality of care should be based on the framework of person-centred care, which implies that qualified staff with knowledge of dementia should treat people with dementia with respect, as well as be aware of their dignity and respect their autonomy.

Care for people with dementia and how the Dementia Plans have changed access to services

In this section, a general description of the care provided to people with dementia will be outlined. When the first Dementia Plan was launched in 2007, a national survey was carried out, capturing all kinds of services specifically tailored for people with dementia, and was subsequently repeated in 2014/15 [3]. The results of these surveys are available in English at http:www.aldringoghelse.no using the search title *Aim wide and hit straight*.

Assessment of dementia

Like in other countries, a large proportion of people with significant signs of dementia are not assessed and do not receive a diagnosis of dementia. It is not known exactly how many people with signs of dementia have no dementia diagnosis at present, although it was reported previously that in 2005, about 50% of people with dementia did receive a diagnosis [4]. Currently, people with MCI and dementia of mild severity are usually referred to memory clinics or outpatient clinics in geriatric medicine, geriatric psychiatry, or neurology in specialized healthcare. A comprehensive assessment is conducted, including neuropsychological evaluation and use of biomarkers and imaging such as MRI, positron emission tomography (PET), and CSF examination in many of these clinics [5]. Today, there are 32 clinics that use a standardized examination protocol and record their data in a dementia research and quality register. About 40% of patients have received a diagnosis of a specific dementia disorder, 40% a diagnosis of MCI, and the remaining 20% either no diagnosis or a psychiatric diagnosis.

People with signs of moderate or severe dementia are usually assessed and diagnosed by family doctors, often with the support of municipality dementia teams. Primary care assessments are less comprehensive, and patients are usually tested with the MMSE and the clock drawing test. The Directorate of Health and the Norwegian National Advisory Unit on Ageing and Health have developed a standardized examination protocol, which can be retrieved from http://www.aldringpoghelse.no (in Norwegian). Not all family doctors are trained to perform dementia-specific assessment and diagnosis, so there is still room for improvement [6].

Post-diagnosis follow-up

People with a dementia diagnosis are usually followed up by their family doctors, who can prescribe anti-dementia drugs. The number of dementia-diagnosed patients with regular follow-ups is not known, but we believe that this number could vary, depending on family doctors' practice, because many family caregivers complain about some family doctors with little interest in following up patients with dementia. Very young people, and especially those with challenging behaviour, such as people with frontotemporal dementia and Lewy body dementia, are usually followed up in specialist healthcare. At present, development projects are in progress to evaluate the usefulness of providing a 'link person' to each patient following their diagnostic assessment. In most cases, dementia coordinators, or dementia teams, will be designated as 'link persons'.

Dementia coordinators and teams

One of the aims of the Dementia Plan 2007–2015 was to establish dementia coordinators and dementia teams in all municipalities. A coordinator is defined as a person who is responsible for supervising people with dementia and informing them and their families of how to get help, as well as guiding health professionals in their service provision to people with dementia. A dementia team consists normally of two or more health professionals, often nurses and occupational therapists, with specialist expertise in dementia. Some teams also include doctors in a consulting role. The team has two roles: (1) to assist family doctors in the diagnostic assessment by conducting home visits and (2) to follow up people with dementia. It is a low-threshold service. All citizens can contact a dementia team for advice and help, including before a dementia assessment is performed. In 2007, 25% of municipalities had either a team or a coordinator, or both, reaching 78% in 2015 [3].

Day care activities

As there are more than 43,000 people with dementia living at home, there is a huge need for day care activities. This service is expensive (transport, food, activities), and for this reason, many municipalities have been reluctant to offer day care services. In 2007, only 30% of municipalities offered day care activities to people with dementia, although this increased to 71% of municipalities in 2015. However, in 2015, only 6000 people with dementia living at home were offered day care activities, so there is some way to go in offering day care services to all people with dementia living in their own home. The Norwegian parliament has agreed that by 2020, it would be mandatory for all Norwegian municipalities to offer day care activities for people with dementia.

Furthermore, the Norwegian Health Association, a volunteer organization that incorporates the Norwegian Dementia Association together with 150 local clubs in its activities, runs a programme called 'Being a Dementia Friend'. Thus, volunteers are recruited to spend 2 hours each week, or every other week, with a person with dementia. It is an ongoing project, and recruitment of volunteers has proven easy.

Special care units in nursing homes

All Norwegian municipalities provide residential care to people with severe disabilities. This therefore explains the fact that 80% of nursing home residents in Norway have dementia. SCUs designed for people with dementia were established at the beginning of the 1980s as small units that could accommodate 6–12 residents. In 2007, 26% of residential places available in nursing homes were allocated to SCUs, and this increased slightly to 28% in 2014 [3].

Family caregivers' dementia schools

One of the most successful initiatives included in the Dementia Plan 2007–2015 has been the establishment of an educational programme for family caregivers that provides 5–6 evening classes, each lasting 3 hours. This programme is organized by the local dementia club, together with the dementia team/coordinator from the municipality, and all programme costs are covered by the Ministry of Health. In 2014, 74% of municipalities offered this programme, compared to 11% in 2007 [3].

ABC Dementia—an educational programme for health professionals

ABC Dementia is a 2-year educational programme for health professionals. Participants have to study booklets or audio books on specific aspects of dementia such as the course of AD, challenging behaviour, person-centred care, ethics of caring for people with dementia, and similar topics. Groups of 6–10 health professionals from different backgrounds and with different training and expertise meet every 2 weeks for group discussions and reflections centred on the study theme and on case examples from their own clinical practice, with sessions lasting about 2 hours. ABC Dementia stands as the biggest success of the Dementia Plan. To date, 26,000 health professionals either have completed or are enrolled in the programme.

Raising awareness of dementia

Information on dementia is accessible via the home page of 60% of Norwegian municipalities, which have also included dementia care in their healthcare plan. In addition, the Norwegian Health Association has been working on raising general awareness of dementia and runs a telephone helpline which is used by more than 3000 people annually. Moreover, the association supports dementia research programmes and raises funding for dementia research. It is also regularly involved in lobbying politicians in the parliament for better care for people with dementia.

Research

As part of the Dementia Plan 2007–2015, the Norwegian Research Council has funded several research projects on how to develop and evaluate new care services for people with dementia living at home or in institutions. Observational studies and randomized controlled trials (RCTs) have been carried out, and projects including those focused on person-centred care have been prioritized. The Norwegian Health Association has also supported basic dementia research.

Challenges

Although we have witnessed an improvement in dementia care in Norway, not all municipalities deliver high-quality services, and therefore, extension of the first Dementia Plan is welcome. We still need to increase awareness of dementia, not only among the general public to help develop a dementia-friendly society, but also among health professionals and family doctors, as well as in hospitals for dementia-friendly hospitals. More people with dementia should have access to day care activities, and the goal is still that all municipalities should offer a range of services to people with dementia. It is not good enough that only 70% of municipalities offer high-quality services. Every person with dementia, regardless of age, gender, ethnicity, and place of living, should be offered high-quality services.

References

1. **Engedal K.** The Norwegian Dementia Plan—making most of the good days. *International Journal of Geriatric Psychiatry.* 2010;**25**:928–30.
2. **Norwegian Ministry of Health and Care Services.** *Dementia Plan 2015.* Publication number I-1129 E. Oslo: Norwegian Ministry of Health and Care Services; 2007.
3. **Gjøra L.** *Å favne bredt og treffe rett.* Toensberg: Aldring og helse; 2015.
4. **Lystrup LS, Lillesveen B, Nygard AM, Engedal K.** Public social health services to demented persons living at home in Norway. *Tidsskrift for Den norske legeforening.* 2006;**126**:1917–20.
5. **Braekhus A, Ulstein I, Wyller TB, Engedal K.** The memory clinic-outpatients assessment when dementia is suspected. *Tidsskrift for Den norske legeforening.* 2011;**131**:2254–7.
6. **Engedal K, Gausdal M, Gjøra L, Haugen PK.** Assessment of dementia by a primary health care dementia team cooperating with the family doctor—The Norwegian model. *Dementia and Geriatric Cognitive Disorders.* 2012 **34**: 263–70.

Chapter 29

Portugal

Manuel Gonçalves-Pereira and António Leuschner

Summary

Dementia care in Portugal presents a mixed balance of strengths and important problems and challenges. This chapter begins by highlighting the scarcity of health service data on dementia, within a rapidly changing and complex array of health and social care systems. Public, private, and third-sector services are not integrated enough to fully meet the needs of people with dementia and their families. Despite examples of good standards in dementia care, some complex challenges still need tackling. Portugal does not have a National Dementia Plan, although formal efforts are being made and a general strategy has been proposed. The chapter briefly discusses leading issues, while highlighting that any selection of goals and the feasibility of achieving them are constrained by a shortage of resources. Taking the need to improve timely diagnosis and integrated formal services as an example, the exact role of primary care is one of the primary topics for discussion.

In short, there are three aspects which Portugal does well in terms of dementia care: (1) every person with dementia has access to emergency services and, in principle, to primary care services within the public National Health Service; (2) there are examples of high-quality standards in clinical dementia care, mainly in urban centres, and an increasing interest from the social sector, non-governmental organizations, and private institutions in community or institutional social care; and (3) there are developments in dementia-related service research, as well as in psycho-geriatric training. For the future, first, primary care should be more involved in early diagnosis of dementia and its appropriate disclosure, as well as in other areas, e.g. treatment monitoring in collaboration with specialized care, counselling and support, and monitoring caregivers' health. Second, the complex bio-psycho-social needs in dementia should be better met through improvement of: timely access to community formal services or specialized accommodation when necessary; 'dementia-friendly' communities and health/social units (e.g. general hospitals, given the multimorbidity in people with dementia); management of behavioural and psychological symptoms of dementia (with more emphasis on non-pharmacological approaches, and less on antipsychotics); informal caregivers' support, ensuring minimum standards of information, counselling, psycho-education, and other family interventions; and legal procedures, access to new technologies, and decent end-of-life care. Finally, gaps should be bridged between health and social care, fostering care coordination and case management in every phase of dementia (with standardization of dementia care processes, e.g. definition of the roles of professionals).

Setting the scene

Epidemiological data

The total population in Portugal was 10,562,178 in 2011, including 19% of people aged 65 years and above. The ageing index rose from 102 in 2001 to 128 in 2011 [1]. Epidemiological data on dementia in Portugal can be summarized here. An initial study found a prevalence rate of 2.7% [95% confidence interval (CI) 1.9–3.8] of dementia, as defined by the Diagnostic and Statistical Manual of Mental Disorders, fourth edition (DSM-IV), in population samples from northern Portugal [2]. In addition, a recent survey reported a prevalence rate of 9.2% (95% CI 7.8–10.9), using the 10/66 Dementia Research Group diagnostic algorithm [3, 4] and excluding nursing home residents [4]; this result probably reflects more accurately the dementia burden among old age community-dwelling Portuguese (illiteracy rate of approximately 20%) [1, 4]. The number of people with dementia has been estimated to be 182,526 among those aged 65 years and above [5] and 160,287 among those aged 59 years and above [6]. However, these estimates are likely to be exceeded using the '10/66' results in Portuguese samples [4].

Overview of health and social care systems

All residents in Portugal have access to the mainly tax-funded National Health Service (NHS), with 25% of healthcare costs also covered by health subsystems and/or voluntary insurance [7]. Public care provision predominates, and users have a limited choice of specialist providers, notwithstanding changing access regulations [8]. Non-public care provision includes physicians' private practice [7] and private hospital care delivery, but this is not affordable to most people.

The social sector supports home care, day care, and long-term care in institutions. The National Network for Integrated Long-Term Care [Rede Nacional de Cuidados Continuados Integrados (RNCCI)] aims to improve care pathways for elderly and dependent people through primary care, hospital care, and long-term care, intersecting health and social services and public, private, and third-sector providers.

Towards a Portuguese dementia policy?

There is no dementia policy in Portugal,[1] despite formal (Resolutions 133-134/2010) and societal calls for action [9].[2]

Recent changes included the RNCCI (2006) and primary healthcare reforms (2007) [7, 10]. Significant efforts have helped to improve the quality/efficiency of primary care and hospital care [11]. However, dementia is not specified in official documents, including the National Health Plan 2012–2016. The National Mental Health Policy and Plan 2007–2016 (Council of Ministers Resolution 49/2008) defined its general aims, including ensuring equal access, protecting human rights, reducing the impact of mental disorders, decentralizing services, and integrating mental health into general healthcare. Although frail elderly people were recognized as a vulnerable group, there was no mention of dementia [12]. Community orientation faced finance/management difficulties [13], and recent evaluations of the Plan's implementation recommended community approaches to risk groups, but again without any specific mention of dementia [14].

In the aftermath of the economic crisis [15], a National Dementia Plan is set to be developed. The Directorate General of Health is facilitating a debate among academics, clinicians, and relevant stakeholders. A preliminary document was produced in 2013, and a work group set up in 2016 under the aegis of the Ministry of Health.[2]

....

[1] According to Alzheimer's Disease International (https://www.alz.co.uk/alzheimer-plans), a *dementia strategy* is generated by private, non-governmental groups aiming to persuade governments to create plans, whereas a *dementia plan* is a policy by which 'a government holds itself accountable for the accomplishment of specific objectives and policy changes', even if this depends on non-governmental collaborators.

[2] At time of writing, a national dementia strategy had not been approved (Decree-Law 116/2018, 19 June).

Good examples in dementia care

The NHS ensures universal healthcare coverage, which may be (almost) free at the point of use. In principle, every person with dementia has access to emergency services and primary care within their home area. GPs are pivotal health professionals [7, 16], although there is still a shortage regionally.

There are examples of high-quality standards in dementia care, mainly in urban centres. Some neurology services are referral centres of excellence, providing clinical diagnostic workup or follow-up for cognitive disorders. Community-oriented care is provided by a small number of mental health teams with expertise in psycho-geriatrics, while isolated hospital psycho-geriatric services also exist [16]. Some high-quality institutions (e.g. within the RNCCI) offer inpatient services to manage challenging behavioural symptoms in people with dementia, as well as to provide long-term or respite care. There is now an increasing interest from private institutions/NGOs in community or institutional social care. In addition, Alzheimer Portugal provides practical support, raises awareness of dementia, and serves as an advocate of patients' and families' rights. For instance, advance directives, which did not exist prior to 2012, have become legally binding since then.

Developments in dementia-related clinical or services research have also been acknowledged. Geriatric medicine was finally recognized in 2014 as a clinical competence. Psychiatry residents and other health professionals now have improved knowledge of cognitive disorders [17, 18], and formal caregivers have better training in this field [19]. Primary topics in geriatric medicine are now included in some medical schools' curricula [17].

Current challenges in dementia care

People with dementia and their families have unmet needs

Even in specialized care settings, complex bio-psycho-social needs are often unmet [20], and most relate to the following issues.

Cost estimates for anti-dementia drugs suggest that not all patients with AD are taking specific medications [6], indicating that under-diagnosis is possible, alongside financial burden on people with dementia and barriers to follow-up prescriptions (which must be issued by neurologists/psychiatrists to ensure maximum partial reimbursement). Diagnosis disclosure is frequently postponed, unsupported, or restricted to caregivers (with stigma, as well as a lack of binding guidelines, as barriers to disclosure), thus raising ethical issues.

GPs should recognize early symptoms of dementia, ensure diagnosis disclosure, monitor treatment in collaboration with specialist care, provide counselling and support, and monitor caregivers' health [21]. However, there are disparities of dementia knowledge and skills among GPs, along with inadequate support from neurologists, psychiatrists, and non-medical staff. The gatekeeping role of GPs may actually contribute to delayed diagnosis; most patients, when referred to neurology or psychiatry, already have moderate or severe dementia [16].

Adequate and timely formal community-based care is lacking. Early institutionalization may ensue, a trend sometimes counterbalanced by a lack of access to overcrowded or unaffordable institutions. Behavioural and psychological symptoms of dementia (BPSD) are often badly managed, due to either a lack of resources or emphasis on pharmacological approaches, namely antipsychotics.

Regarding informal caregiving, around 80% of people with dementia live at home, either alone or with their family [22]. There is a strong (albeit changing) culture of family members caring for dependent old age people, but little information on the number of family caregivers and their characteristics is available. A survey of 544 caregivers was conducted with the collaboration of Alzheimer Portugal, and the following demographic data were obtained from respondents: mean age 60 years, 70% were female, 50% were spouses, and 34% were children of care recipients [23]. Despite a few exceptions (e.g. Alzheimer Portugal's initiatives/partnerships, Alzheimer cafés), there are no structured health and social services that provide information, counselling, or continuing psychoeducation. Family interventions are recommended [24] but are not routinely available. Public service support and psycho-educational groups are virtually non-existent, and families have almost no access to systemic therapy. Efforts by NGOs or municipal projects are sometimes linked to academic research [25].

Among other civil and social issues, obtaining legal guardianship can be a lengthy process, but without it, families'/caregivers' decisions on behalf of people with dementia are often illegal, even when taken in good faith. Although Alzheimer Portugal's efforts in raising awareness of this issue are acknowledged, information on legal procedures is lacking and mental incapacity orders are regarded as a social punishment to people with dementia [26]. There are no paid Public Authority Guardians and no social security compensation transfers ('care allowances'), and caregivers are not entitled to tax benefits or time off work.

Access to, and use of, health and social services by people with dementia

Although difficulties with timely access to, and use of, formal care have been recognized, access to formal care is still not standard across Portugal, despite improvements and some good initiatives. The evidence was recently reviewed

Table 29.1 Number of cases of dementia as a secondary diagnosis at hospital discharge—mainland Portugal (2010–2014)

	2010	2011	2012	2013	2014
Discharged patients	14,281	14,522	15,493	16,690	15,708
Deaths	2526	2519	2863	2845	2720

ICD-9-CM diagnosis codes 290, as secondary diagnosis.

Reproduced from DGH. *Portugal: Saúde Mental em Números 2015—Programa Nacional para a Saúde Mental*. Lisboa, Portugal: Directorate General of Health; 2016.

as part of the European Union's JPND project ACcess to TImely Formal Care (Actifcare), as summarized [27].

In primary care, dementia ranks third among mental health/neuropsychiatric disorders, after depression and anxiety. The proportions of primary care users with a diagnosis of dementia range between 0.49% to 1.01% across Portugal, with an increase in numbers observed between 2011 and 2014 [14].

In 2014, there were a total of 722 patients discharged from NHS hospitals with a primary diagnosis of dementia, representing a total of 14,077 days of hospital admission (mostly to medical and surgical wards). Table 29.1 shows the number of cases of dementia as a secondary diagnosis at hospital discharge.

Dementia specialists are available in hospitals, but with striking disparity across regions in Portugal. Neurologists have traditionally been viewed as being primarily in charge of people with dementia. Multidisciplinary work is incipient, although neuropsychologists often support diagnostic or cognitive interventions. In psychiatric services, little time is devoted to old age users [16], but their involvement in dementia care may be changing. Specialists in neurology and psychiatry both act as consultants in the management of dementia, although liaison with primary care is inadequate. Long waiting times (in the public sector), out-of-pocket payments (mainly in private care), and travel distances are barriers to access to care services, and few patients/families can opt for care by private specialists. Very few psychiatric services provide specific day care for dementia patients. Specialized services are less involved in community and social care overall, whereas social services often are provided without a formal diagnosis of dementia.

In 2007, a total of 71,663 individuals received formal care at home (although, of these, the proportion of people with dementia is unknown). Home care is provided by public/semi-public and non-profit services, as well as by some private providers. There is a mix of concerns and positive developments in this area. In 2011, 0.9% of old age people received long-term institutional care, while only 0.2% received home care [27, 28]; however, home care provision is increasing

[10]. Respite care is also becoming more accessible (provided by the RNCCI) but is limited to 30 days per year. The few existing dementia-specific day centres (in the social sector) rely on the involvement of multidisciplinary teams.

There were 4094 long-term RNCCI beds nationwide in 2014 (with 96% occupancy) [29], but long-term care is also offered by other institutions. Most institutional care is provided through residential structures for the elderly (ERPIs), which numbered a total of 1583 in 2007. These institutions are run by non-profit/private organizations, and sometimes with state funding; however, they lack full 24-hour nursing support [30]. It is estimated that people with dementia account for 29–78% of ERPI residents [9, 14, 19], but the evidence base is poor.

Some designations within the Portuguese formal care setup do not match exactly those in other countries. ERPIs and nursing homes fall under the umbrella term 'care home', providing higher levels of care than 'residential houses' (which are rare in Portugal). Nursing homes are generally not specifically for people with dementia, but NGOs (e.g. Misericórdias Portuguesas, religious orders) or private institutions run a few units specialized in long-term dementia care or psycho-geriatrics [23].

Overall, adequate approaches to dementia are lacking at every level of the hierarchical organization.

A tentative summary of current challenges

Relationships between health and social care systems are complex, and boundaries overlap (see Fig. 29.1). Regulations change frequently, but in recent decades, health and social sector administrations have been separate, turning truly integrated care into a titanic endeavour. For instance, public network health and social home care have different funding sources (from the Ministry of Health and Ministry of Labour and Social Solidarity, respectively), while social services also depend on co-payments or membership fees [10]. Moreover, case management does not exist in community dementia care, which means patients and caregivers may be lost in the system without a compass.

Based on the OECD/WHO framework [31] and findings of the World Alzheimer Report 2016 [32], issues regarding dementia care in Portugal can be outlined as follows: (1) despite current public health efforts, cardiovascular risk (which impacts dementia risk) in the population remains high; (2) there are barriers to early diagnosis and appropriate diagnosis disclosure to patients and families—an area in which primary care should be involved; (3) communities are still not 'friendly' enough towards people with early dementia; (4) there are significant difficulties with timely access to community health/formal social services and to specialized accommodation when it becomes necessary; (5) there is a long way to go in addressing the complex needs and multimorbidity

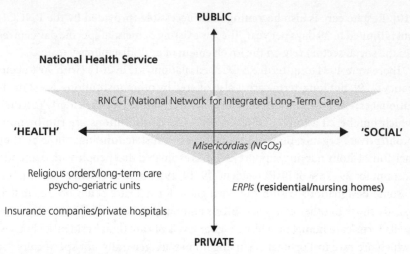

Fig. 29.1 Portuguese health and social care systems sharing complex relationships.

of people with dementia (e.g. in general hospitals), in improving legal proced-ures, and in enhancing access to new technologies or good-quality end-of-life care; (6) there is inadequate formal, as well as informal, support for caregivers and families; and (7) there is a dearth of proactive close-to-home care coordin-ation or case management (with no current standardization of dementia care processes, e.g. definition of the roles of health professionals).

What about the future?

As in other countries, quantifying the growing financial costs of dementia care remains a challenge [31], but it undoubtedly represents a huge burden in Portugal. We have described positive experiences and improvements, as well as major concerns and challenges, in dementia care.

At the time of writing, a workgroup has been set up by the Ministry of Health to draft a possible inspiration for a national dementia policy. Some challenges are being discussed, along with proposals of how to address them. We will not enter into this discussion here, as official outputs will soon be available.[2]

Portugal is one of the participating countries in the Actifcare project, an on-going European research programme on access to timely formal care in commu-nity services (e.g. home care, day care) [33], exploring barriers and facilitators,

---

[2] Ibid.

as well as inequalities, in various countries. This will also produce national best practice recommendations for access to services.

One mainstay of a successful Portuguese policy for dementia should be improved cooperation between, and integration of, health and social services, while case management implementation could also help. A debate has begun on shifting focus from hyper-specialized perspectives towards primary care, by considering task-shifting possibilities [32]—these are contentious, but seminal, issues, and not just for low- and middle-income countries. Guidelines on clinical management of cognitive disorders [24] should be implemented, and guidelines on how to approach people with dementia in general medical care produced. While the WHO calls for evidence-based approaches in dementia [34], targeted epidemiological, clinical, and services research must guide planning and monitoring. As for data governance and the role of big data in gathering evidence, challenges are huge at the consent and funding levels, as well as in international data sharing [31]. Last but not least, caregiver status is now socially recognized, and its official recognition will hopefully occur in the near future, along with a definition of corresponding benefits.

Despite the difficulties, the perspective in Portugal is to approach the challenges in dementia care in cost-effective ways. (Inter)national progress will continuously influence clinical and social practices, with regional and service differences. We are witnessing developments in neurobiology (e.g. biomarkers) and new technologies (e.g. safety alarms, monitoring systems), while valuing bio-psycho-social, person-centred humanistic approaches.

In the short term, a dementia policy should focus on improving the lives of patients and families [31]. Decisive inputs should come from governmental decisions, but also from personal and societal initiatives. Intergenerational solidarity will not be established by decree, and it is partly up to us to build dementia-friendly communities and foster support for daily living. While family interventions are hardly ever implemented due to financial issues, how many of us have helped our own neighbour with dementia or the caregiver next to them? There are economic arguments for doing so, but mainly ethical ones. Comprehensive dementia care goes beyond national strategies or plans to the point of changing individual attitudes. We see this as a core issue in our country, and in today's world.

References

1. **Instituto Nacional de Estatística**. *Censos 2011 resultados definitivos—Portugal.* Lisboa: Instituto Nacional de Estatística; 2012.
2. **Nunes B, Silva RD, Cruz VT, Roriz JM, Pais J, Silva MC.** Prevalence and pattern of cognitive impairment in rural and urban populations from Northern Portugal. *BMC Neurology.* 2010;**10**:42.

3. Gonçalves-Pereira M, Cardoso A, Verdelho A, *et al.* [Implementing a prevalence study of dementia and geriatric depression in Portugal: the 10/66 DRG methodology]. *Revista Portuguesa de Saúde Pública.* 2016;**34**:134–43.

4. Gonçalves-Pereira M, Cardoso A, Verdelho A, *et al.* The prevalence of dementia in a Portuguese community sample: a 10/66 Dementia Research Group study. *BMC Geriatrics.* 2017;**17**:261.

5. Alzheimer Europe. *Prevalence of dementia in Europe.* Luxembourg: Alzheimer Europe; 2013. Available from: http://www.alzheimer-europe.org/Research/European-Collaboration-on-Dementia/Prevalence-of-dementia/Prevalence-of-dementia-in-Europe [accessed 3 August 2018].

6. Santana I, Farinha F, Freitas S, Rodrigues V, Carvalho Á. [The epidemiology of dementia and Alzheimer disease in Portugal: estimations of prevalence and treatment-costs]. *Acta Médica Portuguesa.* 2015;**28**;182–8.

7. Barros PP, Machado SR, Simões JA. Portugal: Health system review. *Health Systems in Transition.* 2011;**13**:1–156.

8. Joumard I, André C, Nicq C. *Health care systems: efficiency and institutions.* OECD Economics Department Working Papers, No. 769. Paris: OECD Publishing; 2010.

9. Alzheimer Europe. *Portugal—national dementia strategies.* Luxembourg: Alzheimer Europe; 2009. Available from: http://www.alzheimer-europe.org/Policy-in-Practice2/National-Dementia-Strategies/Portugal?#fragment1 [accessed 3 August 2018].

10. Genet N, Boerma W, Kroneman M, Hutchinson A, Saltman R. *Home care across Europe: current structure and future challenges.* European Observatory on Health Systems and Policies; 2012. Available from: http://www.euro.who.int/__data/assets/pdf_file/0008/181799/e96757.pdf [accessed 3 August 2018].

11. **Organization for Economic Cooperation and Development.** *OECD reviews of healthcare quality: Portugal 2015—raising standards.* Paris: OECD Publishing; 2015.

12. **Comissão Nacional de Reestruturação dos Serviços de Saúde Mental (CNRSSM).** *Relatório: Proposta de Plano de Acção para a Reestruturação e Desenvolvimento dos Serviços de Saúde Mental em Portugal 2007–2016.* 2008. http://data.dre.pt/eli/resolconsmin/49/2008/03/06/p/dre/pt/html [accessed 23 August 2018].

13. **Comissão Técnica de Acompanhamento da Reforma da Saúde Mental.** *Relatório da Avaliação do Plano Nacional de Saúde Mental 2007–2016 e propostas prioritárias para a extensão a 2020.* 2017. Available from: https://www.sns.gov.pt/wp-content/uploads/2017/08/RelAvPNSM2017.pdf [accessed 23 August 2018].

14. **Directorate General of Health.** *Portugal: Saúde mental em números 2015—programa nacional para a saúde mental.* Lisboa: Directorate General of Health; 2016.

15. Legido-Quigley H, Karanikolos M, Hernandez-Plaza S, *et al.* Effects of the financial crisis and Troika austerity measures on health and health care access in Portugal. *Health Policy.* 2016;**120**:833–9.

16. Firmino H. The practice of dementia care: Portugal. In: **Burns A** (ed). *Standards in dementia care.* Oxford: Taylor and Francis; 2005. pp. 99–103.

17. Ribeiro O, Fernandes L, Firmino H, Simões MR, Paúl C. Geropsychology and psychogeriatrics in Portugal: research, education and clinical training. *International Psychogeriatrics.* 2010;**22**:854–63.

18. **Wang H, Fernandes L, Oster S, Takeda M, Brodaty H, Mintzer JE.** The state of psychogeriatrics in different regions of the world: Challenges and opportunities. *International Psychogeriatrics.* 2013;**25**:1563–9.

19. **Caldas de Almeida M,** *et al. Projecto VIDAS—Valorização e Inovação em Demências (POPH/QREN 2013–15).* 2015.

20. **Fernandes L, Gonçalves-Pereira M, Leuschner A,** *et al.* Validation study of the Camberwell Assessment of Need for the Elderly (CANE) in Portugal. *International Psychogeriatrics.* 2009;**21**:94–102.

21. **Stoppe G.** Primary care: fit for the dementia challenge? In: **Burns A** (ed). *Standards in dementia care.* Oxford: Taylor and Francis; 2005. pp. 185–9.

22. **Alzheimer Europe.** *European Collaboration on Dementia (EuroCoDe) Technical Report (2006–2008).* Luxembourg: Alzheimer Europe; 2008. Available from: http://ec.europa. eu/health/ph_projects/2005/action1/docs/action1_2005_frep_10_en.pdf [accessed 3 August 2018].

23. **Instituto da Segurança Social.** *Situação social dos doentes de Alzheimer: um estudo exploratório.* Fundação Montepio Geral; 2005.

24. **Directorate General of Health.** *Abordagem Terapêutica das Alterações Cognitivas.* Lisboa: Ministry of Health; 2011.

25. **Gonçalves-Pereira M, Sampaio D.** [Family psychoeducation in dementia: From clinical practice to public health]. *Revista Portuguesa de Saúde Pública.* 2011;**29**:3–10.

26. **Firmino H, Carvalho PS, Cerejeira J,** *et al.* Practice of competence assessment in Portugal. In: **Stoppe G** (ed). *Competence assessment in dementia.* Wien: Springer-Verlag; 2008. pp. 117–19.

27. **Bieber A, Broda A, Verbeek H, Stephan A, Meyer G; on behalf of the Actifcare Consortium.** *Structural aspects of access to formal dementia care services across the European countries.* Internal report of the Actifcare Project. 2015. Available from: http:// actifcare.eu/wp-content/uploads/2018/04/ActifCare_Deliverable-2.1_2018-03-29.pdf [accessed 3 August 2018].

28. **Organization for Economic Cooperation and Development.** *Health at a glance: Europe 2012.* Paris: OECD Publishing; 2012.

29. **Administração Central do Sistema de Saúde (ACSS).** *Monitorização da Rede Nacional de Cuidados Continuados Integrados (RNCCI) 2014.* Lisboa: ACSS; 2015.

30. **Joël ME, Dufour-Kippelen S, Samitca S.** *The long-term care system for the elderly in Portugal.* ENEPRI (European Network of Economic Policy Research Institutes) research report no. 84. 2010. Available from: https://www.ceps.eu/publications/long-term-care-system-elderly-portugal [accessed 3 August 2018].

31. **Organization for Economic Cooperation and Development.** *Addressing dementia: the OECD response.* OECD Health Policy Studies. Paris: OECD Publishing; 2015.

32. **Prince M, Comas-Herrera MA, Knapp M, Guerchet M, Karagiannidou MM.** *World Alzheimer Report 2016: improving healthcare for people living with dementia—coverage, quality and costs now and in the future.* London: Alzheimer's Disease International; 2016.

33. **Kerpershoek L, de Vugt M, Wolfs C,** *et al.* Access to timely formal dementia care in Europe: protocol of the Actifcare (ACcess to Timely Formal Care) study. *BMC Health Services Research.* 2016;**16**:423.

34. **World Health Organization.** *First WHO ministerial conference on global action against dementia.* Geneva: World Health Organization; 2015.

Chapter 30

Romania

Adriana Mihai, Geanina Ilinoiu,
and Maria-Silvia Trandafir

Summary
In Romania, dementia care has gradually improved in the last
decade. Accessibility of psychiatric services and availability of
psychiatric and/or psychotherapeutic treatment have been
significantly enhanced by new legislations and regulations.
Public and private sectors of home care for the elderly have also
been developed. Despite these changes, the management of
dementia remains challenging because of delay in diagnosis
and/or inappropriate treatment. Dementia care in the future in
Romania should adopt a professional approach by improving
education and training, as well as changing attitudes, not only
among doctors (general practitioners, psychiatrists, neurologists,
etc.), but also among all those involved in care (nurses, social
assistants, relatives, etc.) and the general population. Reducing
stigma and discrimination will contribute to early diagnosis and
appropriate treatment. Collaborative efforts from a medico-social
and community perspective, with the support of government
authorities, could provide a source of new funding, which
should be distributed according to the needs of each county in
Romania. Individualized complex treatment plan should be done
for each patient as early as possible, for assuring access to all
resources available in collaborative manner with patients' family
and community. Dementia care challenges health specialists
and organizations more and more every year. The social and
economic burden of this disease is highly significant. Quality care
for patients with dementia represents a challenge for specialists
and mental health care organizations whereas there are a rapidly
growing number of individuals in need of assistance. In Romania,
270.000 people are thought to be suffering from dementia and

only around 35.000 of them are diagnosed. The patients with dementia are most often diagnosed in late clinical stages (1).

Achievements and challenges in dementia care in Romania

The National Dementia Strategy

The elaboration of the National Dementia Strategy 2014–2020 represents one of the main goals of the Romanian Alzheimer Society [1]. The need for an action plan appears in the context of recommendations of the European Parliament [*2011 European initiative on Alzheimer's disease and other dementias (2010 to 2084—INI)*] and the WHO (*2013 Action plan on mental health*). The European Union (EU) Commission recommendations underline the need for EU state members to set strategic objectives and an action plan for a dementia strategy, reinforce and adjust policies, develop medical diagnostic and treatment facilities, and upgrade family and community support systems.

Taking into consideration the increase in population of those aged over 60 years in Romania (in 2012, this group represented 20.8% of the population), the Ministry of Health elaborated a National Strategy for Health. The Action Plan 2014–2020 in the National Strategy included the indicator 'OS 4.6: increasing access to high-quality rehabilitation, palliative, and long-term services, adapted to demographical phenomena of the ageing population and specific epidemiological morbidity profile'. This plan aims to revise the norms regarding the organization, financing, and delivery of long-term medical services, to reorganize the medico-social assistance and hospital network for chronic disorders, and to diversify financial sources [2].

Psychiatric care in Romania has gradually improved, following new legislation which enhanced accessibility to psychiatric services and openness towards the community, as well as availability of pharmacological and/or psychotherapeutic treatment [3]. Mental health legislation was significantly changed in Romania in 2002 upon approval of the Mental Health and Protection of Persons with Mental Disorders Law (Law 487/2002).

Elderly care

Over the last few years in Romania, multiple changes have been implemented in the elderly care system. Before 2000, patients with dementia received medical care from GPs. In 2002, the number of patients admitted to psychiatric hospitals and diagnosed with dementia increased ten times, as compared to the previous year [4]. This change took place after the implementation of Law 519/2002 concerning special protection and employment of people with disabilities (Official Monitor, 555/2002), which granted financial help to those with a diagnosis of dementia.

In 2004, the number of people aged over 65 years in Romania was almost 3.2 million. Long-term facilities for older people were poorly represented in the mental healthcare structure [3]. In the same year, the Ministry of Health rated mental health as a priority and took 'measures for rehabilitation of the care system concerning mental health in Romania' through planning to develop accessible and quality mental health services with a less restrictive environment, as well as more programmes for promotion, prevention, and education in mental health. In 2006, there were 80 outpatient settings specifically for patients with dementia.

The private sector of home care for the elderly was also developed. However, retirement pensions alone are inadequate to cover out-of-pocket expenses incurred in private care. Accessibility of private home care was thus limited due to unaffordability. The main limitation of the private sector was a lack of qualified workforce. The salary offered was much lower, compared to salaries offered abroad for the same line of work. A lack of knowledge of dementia among unqualified personnel was apparent in their attitudes and expectations towards users of private care services. Moreover, there are private, or even state, facilities which refuse admission of those who have a diagnosis of dementia.

In the last few years, the number of elderly individuals who needed care and social assistance increased and they were repeatedly admitted to medical hospitals at the request of their families. Under these conditions, the government changed the status of more than 30 hospitals from medical care facilities to home care facilities. In 2011, the Ministry of Health approved a national programme for the development of a national network of home care for elderly people (HG212/2011) [3]. These changes were debated in the media, and this was viewed by some as a means of sending our elderly people away from society into medico-social units with poor care availability.

Legislation OG102/1999 also allowed patients with severe mental disability who are not able to take care of themselves to benefit from provision of a paid caregiver. Because of a lack of qualified personnel in this area, usually a family member would be the paid caregiver. However, the number of patients who benefit from this opportunity is limited because of resource scarcity.

The first memory clinic

In 2000, the Memory Centre, the first service in the country for early detection, diagnosis, and treatment of cognitive disorders, was established in partnership with the Prof Dr Al Obregia Psychiatry Hospital in Bucharest. The multidisciplinary team at the Centre, which consists of psychologists, psychiatrists, and neurologists, have drawn up specific investigation protocols and use validated neuropsychological instruments (e.g. Addenbrooke's Cognitive Examination, a battery of tests for geriatric mental state). This service provided more than 8000 consultations in 2014. The Centre also offers family counselling and support groups for families, operates a phone line for counselling, and provides educational activities for students in medicine and psychology.

In 2009, the National Centre of Mental Health and Fight Anti-Drugs was established (OG1424/2009). The current 'Guidelines for dementia diagnosis and treatment' was approved by the Ministry of Health and published in 2009. These guidelines were developed by neurologists and psychiatrists. The National Health Insurance system has also approved a series of assessments that need to be carried out when making a diagnosis of dementia. These include neuropsychological tests, CT or MRI scans, and laboratory tests. The current mental health services available provide interventions aimed more for identification, diagnosis, and treatment of mental health problems and are less focused on preventive measures.

The actual goal of current health services is to improve access to diagnosis and management of early-stage dementia for elderly people living in urban and rural areas. International guidelines suggest that most patients with dementia can be assessed and managed adequately by their primary care physicians, but a number of studies have raised concerns about GPs' confidence in diagnosing dementia, the adequacy of their training, and their access to resources for the diagnosis and management of dementia. In Romania, current legislation states that only psychiatrists, neurologists, and geriatricians can initiate and continue treatment for dementia. Pharmacotherapy costs are covered by the National Insurance scheme. The role of GPs is to identify patients and refer them to specialists involved in their care. The care pathway, however, presents with difficulties in finding appropriate services to meet the specific needs of each patient, which results in multiple consultations in different care services.

Treatment of psychiatric and medical comorbidities in patients with dementia remains a problem, because of difficult access to specialized services, risk of polypharmacy, and a lack of coherent case management and treatment plan. Low budgeting is an issue, along with an insufficient number of psychiatric hospitals and a lack of qualified staff. There are also inequalities in workforce distribution and bed numbers across different counties.

The future direction in improving dementia care

The rapid changes that characterize the contemporary society in Romania bring along the need to be informed and adapted to the newest demands in all

population groups. People with dementia have specific needs for care and demand special attention and resource allocation (see Table 30.1).

The proportion of patients with dementia is much higher than those who
actually receive a formal diagnosis and treatment for dementia. This is as a result of patients avoiding to be diagnosed because of associated stigma and also
because of a lack of knowledge of dementia among the community [5]. The

Table 30.1 Current challenges in dementia and measures to be taken

Current challenges in dementia	Measures to be taken
Stigma and discrimination	Changing beliefs and attitudes towards the elderly both among the general population and medical staff (educational programmes, media involvement, community exposure to specific needs of this population group, etc.) Distribution of informative materials: books, brochures with information on the disease, memory magnet, post-it notes, and personalized balloons, bookmarks, etc.
Early diagnosis	Access to training programmes both for GPs and specialists Access to novel tests for early diagnosis Intervention for at-risk populations
Access to qualified services	Improve access to services by approving specialist home consultations for those with mobility difficulties Direct communication with specialists ready to answer questions and perform cognitive evaluations Availability of qualified personnel Training programmes for those involved in care
Individualized complex treatment plan	Considering comorbidities Evaluation of individualized needs of each patient
Family and community support	Support programmes for families Training programmes for those involved in care Community intervention for solidarity in helping the elderly
Financial issues	More involvement of government authorities in supporting and protecting patients with dementia New sources of finance, not only for medical services, but also social and community budgets Fair distribution across different counties
Better prevent than treat	Prevention measures Remaining active, preserving autonomy, and being involved in community life Healthy ageing by maintaining physical and mental health Using modern technologies and Internet facilities for special needs and demands

population did not request for mental healthcare services in dementia because they did not know that they could be helped.

Management of dementia can often be challenging. Changes in personality and an inability to perform daily activities can lead to dependence. As the disease progresses, healthcare resource utilization increases until patients eventually become institutionalized. To ensure maximum treatment efficacy for each patient, there is an emerging need for individualized therapies as part of case management. The needs of, and specific resources required for, each patient should be addressed. Case management is a way of improving the quality and cost-effectiveness of care for patients with dementia.

Mental health services need to change paradigms from treating to preventing psychiatric disorders. In the future, these services should be more focused on providing information on how to live longer with a lower risk for developing mental health problems.

Recent studies on the effects of physical exercise and nutrition showed that these interventions impact brain functioning and changes associated with normal ageing. Much suffering as a consequence of dementia can be prevented or alleviated by training the elderly to understand the changes they are going through and helping them to adapt and continue to function while staying closely connected with their surrounding reality. Such strategy would not only benefit from the contribution of mental health professionals, but also from other healthcare professionals, including GPs, nutritionists, kineto-therapists, social assistants, and physicians from different specialties (geriatricians, neurologists, cardiologists, etc.). Physical trainers and alternative therapists (music therapists, art therapists, dance therapists, vocational therapists, etc.) should team up in efforts to prevent somatic and mental health disorders. Modern technologies could be useful in helping people cope with age-related decline in mobility, sensory functioning, speech, communication, etc. More funding should be allocated to this research field. Internet use offers the possibility of an easier connection for those with difficulties with their mobility, as well as easier access to different services (including medical surveillance, communication with family members living abroad, networking, online shopping, and games or exercises for memory or attention stimulation). Mental health services have to be more focused on people's well-being and on the prevention of mental health disorders.

References

1. **Romanian Alzheimer Society**. *National Dementia Strategy 2014–2020*. Available from: http://www.comunicatemedicale.ro/upload/docs/2613.pdf [accessed 22 December 2015].

2. **Ministry of Health**. *National Strategy for Health. The Action Plan 2014–2020*. Available from: http://www.ms.ro/strategia-nationala-de-sanatate-2014-2020/ [accessed 20 August 2018].

3. **Mihai A, Botezat-Antonescu I**. Romania. In: **Samele C, Frew S, Urquía N**. *Mental health systems in the European Union member states, status of mental health in populations and benefits to be expected from investments into mental health: European profile of prevention and promotion of mental health (EuroPoPP-MH)*. European Commission; 2013. pp. 397–406.

4. **Mihai A, Taran L, Nirestean A**. *The implication of legislation in process of psychiatric diagnosis* (abstract). London: Maudsley Forum; 2013.

5. **Tataru N**. Romania. In: **Ames D, Burns A, O'Brien J** (eds). *Dementia*, 3rd ed. Boca Raton, FL: CRC Press; 2005. pp. 296–9.

Chapter 31

Russia

Nikolay Neznanov and Natalia Zalutskaya

Summary

Dementia is an important medical and social problem in the
Russian Federation. Since 1999, Russia has begun to develop
its geriatric services into an integrated system of care for the
elderly, in whom cognitive impairment has been recognized as an
important problem. Currently, each region of Russia has a basic
geriatric centre which includes an age psychiatry department that
provides organizational and methodological guidance for medical,
social, and health institutions involved in care provision for the
elderly population. However, there are a significant number of
financial, medical, social, and community problems that create
barriers to achieving optimal quality of care. Therefore, to address
these problems, the 'Strategy of action for senior citizens in the
Russian Federation until 2025' was launched by the government
of the Russian Federation, which aims to identify new areas of
state and public policy relating to senior citizens and their families,
as well as social institutions interacting with this population group,
including people with cognitive impairment.

Epidemiology

In Russia, the progressive increase in the elderly population and the continued
relatively low life expectancy (76.47 years for women and 65.29 years for men)
[1] constitute important demographic trends causing a natural increase in the
prevalence of specific late-life diseases, in particular cognitive disorders. In
2015, people aged over 65 years accounted for 13.5% of the Russian population
[2]. The exact number of people with dementia in Russia is not known. Age and
gender indicators of AD were determined in a population-based study conducted in one region of Russia. The data obtained were extrapolated to determine the gender and age structure of patients with AD in the general population.

In so doing, it was possible to estimate the number of people suffering from AD in Russia to be approximately 1,248,000 people, accounting for 4.5% of the population older than 60 years, with late-onset AD accounting for almost half of the cases of dementia in elderly people [3]. By 2020, the number of people with AD will increase to 1,354,000 and will constitute 1% of the total population of Russia, with 1,035,000 people, or 0.8% of the total population, with dementia of vascular aetiology [3]. The exponential growth of the prevalence of AD is associated with increasing age and higher rates of age-specific morbidity in women, compared to men. Thus, the prevalence of dementia is significantly different in Russian regions with a high life expectancy (e.g. Ingushetia where the average life expectancy is 76.35 years for men and 81.99 years for women), compared to those with a low life expectancy (e.g. Tyva Republic where the average life expectancy is 56.63 years for men and 67.22 years for women) [1].

Elderly care

When the Ministry of Health launched the Ministry order 'On improvement of medical care for elderly citizens in the Russian Federation' in 1999 [4], geriatric services began to develop as an integrated system of care for the elderly in whom cognitive impairment has been recognized to be a significant problem. Currently, each region of Russia has a basic geriatric centre, which includes an old age psychiatry department, providing organizational and methodological guidance to medical, social, and health institutions involved in care provision for the elderly population. A number of regions also have outpatient clinics which run memory rooms, as well as specialized departments of health and social care set up with particular emphasis on home care provision for elderly and disabled people. Moreover, inpatient centres of gerontology and gerontopsychology operate within the network of institutions that provide medical and social services. Specialized departments of social and health home care for elderly and disabled people are organized in small localities which do not have specialized gerontological centres. In order to compensate for the lack of permanent home-based social and socio-medical care for older people living in small and remote communities in some parts of the country, mobile social services are organized, which are provided by various health professionals, including, for example, physicians and nurses. The aims of these above-mentioned structural units include the solution of problems of diagnostics of cognitive impairment and provision of assistance to people with dementia [5].

In 2016, the government of the Russian Federation approved and launched the 'Strategy of action for senior citizens in the Russian Federation until 2025' [2], which aims to identify new areas of state and public policy relating to senior citizens and their families, as well as social institutions interacting with this population group, including people with cognitive impairment. The main priority of the Strategy is the development of geriatric services as an integrated interagency system of individual medical and social services for elderly people based on assessment of their needs and requirements. The Strategy provides guidance for the implementation of targeted programmes to address the problems of organization of assistance for people suffering from cognitive disorders and dementia and makes recommendations for an increase in the number of day care centres and other forms of community care, as well as the introduction of unified state standards of diagnosis, treatment, and quality control of multi-level care. Of particular importance is the creation of organizational variants of medical and social care, working on the principle of continuity of care, namely, dispensary care–day clinic care–hospital care.

Psychiatric guidelines

In 2013, the Russian Society of Psychiatrists approved the 'National guidelines for the diagnosis and treatment of Alzheimer's disease' [6]. The 'standard of primary healthcare in dementia' [7] was established to standardize the medical process of dementia diagnosis, the range of laboratory methods and instruments available for assessment, medical services, non-pharmacological methods of prevention, treatment, and rehabilitation of people with dementia. A list of drugs approved for use in the treatment of AD in Russia is also available. A number of drugs for the treatment of dementia are included on the list of vital and essential drugs approved for medical use in Russia, and, in accordance with the Federal Law 'On state social assistance' [8], patients in the disability category receive anti-dementia medications free of charge.

Moreover, every Russian citizen is entitled to independently approve an additional list of free medicines issued to patients. Regional programmes on free supply of medicines can extend the list of anti-dementia drugs, as well as the group of patients eligible to receive free medicines—the extension allowed is determined based on the regional income. Caregivers of working age who had to stop working because of their relative's illness receive some state monetary compensation. Patients with dementia are eligible to receive free absorbent underwear and other means of care. An important milestone in the organization of care for people with dementia in Russia was the establishment of the organization 'Help for Alzheimer's Disease Patients and their Families', uniting health professionals and patients and their relatives. Its main goals are to improve the quality of care for people with dementia and their families, insofar as the current developments of medical science would allow, to provide information to patients and their relatives on opportunities of dementia care, to change public attitude towards dementia, to promote respect for people with dementia in society, and to raise awareness among the general public of dementia as pathological ageing. The organization aims to gain the attention of the entire medical community to the problem of cognitive impairment in elderly people.

Dementia care

However, despite these positive achievements in the field of dementia care, there are still a significant number of financial, medical, social, and community problems in Russia that create barriers to achieving optimal quality of care. Full implementation of the concept of organizing care for people with dementia as a system of long-term medical and social support for patients has not been achieved because of difficulties with ensuring care continuity between the different institutions within the healthcare system, as well as between health services and social services. Lack of geriatric offices and geriatric departments in hospitals significantly reduces care accessibility for elderly people with dementia. In addition, there are no large-scale epidemiological studies on the prevalence of dementia in the Russian population. There are also no data on the number of patients who have been given a diagnosis of dementia as well as the stage/severity of their disease. The current setup in dementia management is that patients with mild to moderate dementia are managed by neurologists and those with moderate to severe dementia by psychiatrists, which leads to difficulties in keeping accurate statistical records and, in turn, in obtaining the actual number of patients registered as having a dementia diagnosis. Another problem is the lack of awareness among physicians, primarily those practising in outpatient healthcare settings, of cognitive impairment in elderly patients, which thus results in delay in dementia diagnosis.

The difficulty exists in providing an adequate level of assistance in accordance with accepted standards for people living in remote regions and small settlements, as well as in the full implementation of existing recommendations for the diagnosis of dementia. Difficulties in the organization of aid to people with dementia are due to an insufficient number of beds in inpatient facilities providing social and health services, and a lack of information about the cost of health and social aid and care for different stages of dementia and dependence of these parameters on the diagnostic affiliation of the patient, as well as problems with the assessment of the quality of life of patients in nursing homes and medical and social establishments providing extended stay for seriously ill patients with mental disorders, who cannot do without external help, and interaction of social services with hospitals. Also, the treatment process in dementia can be significantly impaired by low patient compliance. Another problem is the narrow range of non-pharmacological interventions offered to patients and their families. A particular challenge is the organization of palliative and end-of-life care for patients in the terminal stages of dementia. Compensatory payments to caregivers that are not commensurate with their actual social circumstances also represent another problem. And, of course, the most important challenge is to assess the levels of preparedness of the health and social care systems to meet the needs of the predicted increase in the number of people suffering from dementia.

Future plans

Resolution of these issues should be achieved by realization of the approved 'Strategy of action for senior citizens in the Russian Federation until 2025' [2], by ensuring the exclusion of discrimination against elderly people, enhanced access to targeted and timely assistance for elderly people, a differentiated approach to the choice of forms of social support, and the development of a system of evaluation of care needs; by promoting public and private partnerships in the provision of healthcare services for the elderly, as well as community involvement (volunteer, non-profit organizations) in the organization of various forms of care for the elderly; by encouraging scientific research in the prevalence of dementia, drug supply, cost-effectiveness of dementia treatment, and quality of life in long-stay institutions; and by creating a unified system of professional training, as well as additional professional education to specialists, for improved provision of medical and social support to elderly people with cognitive impairment. The Strategy emphasizes on the involvement of civil society in addressing the problems of elderly people with cognitive impairment and in creating dementia-friendly infrastructures and environments.

Dementia prevention

One of the most promising approaches to addressing the problem of dementia lies in its prevention, especially of the vascular risk factors. The Federal Law 'On the protection of public health from exposure to environmental tobacco smoke and the consequences of tobacco consumption' [9] stipulates emphasis on preventive measures. Moreover, the 'Strategy of action for senior citizens in the Russian Federation until 2025' [2] makes provision for improved accessibility of sports facilities and promotes physical sports and an active lifestyle, including through the involvement of sports, cultural, and social organizations to provide appropriate conditions to encourage uptake of sports and recreational activities among elderly people, as well as ensures the availability of cultural activities designed to meet the creative needs of senior citizens. Another important strategy for dementia prevention is to provide elderly people with opportunities to continue paid working on their own free will. There are increasing arguments in favour of initiating therapeutic interventions in the early stages of dementia. In this regard, evaluation of diagnostic and differential diagnostic criteria for early-stage dementia is of particular scientific and practical significance.

References

1. **statdata.ru.** [*Life expectancy at birth by regions of Russia (expected) for 2014 (updated 2016)*]. Available from: http://www.statdata.ru/spg_reg_rf [accessed 7 August 2018].
2. **Government of the Russian Federation.** [*Strategy of action for senior citizens in the Russian Federation until 2025*]. Available from: http://government.ru/docs/21692/ [accessed 7 August 2018].
3. **Belousov YB, Zyryanov SK, Belousov DY, Beketov AS.** Clinical and economic aspects of the treatment of Alzheimer's disease in Russia. *Good Clinical Practice.* 2009;**1**:3–28.
4. **Ministry of Health.** [*On improvement of medical care for citizens elderly in the Russian Federation*]. Available from: http://base.garant.ru/4176179/ [accessed 20 August 2018].
5. **Shabalin VN.** Organization of geriatric services in a progressive demographic aging of the population of the Russian Federation. *Advances in Gerontology.* 2009;**22**:185–95.
6. **The Russian Society of Psychiatrists.** [*Diagnosis and treatment of Alzheimer's disease. National clinical guidelines*]. Available from: http://psychiatr.ru/news/174 [accessed 20 August 2018].
7. **Ministry of Health.** [*Standard of primary healthcare in dementia*]. Available from: http://psychiatr.ru/news/299 [accessed 7 August 2018].
8. **Federal Law of Russian Federation.** [*On state social assistance*]. Available from: http://zakonrf.net/o_gosudarstvennoy_sotsialnoy_pomoshchi/ [accessed 7 August 2018].
9. **Federal Law of Russian Federation.** [*On the protection of public health from exposure to environmental tobacco smoke and the consequences of tobacco consumption*]. Available from: http://docs.cntd.ru/document/499002954 [accessed 7 August 2018].

Chapter 32

Scotland

Seamus V McNulty and Graham A Jackson

Summary

Scotland is a small nation which has a devolved legislature, while still remaining part of the United Kingdom (UK). As the health service has become increasingly divergent from that of the remainder of the UK, more innovative approaches to dementia care have been allowed to develop. The Scottish Dementia Strategy, now in its third iteration, is unique in that it adopts a human rights-based method of dementia care, an approach that has subsequently been followed by other European countries. The Strategy is in continual evolution, with the third Strategy focusing more on care at the end stages of dementia, especially for those in nursing homes or long-term hospital care. Other novel approaches, such as the Dementia Champions programme, have shown benefits in the quality of care for patients with dementia in acute general hospitals, although less so for those in social care settings. Scotland was also a pioneer in enacting incapacity legislation, although this is now under review as shortcomings in the current procedures are becoming unmasked.The challenges of delivering high quality Dementia care to both urban areas with high levels of deprivation and remote and rural areas, including multiple island communities persist. However, the Scottish nation has shown that a pioneering and innovative approach to service development can bring significant benefits to people with Dementia thus raising the standards of care.

Background

Although part of the UK, Scotland has a devolved government that fully administers the health system within the country, as well as other functions of the government.

Scotland makes up approximately one-third of the land mass of the UK but has only 8.4% of the UK population (around 5.3 million). There are five major urban centres, with the most densely populated areas being the post-industrial heartland within the so-called central belt of the country, which includes Edinburgh and Glasgow. There are also areas with very low population densities, including a large number of small islands, where providing services can be particularly challenging.

Scotland has particular public health problems, with higher mortality and higher rates of cancer and cardiovascular disease than most of Western Europe. The reasons for this are not entirely clear but do include poor diet and higher-than-average smoking rates. In 2016, there were an estimated 90,000 people living with dementia in Scotland.

Health and social care

Health and social care, along with some other functions of the government, were devolved from the UK Westminster Government to the Scottish Government when the latter came into being in 1999. Since this point, the two health services in both England and Scotland have diverged markedly, although nominally remaining part of the UK-wide National Health Service (NHS).

Scotland continues to adhere more closely to the founding principles of the NHS, with the Scottish Government Health Department making block grants to each of the seven territorial health boards which subsequently fund, develop, or commission services locally.

Legislation to implement health and social care integration, passed by the Scottish Parliament in February 2014, came into force on 1 April 2016. This brought together NHS and local council care services under one partnership arrangement for each area. Thirty-one local partnerships have been set up across Scotland, and they now manage almost £8 billion of health and social care resources.

Working together, NHS and local council care services are jointly responsible for the health and care needs of patients, to ensure that those who use services get the right care and support whatever their needs, at any point in their care journey.

Dementia as a national priority

Since the identification of dementia as a National Priority by the government in 2007, Scotland's Dementia Strategy has been in continual development. The first Strategy was published in 2010, followed by updated Strategies in 2013 and 2017. A major international policy statement—the Glasgow Declaration—was published by Alzheimer Europe in 2014 and called for dementia to be an international priority and for all European countries to develop a dementia strategy.

The first Strategy has been widely seen as a model, which many other countries have followed. Its particular strength is that it is built upon, and was developed from, the Charter of Rights for People with Dementia [1], which was published by the Scottish Government and developed along with people with dementia, mainly in the form of the Scottish Dementia Working Group. This group, a campaigning group for people with dementia, was set up by, and continues to be supported by, Alzheimer Scotland.

In common with dementia plans developed by other countries, the early stages of the Strategy were largely built around the diagnosis and support for people with early-stage dementia. It was recognized that many people with dementia were being diagnosed in the later stages and were therefore missing out on support. However, the memory clinic model favoured by many other countries, including England, is much less prominent, with diagnosis being made, in the main, within more conventional old age psychiatry services. In spite of this, or perhaps because of this, diagnosis rates in Scotland in general compare favourably with those elsewhere.

Post-diagnosis support

Support after diagnosis in Scotland is particularly well developed, with every person with a new diagnosis of dementia having guaranteed post-diagnosis support from a named individual for at least 1 year. There are different ways of providing this, but normally it is provided by a member of an older people's mental health team or by a Link Worker, a post which has been created specifically with this role in mind. The post-diagnosis support is built around a number of areas, including understanding and self-management of symptoms, planning for the future, peer support, and maximization of the ability of an individual with dementia to remain involved in their community. It is too early to say how effective this will be, and clearly there are challenges in implementing this, but the expectation is that this will enable people with dementia to support themselves in the community for as long as possible, to make plans for the future, and by changing expectations, to delay the need for more expensive social care. Certainly it enables better use of advance planning, with a large increase in the number of people in Scotland appointing a Power of Attorney, someone who will take financial and welfare decisions on the person's behalf if they lose the capacity to do so.

Once dementia has progressed to a level of severity at which an individual requires more support, there has been modelling of a service where each person has access to a dementia practice coordinator. This role is envisaged as being one where the named professional aims to support the individual and their family in order to enable them to live the best life possible with dementia. However, the ability to provide this comprehensively remains a particular challenge in terms of time and workforce resources.

With the third Strategy, there is increased emphasis on care for people with later-stage dementia, particularly those who require ongoing hospital or care home placement. Alzheimer Scotland, after a prolonged consultation, developed the Advanced Dementia Model [2], and the University of the West of Scotland led on the development of a European Best Practice Statement, along with colleagues from six other European countries [3]. Both of these call for an increased recognition of dementia as being a terminal condition and for the development of palliative care services for people with dementia, as well as for an upskilling of the care workforce to deal with the later stages of dementia more appropriately.

As well as better care for people with dementia in nursing homes, there is also a major assessment of how people with dementia are cared for in hospital. It is estimated that between 25% and 43% of people in hospital have dementia [4], and often their care has been seen as less than ideal.

Dementia Champions

The Dementia Champions programme, which began in 2011, is an innovative model which forms part of wider initiatives to support improvements in the care and treatment of people with dementia admitted to, or at risk of, admission to general hospital settings and includes the establishment of Alzheimer Scotland nurse consultants/specialists in each Health Board.

The aim of the programme is to support the development of champions as change agents in improving the experience, care, treatment, and outcomes for people with dementia, their families, and caregivers in general hospitals and at the interface between hospital and community settings. Dementia Champions derive from a variety of professional roles, including nursing staff, allied health professionals (AHPs), social workers, radiographers, dentists, and ambulance personnel.

The programme continues to be delivered, on behalf of NHS Education for Scotland (NES) and the Scottish Social Services Council (SSSC), by the University of the West of Scotland, in partnership with Alzheimer Scotland. Seven cohorts of Dementia Champions, comprising over 700 individuals, had completed the programme by the end of 2016.

An evaluation of the programme [5] showed that there had been some notable improvements, particularly in terms of the skills and knowledge of staff, the care environment, involvement of caregivers, individualization of care, and management of stress and distress. The roles were also demonstrated to have challenged and addressed negative attitudes towards dementia and also to have supported improvements in the attitudes and practices of staff across a variety of professions and settings. However, the positive outcomes were not uniform across the country and had shown limited improvements in care delivery in social care settings.

Increasing scrutiny in Scotland is now being given to the care and support of people with dementia in long-term psychiatric care, following a report from the Mental Welfare Commission (MWC) [6] which highlighted significant deficiencies in, and disparities of, care for such patients.

Subsequent to this, the Scottish Government set up a specific work stream—the Quality and Excellence in Specialist Dementia Care (QESDC)—which was given the remit to assist individual Health Boards improve standards of care for patients in long-term hospital care. A self-assessment tool, based on the Older People in Acute Hospitals (OPAH) inspection, was developed and completed by all NHS Boards, allowing them to undertake a baseline self-assessment of current practices in all dementia care settings. The aim was to enable NHS Boards to identify areas of good practice, but also to determine where improvements could be made. Subsequent to this, in 2016, the Scottish Government commissioned Healthcare Improvement Scotland (HIS) to undertake a Specialist Dementia Unit Improvement Programme.

Scotland has been at the forefront of legislative developments in the management of dementia. The country was the first in the UK to develop incapacity legislation with the passing of the Adults with Incapacity (Scotland) Act 2000. This was, in fact, the first bill enacted by the new Scottish Parliament. It replaced a number of disparate, outdated judicial measures and provided a framework for safeguarding the welfare and managing the finances of adults who lack capacity due to mental illness, learning disability, or a related condition, or an inability to communicate. It was regarded as visionary, rights-based, and modern legislation, and in many respects, it remains so. Particularly important is the fundamental principle that there should be no intervention in the affairs of an adult, unless this would benefit the adult and the benefit cannot be reasonably achieved without the intervention. The Act further stipulates that account must be taken of the past and present wishes of the adult as far as they can be ascertained and that the adult should be encouraged to exercise whatever residual capacity they retain.

Following a review by the Scottish Law Commission in 2014, and a subsequent consultation on this, in 2016, the Scottish Government began considering amendments to the Act.

References

1. **Scottish Government.** *The Charter of Rights for People with Dementia and their Carers in Scotland.* 2011. Available from: http://www.gov.scot/Publications/2011/05/31085414/6 [accessed 6 August 2018].

2. **Alzheimer Scotland.** *Advanced Dementia Practice Model: understanding and transforming advanced dementia and end of life care.* Edinburgh: Alzheimer Scotland; 2016.

3. **Holmerová I, Waugh A, MacRae R,** *et al. Dementia palliare best practice statement, University of the West of Scotland.* 2016. Available from: https://www.uws.ac.uk/research/research-areas/health/dementia-palliare/ [accessed 6 August 2018].

4. **Mukadam N, Sampson EL.** A systemic review of the prevalence, associations and outcomes of dementia in older general hospital inpatients. *International Psychogeriatrics.* 2011;23:344–55.

5. **Ellison S, Watt G, Christie I.** *Evaluating the impact of the Alzheimer Scotland Dementia Nurse Consultants/Specialists & Dementia Champions in bringing about improvements to dementia care in acute general hospitals.* Edinburgh: Blake Stevenson; 2014.

6. **Mental Welfare Commission for Scotland.** *Dignity and respect: dementia continuing care visits. MWC Edinburgh.* 2014. Available from: https://www.mwcscot.org.uk/media/191892/dignity_and_respect_-_final_approved.pdf [accessed 6 August 2018].

Chapter 33

Serbia

Slavica Djukic-Dejanovic and Gorica Djokic

Summary

Serbia is among the demographically older countries in the
world, with 18% of the population aged above 65 years. One
in two persons older than 65 years lives with an old spouse.
The Serbian National Strategy on ageing identified poverty
as a widespread companion of ageing, with a rising poverty
index. In 2007, the first non-governmental organization, called
'Alchajmer', was established in Sremska Kamenica to support
people with Alzheimer's disease and their caregivers. In 2008, the
first Centre for Memory Disorders and Dementia was established
as part of the Neurology Clinic at the Clinical Centre of Serbia
in Belgrade. A National Guide for Alzheimer's disease was
published in 2013. The Serbian health insurance scheme covers
care costs for people with severe dementia through its support
programme called Advanced Home Help, which includes provision
of geriatric housekeepers from the palliative care programme,
as well as modest financial support in accordance with the
state's financial capabilities. There are over 160,000 people with
dementia in Serbia, comprising approximately 13% of the Serbian
population aged above 65 years, of whom only 4% are prescribed
appropriate pharmacological treatment.The three things which
we did best are: a National guide for Alzheimers disease was
published in the year 2013,and included all aspects of Dementia
care from risk factors, early diagose, therapy, to palliative care and
caregivers support, centers for memory disorders and dementia,
specialized daily care centres and Advanced home help are
available for people with dementia. Public awerness campains
and educational campain focused on family doctors with results
in increased recognition of early simptoms. Three things for the
future include the necessity of forming a Register of patients with
dementia in Serbia; expanding the network of NGO's and Daily
Care centres all over the Serbia for the purpose of reducing social

isolation of the demented citizens and their caregivers and public awareness campains should be reinforced and spread not only to a large cities, but also to rural parts of country.

Demographics

According to the Statistical Office of the Republic of Serbia, the average age of the population in Serbia is 42.2 years [1], with 17% of the population aged over 65 years for the period 2011–2015 based on World Bank data [2] or 18% based on the World Population Data Sheet for 2014—which places Serbia among the demographically older countries in the world. The ageing index in 2014 was 133.16 (male 113.48; female 154.03) [3]

The National Strategy

The National Strategy on ageing in Serbia (2006–2015) identified poverty as a frequent companion of ageing, with the poverty index rising to 19.2% in the population aged over 65 years. A strategy for palliative care, which has been under development since 2005, and the National Strategy on ageing both recognized that one in two persons older than 65 years lives with an old spouse [4–6].

In 2006, the Ministry of Health and the Republic Health Insurance Fund incorporated anti-dementia medications onto the so-called 'positive list' of drugs, which means that anti-dementia drugs can be prescribed by neurologists or psychiatrists for patients diagnosed with AD (ICD-10 diagnostic code G30) and, from 2011, also for patients diagnosed with dementia in AD (ICD-10 diagnostic code F00).

In 2007, the first NGO called 'Alchajmer' was established in Sremska Kamenica to support people with AD and their caregivers, and was the first provider of specialized day care for people with AD. Since then, a few more specialized care centres are now in operation that provide either public or private care services [7].

In 2008, the first Centre for Memory Disorders and Dementia was established as part of the Neurology Clinic at the Clinical Centre of Serbia in Belgrade, with the aim for early detection and diagnosis, treatment, and follow-up of patients with memory disorders. The Centre has a capacity to perform 120–150 patient consultations per month—therefore, there is a waiting list for patients to be seen [8].

In 2010, a second specialized centre in Serbia (and the first in the Serbian province of Vojvodina)—the Centre for Dementia and Memory Disorders—was opened at the Clinical Centre of Vojvodina in Novi Sad. This was followed, a year later, by the opening of the Centre for Cognitive Disorders at the General Hospital in Sremska Mitrovica [9].

With regard to treatment of behavioural and psychological signs and symptoms of dementia (BPSD/BPSSD) in outpatient settings, the Dr Laza Lazarević Clinic for Psychiatric Disorders provides 24-hour emergency care all year round for patients with a diagnosis of dementia, as well as outpatient follow-up on working days [10]. The clinic conducted a total of 1455 patient consultations in 2015.

Meanwhile, several privately run nursing homes specialized for people with dementia have been opened, as well as several government-funded Geriatric Centres for patients with dementia such as the Nursing Home in Futog established in 2011. However, there are very long waiting lists for these government-funded Geriatric Centres.

The National Action Plan

An important milestone in dementia care in Serbia came about in 2011 when the NGO 'Alchajmer' launched its initiative—the National Action Plan and programme for dementia, in collaboration with the Centre for Memory Disorders and Dementia (part of the Neurology Clinic) at the Clinical Centre of Serbia in Belgrade, the Centre for Dementia and Memory Disorders at the Clinical Centre of Vojvodina in Novi Sad, the Centre for Cognitive Disorders at the General Hospital in Sremska Mitrovica, the Nursing Home in Futog, and the Geriatric Centre in Novi Sad. The National Action Plan for dementia was put forward to the Serbian government, including the following key proposals: (1) the necessity for a register of patients diagnosed with dementia in Serbia, (2) the need for national guidance on dementia treatment, (3) the importance of public awareness campaigns on dementia, (4) the need for education programmes about dementia for health professionals, and (5) the development of day care centres for people with dementia, etc. [11].

The National Guide

As a result of the National Action Plan, a National Guide for AD was published in 2013. This National Guide included all aspects of dementia care—from risk factors, early diagnosis, and therapy to palliative care and caregiver support [12].

The Serbian health insurance scheme covers care costs for people with severe dementia through its support programme called Advanced Home Help, which includes provision of geriatric housekeepers from the palliative care programme, as well as modest financial support in accordance with the state's financial budget [6, 13, 14].

There are more than 160,000 people with dementia in Serbia, which comprise approximately 13% of the Serbian population aged over 65 years. There are distressing reports that only 4% of patients diagnosed with dementia are prescribed adequate pharmacological treatment, according to data on anti-dementia drug prescriptions and estimated numbers of patients with AD in Serbia, taking into account recommendations on pharmacotherapy prescribing from the National Guide for AD [11].

Public awareness

The last few years have witnessed an intensification in public awareness campaigns in almost all major cities in Serbia, particularly on World Alzheimer's Day and during World Alzheimer's Month. There is evidence of general public interest in the disease. However, our current challenge is to focus on how to distinguish between physiological ageing and MCI or early-stage dementia, hence on early recognition of clinical/cognitive manifestations of dementia [15].

Of equal importance are educational programmes for family doctors: (1) to raise awareness of dementia, (2) to provide training in early recognition, (3) to disseminate knowledge about how to adopt a rapid diagnostic approach, (4) to educate on the vital importance of adequate treatment, and (5) to provide guidance on how to support patients and caregivers [16–18]. Early results from evaluation of the effectiveness of this educational programme obtained in the Pathways to Dementia Care Study showed increased early recognition of clinical manifestations of dementia by family doctors, with subsequent direct referral to a specialist.

Future plans

Our future plans in Serbia should be oriented towards the goals defined in the National Action Plan. We think that public awareness campaigns should be reinforced and cover not only major cities, but also be run across rural parts of the country, because dementia is a nationwide problem that does not affect large urban areas only.

We believe that expansion of the NGO network, as well as day care centres, all across Serbia could help to reduce social isolation of our fellow citizens with dementia and their caregivers and would make health and care services more accessible.

There is a need for more centres for dementia and memory disorders to meet the needs of the growing population aged above 65 years which comprise a predicted estimate of 13% of people with dementia, based on World Bank data. According to our analysis, we propose to have one centre to cater for a population of 100,000–150,000. Moreover, centres for dementia and memory disorders should be uniformly spread across all Serbian regions, and not restricted exclusively to urban regions and major cities, thus ensuring equal access to available diagnostic interventions and treatments for all dementia patients across the country.

It should be emphasized that the existence of a central register of patients diagnosed with dementia is of crucial importance, to help determine the actual needs of people suffering from AD and other types of dementia. Unfortunately, this kind of register is yet to be set up, so for now, we rely on data derived from the number of visits to primary care (family) doctors and to specialists in neurology, psychiatry, or geriatric medicine for diagnostic criteria that correspond to different types of dementia.

The future of dementia care, in our opinion, should focus on early diagnosis and treatment and on encouraging research in these areas, as well as on ensuring that diagnostic tools become more accessible. In this regard, we propose that patients who have already been screened for dementia or cognitive disorders and diagnosed with MCI should undergo laboratory testing for the plasma biomarker brain-derived neurotrophic factor (BDNF) or PiB PET (Pittsburgh compound B positron emission tomography) scanning to help identify those who are at risk of conversion into AD, i.e. those patients at a prodromal stage of AD. This diagnostic approach may allow use of an increased range of therapeutic options through early intervention [19, 20].

References

1. **Statistical Office of the Republic of Serbia.** [*Demographic Yearbook in the Republic of Serbia, 2014*]. Belgrade: Statistical Office of the Republic of Serbia; 2015.
2. **The World Bank.** *Population ages 65 and above (% of total) 2011–2015*. Available from: http://data.worldbank.org/indicator/SP.POP.65UP.TO.ZS [accessed 6 August 2018].
3. **Population Reference Bureau.** *2014 world population data sheet*. Available from: http://www.prb.org/pdf14/2014-world-population-data-sheet_eng.pdf [accessed 6 August 2018].
4. **Government of the Republic of Serbia.** *National strategy on ageing 2006–2015*. Belgrade: Official Gazette of the Republic of Serbia No. 55/05 and 71/05; 2005.
5. **United Nations Economic Commission for Europe.** *Working group on ageing. Policy on ageing*. 2009. Available from: https://www.unece.org/population/wga.html [accessed 20 August 2018].
6. **Government of the Republic of Serbia.** *Strategy for palliative care*. Belgrade: Official Gazette of the Republic of Serbia No. 55/05, 71/05, 101/07, and 65/08; 2005.
7. **Udruženje građana Alchajmer.** Available from: http://www.infocentarzastarije.org.rs/udruzenja.htm [accessed 20 August 2018].

8. **Neurology Clinic, Clinical Center of Serbia**. *Center for memory disorders and dementia*. Available from: http://neurologija.bg.ac.rs/index.php?option=com_content&view=article&id=249&Itemid=232&lang=en [accessed 6 August 2018].

9. **Clinical Centre of Vojvodina**. Available from: https://www.kcv.rs/ [accessed 20 August 2018].

10. **Clinic for Mental Disorders 'Dr Laza Lazarević'**. Available from: http://ww.lazalazarevic.rs [accessed 6 August 2018].

11. **Akcioni plan i program za Alchajmerovu bolest**. Available from: https://view.officeapps.live.com/op/view.aspx?src=http://www.novisad.rs/sites/default/files/attachment/program_obelezavanja_meseca_alchajmerove_bolesti.doc [accessed 20 August 2018].

12. **Republika Srbija Ministarstvo Zdravlja**. *Vodič za dijagnostikovanje i lečenje Alchajmerove bolesti*. Available from: http://www.zdravlje.gov.rs/showpage.php?id=145 [accessed 6 August 2018].

13. **Gradski Zavod za Gerontologiju i Palijativno Zbrinjavanje**. *Kućno lečenje, nega i palijativno zbrinjavanje*. Available from: http://www.gerontology.co.rs/kucno_lecenje.htm [accessed 6 August 2018].

14. **Republički Fond za Penzijsko i Invalidsko Osiguranje**. *Naknada za pomoć i negu drugog lica*. Available from: http://www.pio.rs/lat/novcane-naknade.html [accessed 6 August 2018].

15. **Lepota & Zdravlje**. *Šetnjom podrške obeležen Svetski Dan Alchajmerove bolesti*. 2014. Available from: http://www.lepotaizdravlje.rs/zdravlje/prevencija-i-lecenje/setnjom-podrske-obelezen-svetski-dan-alchajmerove-bolesti/ [accessed 6 August 2018].

16. **Dom Omladine Beograd**. *Tribina: ne zaboravimo one koji zaboravljaju*. 2015. Available from: http://www.domomladine.org/debate/tribina-ne-zaboravimo-one-koji-zaboravljaju/ [accessed 6 August 2018].

17. **Alchajmer Grupa**. Available from: http://www.alchajmergrupa.rs/index.html [accessed 20 August 2018].

18. **Dnevno boravak za stare 'Naše treće doba'**. *Demencije: dijagnoza, klinička slika, terapija, sa osvrtom na ulogu porodice i izabranog lekara*. 2014. Available from: https://neurogoga.wordpress.com/ [accessed 6 August 2018].

19. **Hwang KS, Lazaris AS, Eastman JA**, *et al*. Plasma BDNF levels associate with Pittsburgh compound B binding in the brain. *Alzheimer's and Dementia*. 2015;1:187–93.

20. **Tifratene K, Robert P, Metelkina A, Pradier C, Dartigues JF**. Progression of mild cognitive impairment to dementia due to AD in clinical settings. *Neurology*. 2015;**85**:331–8.

Chapter 34

Spain

Manuel A Franco-Martin and Raimundo Mateos

Summary

In Spain, dementia care varies widely in different regions of the country. Since each region is also autonomous to develop their own health and social service planning, it is difficult to achieve a general model of dementia care in Spain. Moreover, there is no National Dementia Plan to improve inter-professional and inter-regional coordination, thus resulting in a lack of harmonization and implementation of comprehensive treatment plans. Nevertheless, some common features in the country may be identified, including the general methodology for dementia diagnosis and treatment which consists of symptom detection, initial assessment, diagnosis, pharmacological and non-pharmacological treatment, follow-up, and palliative care, several of which are applied similarly in the different regions. The chapter also describes some specific different features such as public foundations for dementia, the National Reference Centre for Alzheimer's disease, and specialized dementia units. The chapter concludes with an overview of the opportunities and challenges in dementia care in Spain.

Introduction

The management and organization of health services in Spain are run in a very distinct manner, because each region is able to lead, manage, and organize its own health services. There are currently 17 different regional health services and 2 authonomous cities with autonomy for managing and organizing the care of people with dementia. In addition, the Spanish government has also developed a basic standard for dementia care that provides minimum assistance and basic interventions for people with dementia. However, since Spain has no National Dementia Care Plan, considerable disparities in dementia care can be identified across the different regions [1]. Therefore, we have divided this chapter into three sections. In the first section, we describe the basics of dementia care shared by all regions. The second section reviews some of the main specific programmes and activities developed by some regions to improve dementia care. And in the final and third section, we draw our conclusions and discuss the unmet needs in relation to the model of dementia care in Spain.

Basic components of dementia care in Spain

In Spain, dementia care can be subdivided into the following components.

Detection of symptoms

In general, progressive memory impairment or an evident change in behaviour are early symptoms considered to be the most useful indicators of the development of dementia, particularly when occurring in the elderly. These manifestations are mainly observed by the individual's family, although sometimes they can be detected by social services if the person receives social support, as well as by GPs, or even specialists in some cases.

Initial assessment

The initial assessment for detecting cases of dementia is generally performed in a primary care centre (PCC), and there is general agreement that the GP, who is more accessible, should be the first health professional to complete an early and timely evaluation as the first step in the diagnostic process [2]. As part of the initial assessment, the GP usually takes a full medical history, including identifying any abnormal behavioural changes, and performs a cognitive and functional assessment [3]. Various screening tools and assessment protocols are commonly applied, including the MMSE and the clock drawing test. Scales to assess basic and instrumental activities of daily living, such as the Barthel index or the Lawton scale, are also commonly used [4]. However, inadequate training of GPs in dementia assessment has been recognized [5, 6].

Diagnosis

When a GP suspects a diagnosis of dementia, the patient is usually referred to a specialist to confirm the diagnosis, although sometimes GP referrals are much delayed [6]. Referrals can be made to three different specialties—neurology, psychiatry, and geriatric medicine, with the choice of specialty depending on the availability and/or accessibility of specialists in specific health areas. Moreover, the choice may also depend on clinical issues. Thus, the oldest patients and/or patients with multimorbidity are commonly referred to geriatricians, whereas patients with behavioural disturbances or neurological symptoms are usually referred to psychiatrists or neurologists, respectively. Notwithstanding, the referral decision may depend on the level of involvement a specific service provider has in terms of dementia care. For example, some mental health services, or even some psychiatrists, avoid taking on the care of dementia patients and may themselves refer these patients to neurologists. In some mental health services, dementia units have been set up, with the involvement of neurologists, psychiatrists, and geriatricians, some on a full-time basis, in the care of dementia patients.

The following assessment techniques are routinely applied to confirm the diagnosis of dementia:

1. Neuroimaging, mainly CT scanning and MRI.

2. Neuropsychological assessments (not implemented in all hospitals) whereby a standard battery of neuropsychological tests are used to determine the patient's cognitive profile, which is particularly important among younger patients.

3. CSF analysis to assess for levels of total Tau (T-Tau), phosphorylated Tau (P-Tau), and Ab42, particularly in patients with focal dementia and MCI, as well as in those with a family history of dementia.

4. Genetic analysis, e.g. for the *APOE* gene, mainly in patients with a family history of dementia.

5. Nuclear medicine investigations: single-photon emission computerized tomography (SPECT), which may be used in patients with atypical clinical syndromes; FDG-PET in patients with atypical clinical symptoms and younger patients, or as part of differential diagnosis workup. Amyloid PET tests are sometimes performed primarily for research purposes.

Specialists are usually responsible for completing the diagnostic process, informing the patient and their family, and developing the treatment plan.

Pharmacological treatment

Pharmacotherapy is usually the first therapeutic intervention to be initiated. In cases of AD, specific treatment includes anticholinesterase inhibitors and/or memantine. All patients with dementia in Spain have access to treatment with these anti-dementia agents. These must be prescribed by psychiatrists, neurologists, or geriatricians, which requires the specific permission of the local department of health, based on a specific diagnosis of AD. Patient follow-up after initiation of pharmacotherapy and monitoring for adverse effects are commonly carried out by GPs. The latter are also in charge of preventive non-pharmacological treatment for cognitive impairment.

Non-pharmacological treatment

In general, the health service is not systematically involved in the development and application of non-pharmacological approaches. Although neurologists, psychiatrists, and geriatricians responsible for the diagnosis and treatment of patients with dementia, and even GPs, commonly recommend non-pharmacological interventions, it is a generic recommendation and these health professionals are not involved in this treatment approach. Deployment of these treatment measures, however, is probably difficult due to a lack of clinical psychologists in many health centres. As a result, although psychosocial strategies are recommended in clinical guidelines, their implementation is not common in Spain [7]. Moreover, some psychiatric departments have limited engagement in these non-pharmacological strategies.

By contrast, non-pharmacological treatments and psycho-social approaches are usually provided by Alzheimer's Family Organizations (including nursing homes and day centres), or non-profit organizations involved in dementia care. However, referral to these establishments is not a systematic and regulated process. Consequently, effective care coordination between pharmacological and non-pharmacological treatment provisions, as well as patient follow-up, is lacking, such that only in exceptional cases is there well-integrated care for patients with dementia.

Follow-up

Patient follow-up is undertaken either in primary care or in specialized centres. However, it is common for specialized centres to have long waiting lists. This results in patients and families often turning to other organizations involved in dementia care or to GPs, as they are more accessible for care provision. Nursing staff in care centres are commonly involved in the follow-up of patients with dementia through following the care plan set up by the team and also carry out assessment and provide early interventions, working alongside caregivers. Organizations involved in dementia care also advocate family caregiving and frequently provide educational programmes and family schools.

In some public health centres dedicated to dementia care in Spain, it is common to apply the methodology of case management focused on continuity of care, to allow effective use of social networks and even to provide adequate financial assistance, where needed, towards patients' living and care expenses. In relation to the follow-up of patients with dementia, one of the most important features linked to high costs and care burden is related to behavioural problems [8]. Studies conducted in Spain reported a very high use of low-dose antipsychotic medications, suggesting that insufficient training in psychosocial interventions contributes to excessive use of sedation in patients with behavioural disturbances.

And finally, during follow-up, functional assessments (e.g. finance management, driving, use of firearms, etc.) are commonly carried out by specialists or GPs to facilitate the patient's application for the disability certificate, so they can access social services or proceed to other applications for obtaining help [9].

In general, a patient's home is considered the most suitable initial setting for dementia care provision (community care), although a long-term care setting is the best option when patients develop higher dependency in activities of daily living [10, 11]. Moreover, the home care setup has been transforming in the last few years; rotation arrangements among family members to provide care for people with dementia are becoming increasingly common—a practice associated with the rejection of placement in long-term care institutions [12]. As a consequence, many relatives have the responsibility of caregiving for people with dementia, despite not receiving adequate support in many regions [13].

Palliative care

This is related to the terminal stage of dementia. In Spain, neurological services tend to have restricted involvement in follow-up, even from early stages, during the course of dementia treatment, and delegate the provision of palliative care to primary care, psychiatric, and/or geriatric services. The rationale is to provide more community support from primary care at this stage of the disease when treatment is less relevant and emphasis should be placed on providing support and better quality of life for the patient with dementia.

Differential features of dementia care in some Spanish regions

The approach applied to the initial phases of dementia care is shared by most regions in Spain, but specialized care and the authority to prescribe pharmacological treatment may vary. Thus, in some regions, only neurological services are allowed to prescribe drugs specifically for AD. In other regions, specialized dementia units are available, which are expected to receive referrals from primary care. These units are run by neurologists, psychiatrists, or geriatricians, frequently involve a multidisciplinary approach, and, as well as using the standard assessments available in the country, provide specialized neuropsychological evaluation of cognitive function. They also commonly provide non-pharmacological treatment and integrated treatment plans. However, the main barrier to accessing care from dementia units is that they are usually located centrally, mainly within tertiary referral hospitals/centres (i.e. far from many users), and not easily accessible from community care. Many nursing homes have also established special care units (SCUs), with personalized approaches specific to dementia patients' needs. However, there is no evidence that they are more efficient than the typical nursing homes, although the number of SCUs is progressively increasing [14].

In addition, there is a State Reference Centre for the Care of Persons with Alzheimer's Disease and other Dementias (CREA) covering the whole country. It is specialized in the neuropsychological assessment of patients with particular diagnostic complexity. It is also specialized in non-pharmacological interventions, but due to limited time availability, lengthy and integrated follow-up treatments are difficult to implement. However, this Centre is intensely involved in research and education on dementia. Similarly, different regions in Spain have well-structured public foundations, outside the national health system, aimed at improving the care of dementia. Their goals and approaches are similar to those of the CREA, although the majority of these foundations, such as the Reina Sofía Foundation or the Pascal Maragall Foundation, have an increased interest in research.

Unmet needs and challenges in the future of dementia care

Some positive features of dementia care in Spain should be underlined, of which one of the most relevant is the development of AD associations and the wide implementation of their services and initiatives. While coordination with the public care network is suboptimal, these associations have contributed largely to the implementation of non-pharmacological approaches.

Another positive feature of dementia care is the national law for supporting all people with unmet dependence needs. Under this law, people with dementia can use resources best suited to their needs and are subsequently reimbursed (either fully or partly) for the costs.[1] While this model is complex and the management difficult, it is working very well in most places in Spain.

On the other hand, one of the challenges to psychiatric services in Spain nowadays is for them to be more involved in the assessment and treatment of disorders traditionally called 'organic', in particular dementia [1]. To some extent, the mental health network has abandoned the care of dementia patients

---

[1] https://www.eurofound.europa.eu/observatories/emcc/case-studies/tackling-undeclared-work-in-europe/law-to-support-care-of-dependent-people-spain

or has taken on the responsibility for treating behavioural symptoms only. This discouraging trend is probably due to several reasons such as poor coordination between healthcare providers, different information according to disease stage, or even unsatisfactory community care from healthcare providers [15]. Indeed, the mental health network, by working more closely with primary care centres than other medical specialties, as is the case for other mental disorders, should help to improve timely diagnosis, the application of comprehensive interventions, the facilitation of home care, and close follow-up of patients, particularly in rural areas that are often deprived of care access in this country.

Furthermore, in Spain, there are only a few specialized care centres, and those that exist usually have long waiting lists or low capacity, a situation which has not improved in the last years [13], despite complaints and the need for such care facilities.

It is also necessary to establish a National Dementia Care Plan to provide, as well as ensure, a minimum standard of care throughout the country and to promote full integration of both pharmacological and non-pharmacological treatment provisions for dementia. Importantly, there should be coordination of activities (care, training, and research) within the CREA,[2] and regional governments should encourage the development of public foundations dedicated to dementia.

Concerning the assessment and diagnostic process of dementia patients, we support a new trend towards reducing the current overemphasis on the biological and somatic aspects of dementia when evaluating patients and focusing more on the psychosocial and neuropsychological aspects, including assessing caregivers' needs, which is done very rarely nowadays. We consider it crucial to document the cognitive profile of patients with dementia, to better design and implement a strategic, integrated treatment plan. Non-pharmacological treatments should be incorporated in the integrated plan, while a reduction in the use of tranquillizers for behavioural disturbances would be a welcome move. Social interventions should also be planned and implemented and certainly include patients' families, which is important when applying non-pharmacological strategies [1]. Similarly, monitoring and adaptation of treatment plans according to the stage of dementia are considered to be very relevant, as well as better implementation of assessments using instruments such as the Rai-Long Care or RAI-Home Care as part of patients' follow-up [16, 17].

Finally, particular emphasis has been placed in Spain on improved provision of information and support to caregivers and on encouraging optimism

---

[2] http://www.crealzheimer.es/crealzheimer_06/centro/presentacion/index.htm

to promote extension of care at home for people with dementia [18]. Three decades after dementia was first highlighted as a major concern by the three main specialties involved in dementia care—neurology, geriatric medicine, and psychiatry, the latter also including the development of a psycho-geriatric model—what has changed the most since has been the general realization of the scale of the 'epidemic of the twenty-first century'.

References

1. Mateos R, Franco M, Sanchez M. Care for dementia in Spain: the need for a nationwide strategy. *International Journal of Geriatric Psychiatry*. 2010;**25**:881–4.

2. Lobo A, Saz P, Quintanilla MA. Dementia. In: Levenson JL (ed). *Textbook of psychosomatic medicine*. Washington: American Psychiatric Press; 2011. p. 115–51.

3. Olazaran J. [Can dementia be diagnosed in primary care?] *Atencion primaria*. 2011;**43**:377–84.

4. Olazaran J, Torrero P, Cruz I, *et al*. Mild cognitive impairment and dementia in primary care: the value of medical history. *Family Practice*. 2011;**28**:385–92.

5. Hallberg IR, Cabrera E, Jolley D, *et al*. Professional care providers in dementia care in eight European countries; their training and involvement in early dementia stage and in home care. *Dementia*. 2016;**15**:931–57.

6. Coll de Tuero G, Garre-Olmo J, Lopez-Pousa S, *et al*. [Perception, attitudes and needs of Primary Care professionals as regards the patient with dementia]. *Atencion primaria*. 2011;**43**:585–94.

7. Vasse E, Vernooij-Dassen M, Cantegreil I, *et al*. Guidelines for psychosocial interventions in dementia care: a European survey and comparison. *International Journal of Geriatric Psychiatry*. 2012;**27**:40–8.

8. Farre M, Haro JM, Kostov B, *et al*. Direct and indirect costs and resource use in dementia care: a cross-sectional study in patients living at home. *International Journal of Nursing Studies*. 2016;**55**:39–49.

9. Márquez F, Mateos R. Practice of competence assessment in dementia: Spain. In: Stoppe G (ed). *Competence assessment in dementia*. New York, NY: Springer Wien; 2008. pp. 155–69.

10. Risco E, Zabalegui A, Miguel S, Farre M, Alvira C, Cabrera E. [Application of the Balance of Care model in decision-making regarding the best care for patients with dementia]. *Gaceta sanitaria*. 2017;**31**:518–23.

11. Tucker S, Brand C, Sutcliffe C, *et al*. What makes institutional long-term care the most appropriate setting for people with dementia? Exploring the influence of client characteristics, decision-maker attributes, and country in 8 European nations. *Journal of the American Medical Directors Association*. 2016;**17**:465 e9–15.

12. Rivera J, Bermejo F, Franco M, Morales-Gonzalez JM, Benito-Leon J. Understanding care of people with dementia in Spain: cohabitation arrangements, rotation and rejection to long term care institution. *International Journal of Geriatric Psychiatry*. 2009;**24**:142–8.

13. Gil-Gregorio P, Regidor-Garcia J, Arriola-Manchola E, Garcia-Navarro JA, Ruipérez-Cantera I. Concerns of the Spanish Society of Geriatrics and Gerontology regarding

care received by patients with dementia. *Journal of the American Geriatrics Society.* 2007;**55**:1314–15.

14. **Crespo M, Hornillos C, Gomez MM.** Dementia special care units: a comparison with standard units regarding residents' profile and care features. *International Psychogeriatrics.* 2013;**25**:2023–31.

15. **Risco E, Cabrera E, Farre M, Alvira C, Miguel S, Zabalegui A.** Perspectives about health care provision in dementia care in Spain: a qualitative study using focus-group methodology. *American Journal of Alzheimer's Disease and Other Dementias.* 2016;**31**:223–30.

16. **Guthrie DM, Pitman R, Fletcher PC,** *et al.* Data sharing between home care professionals: a feasibility study using the RAI Home Care instrument. *BMC Geriatrics.* 2014;**14**:81.

17. **Lix LM, Yan L, Blackburn D,** *et al.* Agreement between administrative data and the Resident Assessment Instrument Minimum Dataset (RAI-MDS) for medication use in long-term care facilities: a population-based study. *BMC Geriatrics.* 2015;**15**:24.

18. **Contador I, Fernandez-Calvo B, Palenzuela DL, Campos FR, Rivera-Navarro J, de Lucena VM.** A control-based multidimensional approach to the role of optimism in the use of dementia day care services. *American Journal of Alzheimer's Disease and Other Dementias.* 2015;**30**:686–93.

Chapter 35

Sweden

Vesna Jelic, Per-Olof Sandman,
and Lars-Olof Wahlund

Summary

Care for the elderly and people with dementia is an important
part of a general welfare system in Nordic countries, particularly
in Sweden. A specific characteristic of the welfare system is that
it is in the main publicly funded, and care services are also under
government supervision. Another feature of the Nordic model
of care for the elderly is that it has a long tradition of in-home
support services for older people. This chapter gives an overview
of relevant demographics and milestones in the development of
a National Dementia Strategy and current National Guidelines on
the care and nursing of people with dementia, as well as results of
their recent evaluation. The chapter concludes with a discussion of
some future challenges in dementia care.

Background

Sweden is the largest Nordic country and one of the largest countries in Europe,
with respect to the geographical area. The country is sparsely populated, with
a population of about 9.8 million people. The total life expectancy at birth is
81.1 years, well above the average life expectancy at birth of the global population, which makes Sweden among the 'oldest' countries in the world with respect to the mean age of its citizens. Around 20% of the Swedish population is
older than 65 years, and the age dependency ratio (the ratio of people above the
working age of 65 years to the workforce of a country) is 30.4% [1].

As in other developed countries, the contracting type of population pyramid
results in an increasing number of people with dementia. The prevalence of
dementia in Sweden is approximately 180,000, including approximately 10,000
cases with early-onset dementia, and the incidence is about 25,000 cases per

year. Societal costs for dementia care are increasing correspondingly, from about 38 billion SEK in 2000 to about 50 billion SEK in 2005 and 63 billion SEK in 2012 [2].

Milestones in the development of dementia care in Sweden

Municipalities introduced already in 1950 in-home care for the elderly. In 1992, an important reform of the health and welfare system—the Ädel reform (*Ädelreformen*)—made clearer the responsibility for people with long-term and complex needs for healthcare [3]. The reform intended to meet, in a cohesive way, the social and medical needs of this vulnerable group. Municipalities took overall responsibility for healthcare in special forms of accommodation and daily care. Most of long-term care and a large part of home care were transferred to the municipal elderly care, including care for people with dementia. The county council kept responsibility for primary, secondary and tertiary medical care. Due to engagements of municipalities in extended medical care, the time allocated to inpatient specialist ward services has been shortened considerably.

In Sweden today, there are about 90,000 places in various forms of institutional living for the elderly. About 70% of these places are occupied by people with dementia. It is estimated that approximately 25,000 people have access to housing specifically built for the care of people with dementia—so-called group homes. Others are in nursing homes or sheltered accommodation. The annual turnover of these places is about 30%. The medical responsibility for special accommodation generally lies within primary care, but there is a strong desire that physicians with geriatric competence should assume this responsibility. A thorough regular review of medications, aimed at reducing cognitively harmful drugs and optimizing others, is under way in the country.

Over the past 25 years, the number of beds for people with dementia has declined rather sharply, which means that an increasing proportion of these people are cared for in their own homes, with the support of the family and home care services. Some municipalities have special home care teams, established with the sole task of providing services to people with dementia.

With an increased amount of informal care for people with dementia, a great emphasis is placed on the care of relatives. In many places in Sweden, there are consultants and training programmes about dementia illnesses for relatives. There are also opportunities for people with dementia to stay in short-term accommodation to allow their relatives temporary respite from care burden.

During the last decade, a significant change has taken place in that more and more of primary, as well as specialist, care is being transferred to private companies. All care and accommodation for people with dementia are still provided by municipalities. This means that there are two principals responsible for patients with dementia. This is not without its problems, particularly in larger municipalities, and cooperation between the two principals is given high priority in the National Board of Health and Welfare guidelines in order to ensure that the important care chain is not damaged or broken.

National Guidelines

The National Board of Health and Welfare published in 2010 National Guidelines on the care and nursing of people with dementia [4]. This document provides evidence-based guidelines for diagnosis, treatment, care, and nursing. The responsibility for the investigation and pharmacological treatment of people with dementia lies within the county councils. All people with suspected cognitive impairment should undergo a dementia assessment. The first contact normally takes place in primary care where a baseline assessment is carried out. If no diagnosis can be established after a baseline evaluation, or when the investigation is complex, the primary care physician will refer the patient for an extended investigation that takes place at a memory clinic with geriatric expertise.

The guidelines put emphasis on person-centred care where the patient's lifestyle, values, and preferences are in focus, rather than the disease itself. A key principle in the care of dementia patients is that they can live at home for as long as possible, which means that the municipality provides home help, food supplies, opportunities to travel to and from daily activities, and opportunities for short-term accommodation for respite to the relatives. District nurses are responsible for the provision of medications, and it is primary care physicians, in particular, who are responsible for the necessary annual follow-ups.

National Guidelines—evaluation

The National Guidelines have had a major impact. However, there are also shortcomings, both in terms of assessment, treatment, nursing care, and support given [5]. All these issues differ at large across the country. Furthermore, it appears that socio-economic conditions, such as education and country of birth, affect the treatment and care provided.

These are some of the main findings of the Board's evaluation of health and social care for people with dementia:

- Less than half of patients being investigated in primary care undergo a complete baseline dementia assessment, and nearly half have a non-specific dementia diagnosis.

- The number of registered dementia investigations and prescriptions of anti-dementia drugs differ greatly between counties.

- Among people with lower levels of education and those born outside the Nordic countries, there are a smaller number receiving treatment with anti-dementia drugs. However, they are more often treated with antipsychotics.

- County councils and municipalities need to provide regular training and guidance for staff working in health and social care for people with dementia.

- The number of places in special dementia care facilities have increased but varies considerably between municipalities.

The Svedish Dementia Registry (SveDem)

The Swedish Dementia Registry (SveDem) is a national quality registry on dementia disorders. SveDem is financed by the Swedish Association of Local Authorities and Regions and the Swedish Brain Power network [6]. SveDem was launched in May 2007. The aim is for a registry with national coverage. Patients newly diagnosed with a dementia disorder are registered and followed up annually. Age, gender, heredity, body mass index (BMI), MMSE scores, diagnoses, dementia workup investigations, medical treatment, support from the community, and time from referral to diagnosis are examples of parameters that are entered into the web-based registry. The registry, which can be used for open comparisons and research, includes primary care, specialist care, and sheltered housing. It is currently the world's largest registry of its kind.

Until 2014, data on diagnosis, care, and treatment of 47,757 patients with dementia have been recorded from 1100 connected centres throughout the country. More than 90% of all memory clinics in Sweden are currently participating in SveDem.

SveDem has provided a number of quality parameters:

- Time from referral to initiation of workup: aim for 1 month—currently 40 days.

- Time from initiation of workup to diagnosis: aim for 1 month—currently 56 days.

- Over 90% of patients undergoing baseline dementia workup according to national guidelines—currently 78%.

- 90% of patients diagnosed with AD should be treated with cholinesterase inhibitors—currently 76%.

- 100% of patients should be followed up once a year.

- No gender differences in care.

- Almost half of newly diagnosed patients (48%) are living alone.

SveDem will lead to improvement in diagnostics, workup, support, and treatment at local and national levels. Memory clinics adhere well to national guidelines concerning baseline dementia workup, but one challenge is to implement the registry in primary care centres.

Dementia centre

About 5 years ago, a Swedish dementia centre was founded with the purpose of gathering and disseminating evidence-based and best-proven expertise in the field of dementia. An important step has been to start online education for nursing staff, based on the guidelines published by the National Board of Health and Welfare in 2010. In January 2012, nearly 30,000 people had completed the education programme.

Future challenges

While the National Guidelines have harmonized care and nursing of people with dementia in Sweden regarding how evidence-based medical care and nursing should be implemented, there are still issues of concern. An increase in private provision of accommodation and in-home services does not necessarily mean better care. On the contrary, focus on profits has resulted in suboptimal care.

The demographics of Sweden are changing at a fast pace, and dementia care provided by municipalities should be adapted to different cultural backgrounds. There is a need for more formal and continuing education of non-medical personnel providing home care and assistance.

In the future, we will have to focus also on the growing number of patients on the other end of the dementia continuum—those in the early clinical phases of the disease. These patients are most often younger, some even still capable of working to some extent and hence not suitable clientele for daily care. At the moment, neither the healthcare system nor municipalities can offer an individually adjusted programme as compensation for a patient's lost social contact with their working environment during long sick leaves.

Finally, by applying the Diagnostic and Statistical Manual of Mental Disorders, fifth edition (DSM-5) diagnostic criteria in clinical practice, the term dementia will no longer be used. Both the general public and bureaucracy of the healthcare system will have to adapt to new etymology and translate it in each individual case into the need for adequate support.

References

1. **Central Intelligence Agency**. *World factbook 2011*. Washington, DC: Central Intelligence Agency; 2011.

2. **Socialstyrelsen**. *Demenssjukdomarnas samhällskostnader i Sverige 2012*. Article no. 2014-6-3. Stockholm: Socialstyrelsen; 2014.

3. **Socialstyrelsen**. *Ädelreformen: Slutrapport*. Article no. 1996-15-2. Stockholm: Socialstyrelsen; 1996.

4. **Socialstyrelsen**. *Nationella riktlinjer för vård och omsorg vid demenssjukdom 2010*. Article no. 2010-5-1. Stockholm: Socialstyrelsen; 2010.

5. **Socialstyrelsen**. *Nationell utvärdering—Vård och omsorg vid demenssjukdom 2014*. Article no. 2014-2-4. Stockholm: Socialstyrelsen; 2014.

6. **Nationella Kvalitetsregister**. *National Quality Registry for Dementia (SveDem)*. Available from:http://kvalitetsregister.se/englishpages/findaregistry/registerarkivenglish/national qualityregistryfordementiasvedem.2159.html [accessed 22 August 2018].

Chapter 36

Switzerland

Florian Riese

Summary

It is estimated that 110,000 people in Switzerland are affected by dementia. Access to professional dementia care is good. The Swiss mandatory health insurance extensively covers medical inpatient and outpatient treatment and the cost of medicines, as well as nursing care. Due to the decentralized organization of the Swiss political and healthcare systems, variation exists in dementia services across the country and there are no nationwide integrated care pathways and no disease registry. Despite the availability of 36 memory clinics, the majority of dementia cases are diagnosed and treated outside specialized services. In 2013, a National Dementia Strategy was initiated to promote the expansion, improvement, and standardization of services. Dementia research in Switzerland is particularly strong in neurobiology, while clinical and health services research is only recently receiving more attention. There are three aspects of its dementia care of which Switzerland is particularly proud: (1) the healthcare system offers access to high-quality acute and long-term dementia care covered by mandatory health insurance, (2) dementia is widely accepted as a public health priority in the ageing Swiss society, and (3) Switzerland initiated a National Dementia Strategy in 2013 that is currently in its implementation phase. In terms of improvement, dementia care pathways could improve the coordination of care between sectors and reduce regional variation in care. Family members and informal caregivers need to be recognized more and supported in their work, and planning of care could be facilitated by creating epidemiological databases on dementia.

The Swiss healthcare system

In Switzerland, the responsibility for healthcare service planning and delivery lies with the 26 cantons. The cantons are also partly responsible for healthcare funding by subsidizing hospitals and insurance premiums. In contrast, the federal government issues health legislation and regulates the health insurance market [1]. This division of responsibilities and the decentralized management of healthcare make 'top-down' implementation of changes to service provision difficult, which leads to variation in services. Service providers, as well as health insurances, compete on the healthcare market, and the Swiss population has repeatedly voted in favour of retaining consumer choice [1]. The overall performance of the Swiss healthcare system is among the best among OECD (Organization for Economic Cooperation and Development) countries [2].

Most medical and nursing care (including dementia care) is covered by the Swiss mandatory health insurance. This includes hospital treatment, outpatient medical treatment, home care nursing, physical therapy, the cost of medicines, and other treatments. The cost of long-term care in nursing homes is split between health insurance (medical and nursing care) and out-of-pocket payments (housing, food, non-nursing services). So far, there is no insurance specifically for long-term care. The total cost of dementia for Switzerland was calculated to be CHF 6.9 billion in 2009. The direct cost of dementia amounted to CHF 3.9 billion, representing 6.4% of total Swiss healthcare costs in 2009 [3].

The Swiss National Dementia Strategy 2014–2017

An ageing society, the increase of single-person households, international migration, and increasing demands regarding availability and flexibility at the workplace are key challenges for the future of dementia care in Switzerland. Consequently, increasing political awareness of the importance of dementia for the Swiss society led to the creation of a National Dementia Strategy, which was published in 2013 [4]. The Strategy identifies projects in four main fields of action: (1) health competence, information, and participation, (2) demand-oriented services, (3) quality and professional competence, and (4) data and knowledge transfer. Notably, due to the decentralized organization of healthcare and the distribution of political responsibility between cantons and the federal government, the Dementia Strategy is not accompanied by federal project funding. Projects are initiated locally and may only be implemented more widely if they demonstrate success.

Epidemiology of dementia in Switzerland

Because there is no national registry, the exact prevalence and incidence of dementia in Switzerland are unknown. Based on extrapolations of prevalence data from other countries, it is estimated that there are currently 110,000 people with dementia in Switzerland [4]. This number is expected to increase to 190,000 by 2030. However, this projection does not yet account for the recent findings of a decreased dementia prevalence and incidence in several countries [5–7]. In terms of incident dementia, the annual number of cases is estimated to be 25,000 [4]. Similar to the total number of dementia cases, the exact number for special populations, such as early-onset forms of dementia or dementia in intellectual disabilities, is unknown [4, 8].

About half of people affected by dementia in Switzerland live at home [4]. Professional care for this population includes day care centres, day clinics, and home care nursing—which is reimbursed by the mandatory health insurance. However, the majority of care at home is provided by family members, of which more than 50% are older than 70 years [4]. The associated caregiver burden is high, and more than 50% of caregivers want additional support [9]. The Swiss Alzheimer Society and other organizations and institutions organize support groups for caregivers [10]. In Swiss nursing homes, approximately two-thirds of residents either have a dementia diagnosis or are suspected to have dementia [11, 12]. Most nursing homes provide dementia care in mixed units, i.e. residents with and without dementia live on the same floor [13]. However, institutions specialized in long-term care for advanced dementia also exist (e.g. Sonnweid nursing home in the vicinity of Zurich [14]).

Dementia care in Switzerland

The need to create integrated dementia care pathways from early diagnosis to palliative care is recognized in the Federal Council's health-policy priorities ('Health 2020') [15]. Yet, no such care pathways currently exist due to the organization of the Swiss healthcare system. Furthermore, the level of available care varies geographically. By contrast, access to dementia services for the individual patient is usually not limited by financial constraints—due to coverage of most dementia care by the mandatory health insurance.

Mirroring current practice, a consensus paper in 2012 assigned a role for both GPs and specialists (i.e. geriatricians, old age psychiatrists, neurologists) in dementia diagnosis and treatment [11]. Clinical diagnosis of dementia is made according to the International Classification of Diseases, tenth revision (ICD-10), and the Swiss Memory Clinics organization has recently issued guidelines for the diagnostic process [16]. At present, there are 36 memory clinics in Switzerland. They are unevenly distributed among regions and have a diagnostic capacity of only about 5000 cases per year [4]—indicating that only a minority of incident dementia cases are diagnosed in specialized services.

Several inter-professional outreach teams have been set up to provide dementia diagnosis and ongoing treatment at home. Even though there are activities for a wider implementation, these outreach teams currently operate only on a pilot basis.

In Switzerland, dementia itself rarely is a reason for hospital admission. However, about 50,000 patients with dementia are annually admitted to Swiss hospitals for other diagnoses [4]. Since dementia may interfere with the normal proceeding in hospital, this presents a particular, and currently often unresolved, challenge in terms of care provision. At present, palliative care standards for the terminal stage of dementia are not systematically implemented in the outpatient setting or in nursing homes. However, the Swiss National Palliative Care strategy endorses the need for palliative care in this population [17].

With respect to pharmacological treatment, the two types of anti-dementia drugs (cholinesterase inhibitors and memantine) are reimbursed by the mandatory health insurance. However, only about 130,000 packages of these medications were sold in 2009 [4]. Thus, it is very likely that not all potentially eligible patients are treated with anti-dementia drugs. For the treatment of behavioural and psychological symptoms of dementia, guidelines have been recently produced [18]. While the use of antipsychotic medications is discussed critically in these guidelines, these drugs continue to be recommended for the treatment of agitation in dementia. Antipsychotics appear to be used in up to 70% of Swiss nursing home residents with dementia [19]. By contrast, no systematic information is available on the use of non-pharmacological dementia treatments in Switzerland [4].

Dementia research in Switzerland

Dementia research in Switzerland has a strong focus on basic research on neurodegenerative diseases. Clinical research and health services research in the field of dementia have only recently gained more attention, as a consequence of the National Dementia Strategy [4]. Similar to the organization of dementia care, dementia research in Switzerland is decentralized. No national research centre for dementia or AD exists in Switzerland, even though the National Centre of Competence in Research on Neural Plasticity and Repair (NCCR Neuro) was funded at the University of Zurich and the Swiss Federal Institute of Technology Zurich from 2001 to 2013 [20]. Internationally, Switzerland is involved in the European Union's JPND [21].

References

1. **Biller-Andorno N, Zeltner T.** Individual responsibility and community solidarity: the Swiss health care system. *New England Journal of Medicine.* 2015;**373**:2193–7.

2. **Organization for Economic Cooperation and Development (OECD).** *OECD reviews of health systems: Switzerland (2011).* Paris: OECD Publishing; 2011.

3. **Ecoplan.** *Kosten der Demenz in der Schweiz.* Bern: Ecoplan; 2010.

4. **Bundesamt für Gesundheit (BAG), Schweizerische Konferenz der kantonalen Gesundheitsdirektorinnen und-direktoren (GDK).** *Nationale Demenzstrategie 2014–2019,* BAG-Publication no. 2016-GP17. Bern: BAG and GDK; 2016.

5. **Matthews FE, Arthur A, Barnes LE,** *et al.* A two-decade comparison of prevalence of dementia in individuals aged 65 years and older from three geographical areas of England: results of the Cognitive Function and Ageing Study I and II. *The Lancet.* 2013;**382**:1405–12.

6. **Christensen K, Thinggaard M, Oksuzyan A,** *et al.* Physical and cognitive functioning of people older than 90 years: a comparison of two Danish cohorts born 10 years apart. *The Lancet.* 2013;**382**:1507–13.

7. **Satizabal CL, Beiser AS, Chouraki V, Chêne G, Dufouil C, Seshadri S.** Incidence of dementia over three decades in the Framingham Heart Study. *New England Journal of Medicine.* 2016;**374**:523–32.

8. **Wicki MT, Riese F.** Prevalence of dementia and organization of dementia care in Swiss disability care homes. *Disability and Health Journal.* 2016;**9**:719–23.

9. **Moor C.** *Menschen mit einer Demenz zuhause begleiten.* Zurich: Centre for Gerontology, University of Zurich; 2010.

10. **Alzheimer Schweiz.** Available from: http://www.alz.ch [accessed 22 May 2016].

11. **Monsch AU, Büla C, Hermelink M,** *et al.* [Consensus 2012—diagnosis and treatment of patients with dementia in Switzerland]. *Revue Médicale Suisse.* 2013;**9**:838–47.

12. **Anliker M, Bartelt G.** [Resident assessment instrument in Switzerland]. *Zeitschrift für Gerontologie + Geriatrie.* 2015;**48**:114–20.

13. **Saldutto B, Becker S, Imhof A.** *Demenzbetreuung in Stationären Alterseinrichtungen.* Bern: CURAVIVA Schweiz; 2013.

14. **Sonnweid.** Available from: http://www.sonnweid.ch/index.cfm/de/heim/portraet/ [accessed 22 May 2016].

15. **Federal Department of Home Affairs.** *The Federal Council's health-policy priorities.* Bern: Federal Office of Public Health; 2013.

16. **Bürge M, Bieri G, Brühlmeier M,** et al. Recommendations of Swiss Memory Clinics for the Diagnosis of Dementia. *Praxis.* 2018; **107**:435–51.

17. **Bundesamt für Gesundheit (BAG), Schweizerische Konferenz der kantonalen Gesundheitsdirektorinnen und-direktoren (GDK).** *Nationale Strategie Palliative Care 2013–2015.* Publication no. GP 10.12 3000 d 1500 f 30EXT1214. Bern: BAG and GDK; 2012.

18. **Savaskan E, Bopp-Kistler I, Buerge M,** *et al.* [Recommendations for diagnosis and therapy of behavioral and psychological symptoms in dementia (BPSD)]. *Praxis (Bern 1994).* 2014;**103**:135–48.

19. **Lustenberger I, Schüpbach B, Gunten von A, Mosimann U.** Psychotropic medication use in Swiss nursing homes. *Swiss Medical Weekly.* 2011;**141**:w13254.

20. NCCR Neural Plasticity and Repair. Available from: https://www.neuroscience.uzh.ch/en/about/history/NCCR-Neuro.html

21. JPND Research. Available from: http://www.neurodegenerationresearch.eu [accessed 22 May 2016].

Chapter 37

Turkey

Özlem Kuman Tunçel and Hayriye Elbi

Summary

Turkey has a rapidly ageing population, the issues of which
are new to the country. To date, there is no National Dementia
Strategy. The strong tradition of family caregiving in Turkey has
perhaps influenced the demand for access to formal care services.
Informal care provided by families, which includes living together
with the elders and providing the most comfort, is one of the
strongest aspects of dementia care in Turkey. Another positive
aspect is new legal regulation of the social security system for the
elderly. Moreover, there is an increasing awareness of dementia
and dementia care, which will hopefully give new impetus to
further advancements in dementia care. The future of dementia
care in Turkey should ideally include: (1) the development of
a National Dementia Strategy, (2) improvement of informal
care, including support for caregivers, and (3) an increase in
the number, as well as improved quality, of in-hospital geriatric
services.

Dementia care in Turkey

Turkey is a rapidly ageing country. According to 2017 population statistics, the
proportion of the population aged 65 years and over is 8.5% [1], and this is projected to increase to 10.2% by 2023, 16.3% by 2040, 22.6% by 2060, and 25.6%
by 2080 [2]. There has been increasing awareness of health issues relating to an
ageing population in recent years in Turkey, which were first mentioned in the
eighth 5-year development plan (2001–2005). To date, there is a no National
Dementia Strategy. Several objectives for patients with dementia have been incorporated into the National Plan of Action on Healthy Ageing (2015–2020)
[3], including: (1) to access acute and long-term treatment, (2) to help patients with dementia who attend hospital unaccompanied and to allocate a staff

member to assist the patient, (3) to authorize government attorneys to provide shelter and a safe place for dementia patients who are found alone on the streets or who are homeless, and (4) to provide educational programmes and rehabilitation support for the relatives of dementia patients.

Alzheimer Europe estimated the number of people with dementia in Turkey in 2012 to be 331,512, which represents 0.44% of the total population of 74,508,771 [4]. Dementia prevalence was found to be 0.8% in the 15 years and above age group and 5% in the 65 years and above age group, according to the Chronic Diseases and Risk Factors Survey in Turkey (2013), which also found no gender difference in terms of dementia prevalence [5]. In this study, two patients from each family physician list were selected by a random sampling method and were invited to the family healthcare centre. Of note, if we take into account the possible difficulty for patients with dementia to attend the family healthcare centre, this implies that the prevalence obtained in this survey would be lower than the actual prevalence in the community. The proportion of elderly people who died from AD increased from 3.4% to 4.5% between 2012 to 2016 [1]. However, there is no precise National Strategy to decrease it.

Anti-dementia drugs

In terms of pharmacological treatment for dementia, the costs of anti-dementia drugs (donepezil, rivastigmine, memantine, and galantamine) are covered by the Turkish reimbursement system, which does not necessitate any specific examination to be carried out for reimbursement. Anti-dementia drugs can be prescribed by psychiatrists, neurologists, or geriatricians, unless a medical report is available showing a formal diagnosis of dementia, in which case the drugs can be prescribed by any physician.

Nursing home care

In Turkey, there are a total of 350 nursing homes, with an occupancy rate of 80.4%. Of a population of 6,495,239 people aged 65 years and over in 2015, 23,132 were receiving nursing home care [6]. Although there is a shift in family structure away from the extended family to the smaller nuclear family, older people in need of care often live with their family, and institutionalization is very low in Turkey. This applies also to people with dementia. In the early stages of the disease, people with dementia usually compensate for their memory or behavioural problems. They mostly receive a diagnosis of dementia when their wife or husband dies and they move in with their children. Care is mainly provided by family members, mostly the daughters or daughters-in-law. Despite limited support from the government, families do their best to provide the most comfort to their elders. We can be proud of this informal care provided by families. This strong tradition of family caregiving has perhaps influenced the demand for access to formal care services, and seeking for these services is very late in Turkey. Some families who have the financial means employ a caregiver to live either in their house or in a house nearby. Until recently, caregivers in general were not trained in elderly care or dementia care. However, courses on elderly care are now available and provided by some municipalities and private sector organizations, and some universities also offer an Elder Care Associate Degree Programme. Therefore, the overall goal is to build a more qualified, educated, professional caregiving workforce for the elderly, and hopefully for people with dementia, in Turkey.

Most nursing homes in Turkey do not usually accept people with severe mental disorders and dementia, although some elderly people may develop dementia while living there. As part of the ninth 5-year development plan (2007–2013), policies for the promotion and support of care for older people living in their own homes are being developed. The first legislation focusing specifically on home care services came into force in 2005. The first step involved family physicians assuming primary responsibility for the provision of healthcare. This was followed by involvement of hospitals in home care services by 2010. The costs of home care services provided by the Ministry of Health are reimbursed by the social security system. However, excessive workload and abuse of the home care system have been described as major challenges by physicians who provide home care services. Moreover, the extent of home care services is not clearly defined. Therefore, current legislation needs to be changed, so it is compatible with current practice [7]. Despite abuse of the system, there are also patients who really need home care but are not aware of the system, and hence do not benefit from the service. Alternative private home care services are available for patients who have the financial means to afford such services.

The state provides financial support, albeit limited, to patients and families, although it is not easy to gather the necessary documents as part of the application process. If a patient has no income, depending on their disability scores, they (their guardians on their behalf) receive a disability pension. In addition, caregivers (relatives or guardians) are eligible to receive a home care allowance.

Social challenges

Currently, in addition to the challenge of improving home care service provision in Turkey, another challenge lies in the inadequate support for dementia patients' relatives who are caregivers. As mentioned previously, people with dementia mostly live with their family. Providing care for an elderly person with dementia in the long term likely results in care burden for the family caregiver, both physically and mentally, which, in turn, impacts on the care of the patient. To address caregiver burden, day care centres should be made available nationwide. For patients who are bedridden, access to qualified and reliable caregivers should be provided by the government, at affordable costs. Some municipalities have small-capacity dementia centres, but these are rare. Therefore, one of the objectives of the National Plan of Action on Healthy Aging (2015–2020) is to provide education and rehabilitation support for dementia patients' relatives. The effectiveness of the Plan in achieving this objective will be evaluated subsequently through satisfaction surveys of both patients and caregivers.

A further challenge relates to inadequate support provision in crisis situations. One potential solution is the development of a support service specifically for emergency situations; this would help to minimize hospitalization and enable patients to remain at home safely, as well as provide relief to caregivers. Moreover, there is also scarcity of geriatric services which are unevenly distributed across the country.

Preventive care for the elderly is very weak in Turkey. Although we are very close to our elders who also enjoy considerable respect in, and close ties with, the community, our culture does not support active ageing. Our lifestyle mostly consists of inactive daily living, including leisure time. Strategies to encourage older people to participate in sports and physical activity are needed. Accessible and affordable sport facilities, which are appropriately adapted for elderly people, should be established.

References

1. Turkish Statistical Institute. *İstatistiklerle Yaşlılar 2017*. Ankara: Turkish Statistical Institute; 2018. Available from: http://www.tuik.gov.tr/PreHaberBultenleri.do?id=27595 [accessed 17 August 2018].

2. Turkish Statistical Institute. *Population projections 2018–2080*. Available from http://www.turkstat.gov.tr/PreHaberBultenleri.do?id=30567 [accessed 17 August 2018].

3. Public Health Agency of Turkey. *Türkiye Sağlıklı Yaşlanma Eylem Planı ve Uygulama Programı 2015–2020*. Publication no. 960. Ankara: Republic of Turkey Ministry of Health; 2015.

4. Alzheimer Europe. *Dementia in Europe yearbook 2013*. Luxembourg: Alzheimer Europe; 2013.

5. Republic of Turkey Ministry of Health. *Chronic diseases and risk factors survey in Turkey*. Publication No 909. Ankara: Republic of Turkey Ministry of Health; 2013.

6. TurkStat. *Address-based population registration system 2015*. Ankara: Turkish Statistical Institute; 2015.

7. Aksoy H, Kahveci R, Doner P, *et al.* Physicians' attitudes toward home healthcare services in Turkey: a qualitative study. *European Journal of General Practice*. 2015;21:246–52.

Chapter 38

Wales

Bob Woods

Summary

This chapter documents the developments in Wales relating to a National Dementia Vision and Strategy. A new Strategy was promised by December 2016, but was finally published in February 2018. While activity and progress are evident in many areas, much remains to be done. Wales benefits from having an Older People's Commissioner, a statutory voice for older people, including those living with dementia, and from its rich cultural, linguistic, and artistic heritage, with active third-sector organizations. Like many countries, Wales has had well-publicized scandals in relation to quality of care in hospitals and care homes, which have provided learning and impetus for development. Compared with other parts of the United Kingdom, dementia diagnosis rates in Wales appear low and are now the subject of government targets. The new Strategy will need to fully engage with people living with dementia in order to address these challenges, while building on the growing social movement of dementia-friendly communities.

Introduction

Wales is a country of just over 3 million people within the UK. The National Assembly for Wales has had, since 1999, devolved responsibility for health and social care, among other domains. This has opened the way for divergence in policy and practice between Wales and the other UK countries, with the relative strengths and weaknesses of the National Health Service(s) (NHS) in England and Wales becoming politically contentious at times when the Westminster Government is formed by a different political party from that in Wales.

The majority of the population live in the South of the country, an area once an industrial powerhouse built around coal and steel industries, of which only vestiges remain. The remainder of the country is largely rural, with farming and tourism as the major industries. In the North and West of Wales, the Welsh language is widely used and has strong cultural significance. The relative deprivation of large areas of North and West Wales have been recognized in significant inputs from European Union structural funds over many years.

A dementia strategy?

In most countries, it is relatively straightforward to determine whether a dementia strategy exists or not, but in Wales, this has become a contentious issue. Work undertaken for the Welsh Government between 2008 and 2010 took, as its basis, that there were already more than enough strategies—what was required was action and implementation [1]. This work resulted in the publication of a 'National Dementia Vision for Wales' in 2011 [2]. Published under the joint banner of the Welsh Assembly Government and the Alzheimer's Society, the Vision was subtitled 'Dementia Supportive Communities'. The Vision included six commitments:

1. To improve services.
2. To improve information.
3. To raise awareness.
4. To improve training.
5. To support research.
6. To work towards a long-term vision.

Some years later, there is no doubt that actions promised in relation to each commitment have been progressed. In 2010, funding was announced for dementia coordinators in each Health Board and for dedicated services for younger people with dementia. These posts—albeit thinly spread—are still evident and are additional to previous services. Information packs were made available in Memory Clinics for all those newly diagnosed, and selected books for caregivers and people with dementia made available through 'Book prescription' schemes in libraries. Awareness raising, especially through health promotion, has been supported. Training in dementia care has been made more widely available, with Health Boards set ambitious targets for more than half of their staff to have received dementia training at a level appropriate to their role. Research has been supported through, for example, Welsh Government infrastructure funding for NEURODEM Cymru, the Wales Dementias and Neurodegenerative Diseases Research Network (2005–2015), and subsequently the Centre for Ageing and Dementia Research (2015 onwards), a collaboration between the Universities of Swansea, Cardiff, and Bangor.

The commitment regarding a long-term vision contained three distinct goals:

1. Establishing a high-level dementia group to drive change in dementia services.

2. Improving care on general wards for those with dementia.

3. Ensuring that bilingual provision of services for those diagnosed with dementia is planned for.

Of these, considerable work has been undertaken in relation to general hospital wards, as part of the 1000 Lives Plus initiative (see further text), and work has been undertaken to ensure current cognitive assessment measures are available in Welsh (although good normative data are lacking). The 'high-level dementia group' has perhaps been the most difficult aspect to sustain, with driving coordinated change across six Health Boards and 22 Local Authorities (responsible for social care) proving a challenge in a context where much decision-making and prioritization of resources is devolved to a local level. Further tranches of funding for improving dementia care have been made available in the intervening years, e.g. in 2015 for link workers to work between primary care and Memory Clinics and for additional occupational therapy input to inpatient NHS wards, and in 2015, the Welsh Minister for Health signed Alzheimer Europe's Glasgow Declaration, indicating the Welsh Government's commitment to a planned, strategic approach to dementia care, e.g. through specific dementia-related actions in the Government's Mental Health Delivery Plan.

Following a concerted campaign by the Alzheimer's Society for Wales to have a Dementia Strategy, the incoming Welsh Government, elected in May 2016, announced that, by December 2016, it would introduce a dementia strategic plan to cover the period 2017–2019. In the event, after a period of consultation on a draft document, extensive involvement of people living with dementia and caregivers, and a call for a human rights approach to be at the core, the 'Dementia Action Plan for Wales 2018–2022' [3] was finally published in February 2018. This was accompanied by £10 million per annum of additional funding and is intended to set out the actions, with associated outcome measures, to be delivered by the Welsh Government and external partners which will support all those affected by dementia in Wales. It is interesting, but probably a matter of semantics, that the Welsh Government once again shied away from having the word 'Strategy' in the title of its document. Again, what matters is implementation and the establishment of a transparent linkage between strategy, actions, and funding, so that the document is not merely a matter of words. The active involvement of people living with dementia and caregivers in monitoring its implementation offers hope that it will be followed through.

Made in Wales

There are numerous high-quality projects and programmes in dementia care in Wales, but here, three with a distinct Welsh emphasis will be highlighted.

1. *1000 Lives plus* is the major quality improvement programme for the NHS in Wales. It sets out intervention packages to address selected drivers (e.g. improving memory assessment services) and encourages staff to work at a local level in quality improvement circles, collecting relevant data, identifying and implementing local solutions and strategies to improve services, and monitoring performance over time. For the dementia workstream, five drivers were selected in consultation with a forum of people with dementia and their caregivers, and developed with a range of practitioners, with the interventions drawing heavily on the NICE-Social Care Institute for Excellence (SCIE) Guideline on dementia [4], which defined best practice in dementia care for health and social care. The domains selected were:

   • Timely diagnosis—improving memory assessment services.

   • Care of people with dementia in general hospitals.

   • Reduction in the use of antipsychotic medication in people with dementia.

   • Enhanced support for family caregivers.

   • Improved quality of care and family involvement in NHS units for people with dementia.

   A number of resources were provided for local services, including a 'How to Guide' [5], and bilingual feedback surveys for family members. Regular national events and webinars were held to support teams working on these drivers. A number of workshops were held for GPs and care home managers in relation to reducing antipsychotic medication use. Attention to the general hospital domain was encouraged by participation in a UK-wide audit of dementia care in general hospitals, with each Health Board required to have an action plan in place to bring about improvements. Memory Assessment Services also participate in a national audit and meet annually to identify areas of concern and share good practice.

2. *Older People's Commissioner.*

   In 2008, Wales became the first country in the world to appoint a Commissioner for Older People, with a remit to act as an independent voice and champion for older people across Wales, advocating on their behalf. The Commissioner has wide-ranging powers, allowing her to hold to account Health Boards, Local Authorities, and the government in relation to services for older people, including those with dementia, and requiring these agencies to respond to, and act on, their recommendations. Although not specific to people with dementia, extensively researched reports on care of older people in general hospitals [6] and in residential care [7] have provided a perspective on practice, reflecting the views and experiences of those (literally) at the mercy of those providing the services. A recent report [8] seeks to reflect the voice of people with dementia and their caregivers. It concluded that knowledge and understanding of dementia are lacking among both professionals and the wider public, that dementia services in Wales need greater flexibility if they are to be effective in meeting people's needs, and that lack of coordination and cooperation between services results in unnecessary obstacles for people living with dementia and their caregivers. These are challenging conclusions, which the report makes a number of recommendations to address. People with dementia in Wales benefit greatly from having this statutory voice for older people, rather than having to rely only on campaign and advocacy groups, with no direct route into publicly funded services.

3. *cARTrefu.*

The third example of a programme with a distinct Welsh flavour is provided by 'cARTrefu', which engages older people in care homes in a variety of creative arts. cARTrefu is the Welsh word for 'to reside', so cARTrefu aims to embed arts within residential care. The initiative is led by a third-sector organization—Age Cymru, and while not specifically for people with dementia, it is likely that most participants do have dementia, given that the majority of care home residents are affected. Professional artists from four different fields (performing arts, visual arts, words, and music) have 2-month residencies in care homes across Wales, introducing residents to new experiences, as well as offering participation in some more familiar arts-based activities. Over 1000 art workshops were delivered in care homes around Wales (https://www.ageuk.org.uk/cymru/our-work/arts-and-creativity/cartrefu/), and the results of an evaluation were very positive. The aim is for care home staff to develop new skills by working alongside artists and have the confidence to utilize them in their day-to-day interaction and engagement with residents. The approach fits well with the Welsh culture of Eisteddfod where, locally and nationally, there is a tradition of performance and of music, poetry, and other arts, as well as a strong emphasis on involvement of the third sector in innovative service delivery.

Challenges

As is clear from the conclusions of the Older People's Commissioner's (2016) report [8], there remain many challenges to achieve high-quality dementia care services in Wales. A series of disturbing, detailed reports on 'scandals' in, respectively, general hospital care [9], a specific NHS unit for people with dementia [10], and a chain of care homes [11] have highlighted poor practice and instances of a shocking lack of dignity and respect. These reports were surrounded by extensive media coverage, with headlines such as 'Patients kept like animals in a zoo' (http://www.bbc.com/news/uk-wales-north-east-wales-32904599), and subsequent government apologies and reaction. Clearly, despite all the initiatives and action plans, systems have not been robust enough to ensure that people with dementia in Wales can be guaranteed acceptable levels of care either in NHS hospitals or in care home settings. Although training is often seen as the answer to such lapses in standards, the reports make clear that system and culture change are fundamental to ensuring quality care.

A second challenge relates to the perceived low rates of dementia diagnosis in Wales. The Alzheimer's Society has, for several years, published figures showing the number of people entered onto primary care dementia registers expressed as a proportion of the expected number of people with dementia in the locality, estimated from age-specific prevalence rates applied to the local age distribution. Wales has consistently had rates lower than the other UK nations. The rate reported by the Alzheimer's Society for 2014–2015 was 43.4%, compared with 48% for England. However, in England, increasing this rate has been a key target set by the government, e.g. in the Prime Minister's Challenge, and by 2016, the NHS in England was reporting a figure of 67%. The Welsh Government traditionally is generally less inclined to set performance targets but has now expressed the ambition to reach 50% in the 2015–2016 figures. The methodology for establishing these rates may be questioned, but an Alzheimer's Society's report [12] makes clear that there are major gaps in both how the diagnosis is shared and in the provision of post-diagnostic support and information.

Meeting the challenge

The new Dementia Strategy for Wales will doubtless include actions to address low diagnosis rates and improve post-diagnostic support, and Wales can learn lessons from the other UK nations in this respect. Providing good-quality care in hospital and care home settings is likely to continue to pose challenges, not least in view of the need to invest more resources in this endeavour. This is a result of the increasing numbers of people living with dementia in late life, who will have needs related to both their dementia and to a range of other health conditions, and the increased costs of care staff in a UK context where increases in minimum wages have a disproportionate effect on the care sector. This unfortunate reflection on the status of those who provide such valuable care for those people with dementia requiring personal care and support must be addressed in the levels of funding provided for care home placements by Local Authorities and NHS in Wales if the current system is to be sustainable.

More broadly, the new Strategy is likely to continue with the theme of Wales becoming a dementia-friendly nation, and there are certainly already indications across Wales of increasing awareness, with increasing numbers of the general public becoming 'Dementia Friends' and a number of towns and villages and other organizations committing themselves to working towards becoming 'Dementia-Friendly Communities'. The possible cost of increased awareness is shown in the finding from a Welsh Government survey published in February 2016 (http://www.wales.nhs.uk/news/40497) that 76% of people in Wales are worried about developing dementia in later life. This fear may provide an opportunity to engage more younger people in risk reduction, and this has been part of a Welsh Government campaign, encouraging six healthy lifestyle actions, including 'try new things', as well as the usual smoking and weight exhortations.

Self-advocacy by people with dementia is also showing welcome signs of development, with a culture change beginning to be evident where it is no longer acceptable to simply have caregivers of people with dementia on a planning or advisory group. High-profile TV programmes, such as a 2016 BBC Panorama showing the wide-ranging effects of dementia on Chris Roberts and his family living in North Wales, have helped to bring home the complexity of the issues involved and highlight how the person with dementia may well be able to make their own decisions and express their own views. The extent to which the future agenda for improving life for people with dementia and their caregivers is driven by those most affected will be a good guide to the success of the new Strategy and future actions.

References

1. **Woods B.** National Dementia Plan—Wales (commentary). *International Journal of Geriatric Psychiatry.* 2010;**25**:923–4.
2. **Welsh Assembly Government.** *National Dementia Vision for Wales: Dementia Supportive Communities.* Cardiff: Welsh Assembly Government; 2011. Available from: http://gov.wales/docs/dhss/publications/110302dementiaen.pdf [accessed 9 August 2018].
3. **Welsh Government.** *Dementia Action Plan for Wales: 2018–2022.* Cardiff: Welsh Government; 2018. Available from: http://gov.wales/docs/dhss/publications/ 180214dementiaen.pdf [accessed 9 August 2018].
4. **National Institute for Health and Clinical Excellence and the Social Care Institute for Excellence (NICE-SCIE).** *Dementia: supporting people with dementia and their carers in health and social care.* NICE-SCIE: Clinical Guideline 42. London: NICE-SCIE; 2006.

5. **1000 Lives Plus**. *Improving dementia care: how to guide 15*. Cardiff: 1000 Lives Plus (NHS Wales); 2010. Available from: http://www.1000livesplus.wales.nhs.uk/sitesplus/documents/1011/How%20to%20%2815%29%20Dementia%20%28Feb%202011%29%20Web.pdf [accessed 9 August 2018].

6. **Older People's Commissioner Wales**. *Dignified care—the experiences of older people in hospital in Wales*. Cardiff: Older People's Commissioner; 2011. Available from: http://www.olderpeoplewales.com/en/Reviews/dignity-and-respect.aspx [accessed 9 August 2018].

7. **Older People's Commissioner Wales**. *A place to call home: a review into the quality of life and care of older people living in care homes in Wales*. Cardiff: Older People's Commissioner; 2014. Available from: http://www.olderpeoplewales.com/en/reviews/residential_care_review.aspx [accessed 9 August 2018].

8. **Older People's Commissioner Wales**. *Dementia: more than just memory loss*. Cardiff: Older People's Commissioner; 2016. Available from: http://www.olderpeoplewales.com/en/Publications/pub-story/16-03-14/Dementia_More_Than_Just_Memory_Loss.aspx#.V9abJXo-gUM [accessed 9 August 2018].

9. **Andrews J, Butler M**. *Trusted to care*. Cardiff: Welsh Government; 2014. Available from: http://gov.wales/topics/health/publications/health/reports/care/?lang=en [accessed 9 August 2018].

10. **Donna Ockenden Ltd**. *External investigation into concerns raised regarding the care and treatment of patients, Tawel Fan Ward, Glan Clwyd Hospital*. Cardiff: NHS Wales; 2015. Available from: http://www.wales.nhs.uk/sitesplus/documents/861/tawel_fan_ward_ockenden_internet.pdf [accessed 9 August 2018].

11. **Flynn M**. *In search of accountability: a review of the neglect of older people living in care homes investigated as Operation Jasmine*. Cardiff: Welsh Government; 2015. Available from: http://gov.wales/topics/health/publications/socialcare/reports/accountability/?lang=en [accessed 9 August 2018].

12. **Alzheimer's Society**. *Diagnose or disempower: receiving a diagnosis of dementia in Wales*. London: Alzheimer's Society; 2015. Available from: https://www.alzheimers.org.uk/sites/default/files/migrate/downloads/diagnose_or_disempower.pdf [accessed 9 August 2018].

Section 5

North America

Chapter 39

Canada

Serge Gauthier

Summary

Canada has a long tradition of epidemiologic, basic, and clinical research in dementia, with a special interest in the vascular component of late-onset dementia. A National Dementia Strategy for Canada will set standards of care across the country, both for diagnosis and treatment, and will have to be adaptive to new diagnostic technologies and new treatments. Prevention for the lower-risk ageing population through education and healthy lifestyles is a clear path to go, whereas preventive treatments for higher-risk populations is a challenge that we are clearly dedicated to solve within the next decade.

Introduction: a historical perspective

Canada has a long tradition of research in neurological disorders such as AD and Parkinson's disease. The Canadian Study on Health and Aging was an epidemiological population-based study of people aged 65 years and over, linking all medical schools across the country, which gave us prevalence data on MCI (called at that time 'Cognitively Impaired Not Demented' or CIND) and on dementia in 1994, and incidence data after a 5-year follow-up [1, 2]. This study helped to create an academic consortium to facilitate randomized clinical trials in Canada [Consortium of Canadian Centers for Clinical Cognitive Research (C5R)], which has links with similar consortia in Asia, Europe, the United States, and Oceania [3]. The C5R has also interacted with the federal regulatory authorities for drug approval, using consensus meetings [4]. A strong interest in the vascular component of late-onset dementia has been encouraged by Vladimir Hachinski since the definition of multi-infarct dementia and of leukoaraiosis in the 1970s.

More recently, another consortium was created to accelerate research in AD and related dementias—the Canadian Consortium on Neurodegeneration in

Aging (CCNA), led by Howard Chertkow. In its first 4-year cycle, the CCNA put emphasis on translational research through a dedicated knowledge transfer team [5] and an Ethical, Legal, and Social Impact (ELSI) committee, looking, for instance, at the socio-economic impact of new drugs for AD [6]. The CCNA is part of a concerted effort from the Canadian Institutes for Health Research (CIHR) for a Dementia Research Strategy [7].

In terms of clinical practice guidelines, Canada has a tradition of consensus meetings with all stakeholders, including the Alzheimer Society of Canada, patients' representatives, and clinicians in the different disciplines caring for people with dementia. The latest meeting took place in 2012, with emphasis on new diagnostic criteria using biomarkers [8]. The next consensus conference will take place in 2019 and will address the proper use of biomarkers in the diagnosis of dementia and anticipate the needs for optimal use of new disease-modifying drugs in 2020.

Worldwide implication

Canada has been a key participant in the G8 global dementia initiative from 2013 to 2015, hosting one of the meetings in Ottawa. Yves Joanette is the director of the CIHR Institute on Aging and a member of the World Dementia Council, which is following on the First World Health Organization Ministerial Conference on Dementia where more than 90 countries have now signed in. This may facilitate the development of a comprehensive National Dementia Strategy for Canada, through an advisory committee, led by Pauline Tardif and William Reichman, which is currently studying various priorities for research, treatment, and prevention. Implementation of a federal plan will require harmonization between the ten provinces and two territories, which are responsible for medical care.

Future challenges

I am particularly proud of our interdisciplinary approach to dementia research and care, and the steady support of the Alzheimer Society of Canada for training new investigators from different fields—from occupational therapy to basic neurosciences. I am not as happy with the variability in access to diagnostic technology (only one province currently provides access to glucose PET imaging in atypical cases of cognitive decline, a bad omen for access to amyloid imaging in the near future) and the variability in reimbursement of the current symptomatic drugs, also a bad omen for reimbursement of future disease-modifying drugs.

Current challenges are not so much related to access to diagnosis once dementia is clinically manifested, but rather access to personalized and sustained care across the disease stages. Hopefully, the cancer and diabetes care models will prove useful, with well-trained nurse practitioners being available for long-term management. There is also disparity in home care support, even within cities, which will require better planning at the province level.

Conclusion

I have hope that a National Dementia Strategy for Canada will set standards of care across the country, both for diagnosis and treatment, and that it will prove to be adaptive to new diagnostic technology and new treatments. Prevention for the lower-risk ageing population through education and healthy lifestyles is a clear path to go, whereas preventive treatments for higher-risk populations is more of a challenge, which we are clearly dedicated to solve within the next decade.

References

1. The Canadian Study on Health and Aging. Study methods and prevalence of dementia. *Canadian Medical Association Journal.* 1994;**150**:899–913.
2. The Canadian Study of Health and Aging Working Group. The incidence of dementia in Canada. *Neurology.* 2000;**55**:66–73.
3. Gauthier S, Garcia A, Sano M, *et al.* Priorities for research consortia on Alzheimer's disease. *Alzheimer's and Dementia.* 2010;**6**:359–62.
4. Feldman H, Gauthier S, Chertkow H, Conn DK, Freedman M, MacKnight C, for the 2nd Conference on Antidementia Guidelines. Canadian guidelines for the development of antidementia therapies: a conceptual summary. *Canadian Journal of Neurological Sciences.* 2006;**33**:6–26.
5. Cook C, Rockwood K. Knowledge translation: an overview and recommendations in relation to the Fourth Canadian Consensus Conference on the Diagnosis and Treatment of Dementia. *Alzheimer's Research and Therapy.* 2013;**5**(Suppl 1):S6.
6. Tomaszewski S, Gauthier S, Wimo A, Rosa-Neto P. Combination therapy of anti-tau and anti-amyloid drugs for disease modification in early-stage Alzheimer's disease: social-economic considerations modeled on treatments for tuberculosis, HIV/AIDS and breast cancer. *Journal of Prevention of Alzheimer's Disease.* 2016;**3**:164–72.
7. Joanette Y, Gutman G, Muscedere J. Exploring the many facets of research in late-life issues. *Canadian Journal on Aging.* 2014;**33**:220–5.
8. Patterson C, Gauthier S. Diagnosis and treatment of dementia: the Fourth Canadian Consensus Conference. *Alzheimer's Research and Therapy.* 2013;**5**(Suppl 1):S1.

Chapter 40

Mexico

Federico Ramos Ruiz and Amador Ernesto
Macias Osuna

Summary

The world population is ageing at an accelerated pace. It is
estimated there are 900 million people aged 60 years or above
worldwide, and with the rise in life expectancy comes an increased
prevalence of chronic diseases such as dementia. In September
2015, Alzheimer's Disease International reported a total of
46.8 million people with dementia worldwide, which is expected
to increase to 74.7 million and 135.1 million by 2030 and
2050, respectively. Dementia also has a tremendous worldwide
economic impact on health systems. In 2015, the total cost of
dementia care was 818 billion dollars, representing an increase of
35.4% from 2010.

Current dementia care in Mexico

According to the Health and Nutrition National Survey conducted in 2012,
an estimated total of 860,000 people suffer from dementia in Mexico. Several
initiatives have been taken over the few decades to address the problem of
dementia in the country. In 1988, the first support group for relatives—the
Mexican Association of Alzheimer and Related Disorders AC (AMAES)—
was established in Mexico City. In 1993, the Instituto Nacional de Ciencias
Médicas y Nutrición introduced the first programme in geriatric medicine
as part of the training of medical doctors in geriatric medicine. In 2002,
the Alzheimer associations in Mexico were integrated to form the Mexican
Federation of Alzheimer, with the aim to provide families with information
and education about AD and its care. Moreover, in 2003, Mexico became one
of the founding members of Alzheimer Ibero América, an organization with

the purpose of uniting efforts from its member countries in raising awareness of AD in this region, both at the public and government levels. Finally, in
2011, on the occasion of the World Alzheimer's Day, the Health Secretary at
the time (Dr Solomon Chertorivsky) instructed the Director of the National
Institute of Geriatrics (founded in 2008) Dr Luis Miguel Gutiérrez Robledo,
as well as the Mexican Federation of Alzheimer, to develop a National Action
Plan against dementia. This Action Plan, which was presented in 2014, is key
to the federal government's efforts to establish and strengthen links with other
health agencies.

To date, there are 540 certified geriatricians in Mexico, according to the
Mexican Council of Geriatrics. However, Mexico faces a great challenge
because of a lack of healthcare professionals with adequate training in elderly care. According to the American Geriatrics Society, one geriatrician is
needed for every 10,000 individuals aged 75 years or above. However, in
Mexico, this ratio is lower, with only one geriatrician for every 22,000 older
adults.

By 2050, it is estimated that one in every four Mexicans will be 60 years or
older. At present, an estimated total of 860,000 Mexicans are affected by some
type of dementia, most of whom have insufficient access to adequate comprehensive health services and are cared for by caregivers without guidance
or training in dementia care—with detrimental effects in terms of health and
economy, not only for patients, but also for their families and primary caregivers [10]. It is therefore imperative to reinforce the number of well-trained
health providers, so the current and upcoming challenges in the Mexican health
system can be addressed.

The challenge of dementia in Mexico

The world population is ageing at an accelerated pace, and with this rise in
life expectancy comes an increased prevalence of chronic diseases such as dementia. Currently, there are about 900 million people aged 60 years and over
in the world.

In September 2015, ADI reported a total of 46.8 million people with dementia worldwide, which is expected to increase to 74.7 million and 135.1 million by 2030 and 2050, respectively. This means 9.9 million people per year,
which equates to one new dementia case presenting every 3.2 seconds, rather
than every 4 seconds, as previously calculated [1].

In 2010, the total estimated cost of dementia in the world was 604 billion dollars. In 2015, according to ADI, this increased to 818 billion dollars, representing an increase of 35.4% [1].

In high-income countries, informal care (45%), defined as care provided by a family member or friend, and formal care provided by formally trained health staff (40%) account for most of the costs, while the proportional contribution of direct medical costs (15%) is much lower. By definition, direct medical costs may be fixed or variable. Fixed direct costs include building, equipment, technology, laboratory, laundry, environmental control, and administrative expenses. Variable direct costs include expenses related to medicines, food, professional fees, treatments, procedures, surgical procedures, materials, imaging studies, laboratory analyses, and microbiological cultures. By contrast, in low- and middle-income countries, such as Mexico, direct medical costs and formal care costs are lower, while informal care costs predominate. However, population demographic changes in many low- and middle-income countries could lead to a reduction in informal care provision by family members in the decades to come [1–6].

Mexico is no exception when it comes to this growth, and it is estimated that there are approximately 860,000 people with dementia in the country, according to the Health and Nutrition National Survey conducted in 2012. The prevalence of dementia and cognitive impairment without dementia has been reported to be 7.9% and 7.6%, respectively, in the population of those above 60 years [2, 4, 7–9]. Moreover, the prevalence of dementia and cognitive impairment without a diagnosis of dementia in Mexico was also reported, according to years of schooling.

In Mexico, the Instituto Mexicano del Seguro Social (IMSS) (Social Security Mexican Institute) is the main healthcare provider for older adults, providing services to 36.2% of older adults, followed by health centres and hospitals—both state-run—catering for 31.1% of the elderly population, private services 17.6% (of which 26% also involves the collaboration of pharmacies), and the Instituto de Seguridad y Servicios Sociales de los Trabajadores del Estado (ISSSTE) (State Workers' Security and Social Services Institute) 9.1% [7].

As mentioned previously, the first programme in geriatric medicine was introduced in 1993 at the National Institute of Medical Sciences and Nutrition (Instituto Nacional de Ciencias Médicas y Nutrición) [11]. Currently, there are 23 institutions in Mexico offering specialty programmes on geriatrics, including nine hospitals in Mexico City, four in Monterrey, four in the State of Mexico, two in Guadalajara, one in San Luis Potosi, Durango, Leon Guanajuato, and Torreón Coahuila. In 2009, there were 414 professionals specialized in eld-erly care, including 316 specialists in geriatrics and 23 nurses specialized in the care of older adults, with the remainder consisting of other professionals with a Master qualification in Science in Nursing of Older Adults [12]. Currently, there are 540 certified geriatricians, according to the Mexican Council of Geriatrics [13].

In Mexico, by 2050, one in every four Mexicans will be 60 years or older, and currently, there is only one geriatrician for every 22,000 older adults [7, 14]. Thus, it is evident that there is insufficient training of human re-sources specialized in the care of the elderly to adequately meet the needs of the elderly population in the country (one geriatrician is needed for every 6000 individuals aged 75 years or above).

First steps in the creation of an Action Plan for Alzheimer's disease and other types of dementia in Mexico

In Mexico, dementia-related organizations began to appear from 1986 with the formation of the first support group for relatives in Mexico City, which then led to the formation of the Mexican Association of Alzheimer and related dis-orders AC (AMAES) in 1988; in that same year, ADI joined in and extended its services to cover the different states of Mexico. In 2002, the Alzheimer asso-ciations in Mexico were integrated and the Mexican Federation of Alzheimer (FEDMA; https://es-la.facebook.com/federacionmexicanadealzheimer/) was established [15], which is currently represented in 22 Mexican states with at least one support group in each state. Moreover, there are a total of 48 support groups in the country, which aim to provide families with information and edu-cation about AD and its care [15].

In 2003, the Alzheimer Ibero América was established, with Mexico as a founding member. The organization includes Latin American countries, Spain, and the Caribbean. Its goal is to unite efforts of its member countries in raising awareness both at the public and government levels [3, 4, 16].

Subsequently, the 10/66 Dementia Research Group, which is part of ADI, was also integrated. The Group conducted comprehensive cross-sectional surveys in one phase among all residents aged 65 years or older in 14 geographically de-fined catchment areas, reaching a sample between 1000 and 3000 participants for each centre. These surveys were conducted between 2003 and 2007 in ten countries (India, Brazil, Venezuela, Cuba, Mexico, Dominican Republic, China, Peru, Nigeria, and Puerto Rico) [3, 17, 18]

Moreover, another initiative in dementia care in Mexico was the development of the Asociación de Médicos Especialistas en Demencias (Association of Medical Specialists in Dementia), which brings together neurologists, geriatricians, psychiatrists, and psychologists with a special interest in dementia. The goal of the association is to enable discussion among specialists on advances in dementia diagnosis and treatment, as well as promote regional care and research in dementia.

In 2011, on the occasion of the World Alzheimer's Day, the Health Secretary at the time (Dr Solomon Chertorivsky) instructed the Director of the National Institute of Geriatrics (founded in 2008) Dr Luis Miguel Gutiérrez Robledo, as well as the Mexican Federation of Alzheimer, to develop a National Action Plan against dementia. Thus, in that same year, a working alliance was signed between these institutions in a document called *Alzheimer and Other Dementias Action Plan, Mexico 2014*, which was presented in 2014 [19]. This Action Plan is key to the federal government's efforts to establish and strengthen links with other health agencies.

Key objective of the Alzheimer and Other Dementias Action Plan

The main objective of the Alzheimer and Other Dementias Action Plan is to promote the well-being of people with AD and related diseases, as well as their families, by strengthening the response capacity of the Mexican health system, in synergy with all other relevant institutions involved in dementia care [10, 14, 19].

This Action Plan was drafted by a working group composed of the following institutions [10, 14, 19]:

- Instituto Nacional de Geriatría (National Institute of Geriatrics) (http://www.geriatria.salud.gob.mx).
- Instituto Nacional de Neurología (National Institute of Neurology) (http://www.innn.salud.gob.mx).
- Instituto Nacional de Salud Pública (National Institute of Public Health) (http://www.insp.mx).
- Instituto Nacional de las Personas Mayores (National Institute of Older People) (http://www.inapam.gob.mx).

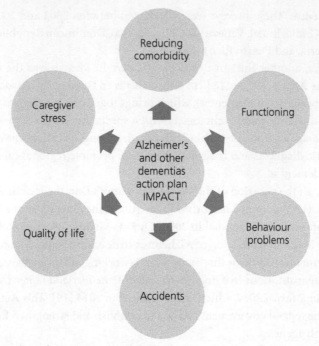

Fig. 40.1 Outline of the National Action Plan.
Source data from Robledo Gutierrez LM, Arrieta Cruz I. *Plan de acción alzheimer y otras demencias, México 2014*. Plan acción alzheimer [Internet]. 2014;79. Available from: http://inger. gob.mx/bibliotecageriatria/acervo/pdf/plan_alzheimer_WEB.pdf.

◆ Federación Mexicana de Alzheimer (Mexican Federation of Alzheimer) (https://es-la.facebook.com/federacionmexicanadealzheimer/).

An outline of the National Action Plan is shown in Fig. 40.1.

The Mexican State, through the Ministry of Health and supported mainly by the Institute of Geriatrics and Neurology, is now focusing on innovative approaches to the prevention and care of dementia. The aim of the National Action Plan against dementia, which addresses dementia not only from a clinical perspective, but also in terms of its social and economic impact, is to promote the development of a national strategy, as well as cooperation with private institutions, to address the problem of dementia in its true dimension.

References

1. **Alzheimer's Disease International**. *World Alzheimer Report 2015: the global impact of dementia*. Available from: https://www.alz.co.uk/research/world-report-2015 [accessed 25 May 2016].

2. **Mejia-Arango S, Gutierrez LM.** Prevalence and incidence rates of dementia and cognitive impairment no dementia in the Mexican population: data from the Mexican Health and Aging Study. *Journal of Aging and Health.* 2011;**23**:1050–74.

3. **Sosa AL, Albanese E, Stephan BCM,** *et al.* Prevalence, distribution, and impact of mild cognitive impairment in Latin America, China, and India: a 10/66 population-based study. *PLoS Medicine.* 2012;**9**:e1001170.

4. **Llibre Rodriguez JJ, Ferri CP, Acosta D,** *et al.* Prevalence of dementia in Latin America, India, and China: a population-based cross-sectional survey. *The Lancet.* 2008;**372**:464–74.

5. **Ham Chande R, Gutiérrez Robledo LM.** [Health and aging in the 20th century]. *Salud Pública de México.* 2007;**49**:s433–5.

6. **Mejía-Arango S, Miguel-Jaimes A, Villa A, Ruiz-Arregui L, Gutiérrez-Robledo LM.** [Cognitive impairment and associated factors in older adults in Mexico]. *Salud Pública de México.* 2007;**49**:s475–81.

7. **Ensanut.** *Ensanut 2012.* Cuernavaca: Instituto Nacional de Salud Pública; 2012. p. 200.

8. **Albala C, Lebrão ML, León Díaz EM,** *et al.* [The Health, Well-Being, and Aging ('SABE') survey: methodology applied and profile of the study population]. *Revista Panamericana de Salud Pública.* 2005;**17**(5-6):307–22.

9. **Guitiérrez Robledo L.** *Grupo de consenso sobre el síndrome de deterioro intelectual y padecimientos demenciales.* México: Fundación Mexicana para la Salud; 1996.

10. **Robledo Gutierrez LM, Arrieta Cruz I.** *Plan de acción Alzheimer y otras demencias, México 2014.* México: Instituto Nacional de Geriatría; 2014. Available from: http://diariote.mx/docs/plan_alzheimer_WEB.pdf [accessed 9 August 2018].

11. **Mora David L, Castro Miguel F, García Carlos B.** La geriatría en México. *Investigación en Salud.* 2006;**VIII**:185–90.

12. **Avila F, Caro E, Negrete M, Montaña M.** La enseñanza de la geriatría en México. *Envejec Hum Una visión Transdiscipl.* 2010; 271–84.

13. **Consejo Mexicano de Geriatría.** Available from: http://consejomexicanodegeriatria.org [accessed 9 August 2018].

14. **Mathers CD, Loncar D.** Projections of global mortality and burden of disease from 2002 to 2030. *PLoS Medicine.* 2006;**3**:e442.

15. **FEDERACIÓN MEXICANA DE ALZHEIMER.** https://es-la.facebook.com/federacionmexicanadealzheimer/

16. **López-Pousa S, Garre-Olmo J, Monserrat-Vila S,** *et al.* [A proposal for a clinical registry of dementias]. *Revista de Neurología.* 2006;**43**:32–8.

17. **Mejia-Arango S, Gutierrez LM.** Prevalence and incidence rates of dementia and cognitive impairment no dementia in the Mexican population: data from the Mexican Health and Aging Study. *Journal of Aging and Health.* 2011;**23**:1050–74.

18. **Prince M, Acosta D, Albanese E,** *et al.* Ageing and dementia in low and middle income countries-Using research to engage with public and policy makers. *International Review of Psychiatry.* 2008;**20**:332–43.

19. **Robledo Gutierrez LM, Stalnikowitz DK.** *Envejecimiento y salud: una propuesta para un plan de acción.* México: Instituto Nacional de Geriatría; 2012. Available from: http://envejecimiento.sociales.unam.mx/archivos/GERIATRIAenvysaludweb.pdf [accessed 9 August 2018].

Chapter 41

United States

Angela M Lunde, Ronald C Petersen, and John A Lucas

Summary

In the United States, the National Alzheimer's Project Act was signed into law in January 2011, and the first National Plan appeared just over 12 months later, with five goals: to prevent and effectively treat Alzheimer's disease by 2025, to enhance care quality and efficiency, to expand support for people with Alzheimer's disease and their families, to enhance public awareness and engagement, and to improve data to track progress. The National Plan has seen a rise in research funding (currently standing at US$1.4 billion). Individual states, at the same time, began discussions about initiatives aimed at addressing personal, societal, and financial implications of Alzheimer's disease. An example is from Minnesota where counselling and support for caregivers are provided, with an estimated saving for the state of Minnesota of US$970 million by 2025. In addition, a number of treatment trials are under way, looking at the effect of monoclonal antibodies on Alzheimer's disease and a series of genetic studies.

Introduction

In 2018, over 50 million people worldwide are estimated to be living with AD or another form of dementia, and many more have milder forms of memory loss or are at risk of developing dementia (Dementia Statistics, 2016) [1]. Overall, the United States is on an ambitious path to address the disease, with coordinated efforts and goals, ranging from preventing and effectively treating the disease to improving the quality of life for those impacted through public engagement, education, and widespread community and organizational change.

Dementia care in the United States has been largely influenced by the National Alzheimer's Project Act (NAPA) that was signed into law in January 2011. The law required the Secretary of Health and Human Services to develop the first National Plan to Address Alzheimer's Disease. The law also required that an Advisory Council be empanelled to counsel the Secretary on the development and revision of the Plan. Once developed, the Plan was to be revised on an annual basis through to 2025 [2]. The first National Plan was published in May 2012 and has five goals (see Table 41.1).

The primary goal of the Plan is to prevent and effectively treat the disease by 2025, and a great deal of effort has been expended with respect to research on the disease. The Plan refers to the term 'Alzheimer's disease' but also includes related disorders such as frontotemporal degeneration, dementia with Lewy bodies, and vascular cognitive impairment and dementia. To assess the state of progress of research and identify gaps moving towards the goal of 2025, several research summits have been held at the National Institutes of Health, as directed by the National Plan. Summits on AD research were held in 2012 and 2015, while summits for AD-related disorders were held in 2013 and 2016. A similar summit to assess the state of progress on care and services was held in late 2017. This first-of-its-kind Care and Service Research Summit convened with a focus on care, services, and supports for people currently living with dementia and caregivers [3]. The Summit sought to identify and later prioritize what research is needed to improve quality of care and outcomes across care settings, including improving the lived day-to-day experience of people with dementia and their caregivers.

These summits have been particularly important in promoting the research agenda. Following each summit, a set of recommendations is generated, which then lead to milestones that can be assessed annually to determine if progress is being made and also supply the substrate for additional funding opportunities from the National Institutes of Health. These have resulted in numerous requests for applications and an expanded research programme for AD and related disorders.

Table 41.1 National Plan for the United States [4]

Goal 1—Prevent and effectively treat Alzheimer's disease by 2025
Goal 2—Enhance care quality and efficiency
Goal 3—Expand supports for people with Alzheimer's disease and their families
Goal 4—Enhance public awareness and engagement
Goal 5—Improve data to track progress

The NAPA law also required that the Advisory Council developed a set of independent recommendations each year, i.e. the Council would determine a set of recommendations for improving research, care, and services for AD, and these recommendations would be transmitted directly to the Secretary of Health and Human Services and to Congress. While the federal members may participate in some of these activities, the ultimate decision regarding the content of the recommendations was made by the non-federal members. This set of recommendations allowed the Advisory Council to express its aspirational goals to accomplish the primary goal of the plan by 2025 [2].

The Advisory Council on Research, Care, and Services that was determined by law comprises approximately 26 individuals, half from the federal government and half from the private sector. The Council is chaired by a non-federal member, and the 12 non-federal members of the Council comprise six categories: care providers, caregivers, patient advocates, state health agencies, advocacy groups, and researchers. The Advisory Council meets face-to-face quarterly in Washington and assesses progress and makes recommendations for the next revisions of the Plan. The Council turns over on a regular basis, and the federal members participate in all of the subcommittee activities. The Council has resulted in increased communication not only among federal agencies, but also among the federal agencies and the private sector [2].

The National Plan to Address Alzheimer's Disease also serves as a catalyst for the Alzheimer's Accountability Act that was passed by Congress in 2014. The Alzheimer's Accountability Act required the National Institutes of Health to generate an annual budget providing the best estimate of the next fiscal year's funding, to enable the research community to reach the goal of the National Plan by 2025. The first professional judgement budget was generated for fiscal year 2016, and the second one for fiscal year 2017 was presented to the Advisory Council in August 2016.

Since the inception of the National Plan to Address Alzheimer's Disease, research funding for AD and related disorders has risen substantially. At the outset of the National Plan in 2011, the federal budget for AD and related disorders research was approximately $450 million. As of fiscal year 2016, that had risen to $991 million and is expected to go higher. Congress recently passed the fiscal year 2017 budget, allocating an additional $400 million for AD research. This brings the current federal budget for research to approximately $1.4 billion. As noted earlier, the recommendations from the Advisory Council have included a statement that the scientific community estimates that the annual federal budget for AD and related disorders should be approximately $2 billion per year to make substantial progress.

The impact of the National Plan thus far has been energizing the field from research through to care and services. Increasing attention is being paid to these disorders, which is absolutely necessary, considering the impact of these conditions on individuals, families, and the healthcare economy. At the same time the NAPA law began its proceedings, individual states were also engaging in strategic discussions and consumer-driven initiatives with overall aims to address the personal, societal, and financial implications of AD and related dementias [3]. More specifically, key priorities for many states now include:

- Diagnosing AD and other dementias earlier and more reliably.
- Improving training and resources in dementia care by paid caregivers and medical practitioners.
- Decreasing stigma by increasing education and public awareness.
- Improving dementia services and access for individuals with dementia and caregivers.
- Reducing the burden of dementia costs on individuals and families.

An example of this progress comes from Minnesota where, in 2009, the legislature charged the Minnesota Board on Aging to establish the Alzheimer's Disease Working Group (ADWG) and to make recommendations for policies and programmes that would prepare Minnesota for the future [5]. Out of this work came Minnesota ACT on Alzheimer's, a state-wide, multidimensional collaboration focused around large-scale social change and building community capacity to transform and respond to AD [6]. Over the past several years, the work has transitioned to implementation (National Alzheimer's and Dementia Resource Center, 2018), including long-term sustainability, with a strong focus in three areas: community engagement, healthcare practice change, and health equity integration [7].

ACT has also provided the foundational model for what is currently called Dementia-Friendly America (DFA), offering support and resources across the United States for communities to strategically identify their unique needs and respond with action. Community-based models, such as ACT, offer opportunities for not only improved dementia care, but also cost savings [8].

The following represents a small example of community-based care interventions taking place in the United States. Each of these has existing or emerging evidence to support their effectiveness:

- New York University Caregiver Intervention: an evidence-based intervention for caregivers [9].
- REACH: a resource for enhancing Alzheimer's caregiver health [10].
- The Savvy Caregiver program: a multi-session programme that helps caregivers better understand the changes they are experiencing and how to best

provide individualized care for their loved ones throughout the progression of AD or dementia [11].

- Partners in Dementia Care: a care coordination programme that enhances access to needed services and strengthens the family care support network [12].

- Mindfulness-Based Dementia Care (MBDC): a programme aimed at teaching meditation techniques to improve caregiver well-being [13].

- TAP (Tailored Activity Program): a home-based intervention that trains caregivers to design and use activities that draw on a person with dementia's interests and abilities [14].

- The National Alzheimer's and Dementia Resource Center (NADRC) resource centre staff provide individualized technical assistance to grantees and AoA/ACL programme staff when requested [7].

- The US Federal Health Resources Services Administration (HRSA) Alzheimer's disease and Related Dementia's Training Curriculum for the primary care workforce training focused on dementia care and helping providers address caregiver needs [15].

Caregiving

In 2016, 15.9 million family and friends provided 18.2 billion hours of unpaid care to those with AD and other dementias—care valued at $230.1 billion. Due to the physical and emotional burden of caregiving, AD and dementia caregivers had $10.9 billion in additional healthcare costs of their own in 2016. Nearly 60% of AD and dementia caregivers rate the emotional stress of caregiving as high or very high, and 30–40% report symptoms of depression (Alzheimer's Association, 2017) [16].

In recognition of the toughness of the caregiving job and the increasing prevalence of dementia, there has been growing interest among public policymakers and within communities and healthcare systems to address the challenges caregivers face. Numerous programmes and initiatives have been undertaken, with reasonable to good outcomes; however, the vital measurement, particularly to policymakers, is the demonstration of overall cost savings [17].

One Alzheimer support programme in Minnesota—known as Family Memory Care—effectively demonstrated an ability to reduce the costs of care associated with AD by focusing on care coordination and community support. The programme is modelled after the New York University Caregiver Intervention (NYUCI) programme. It provides caregivers with sessions of individual and family counselling, a weekly support group, and telephone counselling, as needed, in an effort to keep people with AD in community and home settings. In a study published in Kaiser Health News, researchers demonstrated that if the programme were implemented state-wide, it could save Minnesota nearly $970 million by 2025 [18].

States across the country are also looking at ways to improve and shape the healthcare experience for dementia patients and caregivers. For example, ACT on Alzheimer's developed evidence- and consensus-based practice standards that include practical web-based tools and resources for primary care providers, allied care teams, care coordinators, and community organizations [6]. An critically important issue at this time is on ways to identify and include 'family caregiver' in the medical health records and to recognize that the role of caregiving is associated with increased health risks. In this way, caregivers could be routinely assessed and appropriate treatment plans prescribed.

Further, direct care staff and/or paid caregivers in the United States have difficult jobs, and most do not receive the training necessary to provide good dementia care. Turnover rates are high among direct-care workers, and recruitment and retention are persistent challenges. To address these issues, there has been a great deal of effort across the country on training the workforce who directly care for people living with dementia. Beginning in 2016, Minnesota legislation required care staff to have 8 hours of dementia-specific training prior to interaction with residents, and an additional 8 hours annually. Other states have made similar progress. This alone will not solve the complex problem, but it is a critical piece.

Treatment trials

More than 400 clinical trials are currently looking at new treatments for AD, and many of them are actively recruiting. A number of treatment trials are under way, looking at the effect of monoclonal antibodies on AD and a series of genetic studies. For over a decade, investigators have sought to identify a pharmacologic means of clearing amyloid beta protein (AB) from the brains of people with AD. A large literature initially suggested that brain deposition of AB initiated the onset of AD. Most anti-AB strategies have not worked, and passive immunization against monomers has been ineffective at the stage of mild to moderate AD. A number of prevention studies are being led from the United States. For example:

- A4 study a 3-year double-blind, 1000-person solanezumab study in cognitively normal subjects who show signs of abnormal amyloid on PET scanning [19].

◆ DIAN study: examining the action of solanezumab and gantenerumab versus placebo in unaffected carriers of dominantly inherited genes [20].

◆ ApoE 4 study: examining the long-term impact of two agents on cognition, including an active immunization compound (CAD 106) and a beta secretase inhibitor (CNP520) [21].

◆ Columbian kindred study: using a passive immunization agent (crenezumab) in a large family cohort of asymptomatic carriers of a dominantly inherited AD gene [22].

◆ There have been some anti-Tau treatments, and so far, they too have failed in cohorts of patients who have mild to moderate AD [19]. Further anti-Tau treatments are now under way such as anti-tau passive immunization.

References

1. **Alzheimer's Disease International.** *Dementia statistics 2016.* Available from: https://www.alz.co.uk/research/statistics [accessed 30 January 2018].

2. **Office of the Assistant Secretary For Planning and Evaluation (ASPE).** *National plan to address Alzheimer's disease:2013 update.* Available from: https://aspe.hhs.gov/system/files/pdf/102526/NatlPlan.pdf [accessed 30 January 2018].

3. **Office of the Assistant Secretary For Planning and Evaluation (ASPE).** *Research Summit on Dementia Care.* 2017. Available from: https://aspe.hhs.gov/national-research-summit-care-services-and-supports-persons-dementia-and-their-caregivers [accessed 30 January 2018]. https://aspe.hhs.gov/national-research-summit-care-services-and-supports-persons-dementia-and-their-caregiver.

4. **NIH National Institute on Aging.** *NIA and the National Plan to Address Alzheimer's Disease.* 2016. Available from: https://www.nia.nih.gov/about/nia-and-national-plan-address-alzheimers-disease [accessed 30 January 2018].

5. **Minnesota Board on Aging.** *Preparing Minnesota for Alzheimer's: the Budgetary, Social adn Personal Impacts.* Report to the Minnesota Legislature by The Minnesota Board on Aging on behalf of the Alzheimer's Disease Working Group. Minneapolis, MN: Minnesota Board on Aging; 2011.

6. **ACT on Alzheimer's.** *Minnesotans working together on the impacts of Alzheimer's.* Available from: http://www.actonalz.org/about [accessed 30 January 2018].

7. **National Alzheimer's and Dementia Resource Center.** Available from: https://nadrc.acl.gov/ [accessed 30 January 2018].

8. **Paone D.** *ACT on Alzheimer's evaluation reports.* Minneapolis, MN: Paone and Associates, LLC; 2015. https://aspe.hhs.gov/national-research-summit-care-services-and-supports-persons-dementia-and-their-caregiver

9. **Foldes SS, Moriarty JP, Farseth PH, Mittelman MS, Long KH.** Medicaid savings from the New York university caregiver intervention for families with dementia. *The Gerontologist.* 2018;**58**:e97–106.

10. **National Association of Chronic Disease Directors.** *Implementing a community-based program for dementia caregivers: an action guide using REACH OUT.* Atlanta,

GA: National Association of Chronic Disease Directors; 2009. Available from: http://www.rosalynncarter.org/UserFiles/ReachOutActionGuide.pdf [accessed 31 January 2018].

11. **Rosalynn Carter Institute for Caregiving.** *Savvy caregiver (Ostwald/Hepburn).* 2017. Available from: http://www.rosalynncarter.org/caregiver_intervention_database/dimentia/savvy_caregiver/ [accessed 30 January 2018].

12. **VA Office Research and Development.** *Partners in Dementia Care: A Telephone Care Consultation Intervention Provided to Veterans in Partnership With Local Alzheimer's Association Chapters.* Clinicaltrials.gov; 2016. https://clinicaltrials.gov/ct2/show/NCT00291161 [accessed 1 February 2018].

13. **Manteau-Rao M.** *Caring for a loved one with dementia: a mindfulness-based guide.* Oakland, CA: New Harbinger Publications; 2016.

14. **Gitlin LN, Winter L, Vause Earland T,** *et al.* The Tailored Activity Program to reduce behavioral symptoms in individuals with dementia: feasibility, acceptability, and replication potential. *The Gerontologist.* 2009;**49**:428–39.

15. **Health Resources & Services Administration.** *HRSA Health Workforce. Training curriculum: Alzheimer's disease and related dementias.* HRSA Health Workforce; 2017. Available from: https://bhw.hrsa.gov/grants/geriatrics/alzheimers-curriculum [accessed 30 January 2018].

16. **Alzheimer's Association.** 2017 Alzheimer's disease facts and figures. *Alzheimer's and Dementia.* 2017;**13**:325–73.

17. **AARP Public Policy Institute and National Alliance for Caregiving.** *Caregiving in the U.S. 2015.* Greenwald & Associates; 2015.

18. **Gillespie L.** *Alzheimer's disease support model could save Minn. millions.* KHN Kaiser Health News; 2014. Available from: https://khn.org/news/alzheimers-disease-support-model-could-save-minn-millions/ [accessed 30 January 2018].

19. **Sperling RA, Rentz DM, Johnson KA,** *et al.* The A4 study: stopping AD before symptoms begin? *Science Translational Medicine.* 2014;**6**:228fs13.

20. **Bateman RJ, Benzinger TL, Berry S,** *et al.*; **DIAN-TU Pharma Consortium for the Dominantly Inherited Alzheimer Network.** The DIAN-TU Next Generation Alzheimer's prevention trial: adaptive design and disease progression model. *Alzheimer's and Dementia.* 2017;**13**:8–19.

21. **Gauthier S, Feldman HH, Schneider LS,** *et al.* Efficacy and safety of tau-aggregation inhibitor therapy in patients with mild or moderate Alzheimer's disease: a randomized, controlled, double-blind, parallel-arm, phase 3 trial. *The Lancet.* 2016;**388**:2873–84

22. **Ringman JM, Goate A, Masters CL,** *et al.*; **Dominantly Inherited Alzheimer Network.** Genetic heterogeneity in Alzheimer's disease implications for treatment strategies. *Current Neurology and Neuroscience Reports.* 2014;**14**:49.

Section 6

South America

Chapter 42

Argentina

Fátima González Palau and Tatiana
Castro Zamparella

Summary

In 2000, the United Nations placed Argentina among the
countries with the oldest populations in Latin America. Ageing
of the Argentinian population has progressed steadily over the
decades, alongside a rise in the prevalence of dementia. In 2011,
findings from the first Central Registry of Cognitive Pathologies
were published, which showed that among all dementia
types, Alzheimer's disease, in any of its forms, was diagnosed
in 70.5% of subjects. Regarding treatment, findings from the
study also showed the considerable importance given to the
specific treatment of behavioural and psychological symptoms
of dementia. Non-pharmacological treatment is usually based on
interventions directed to patients and families. In Argentina and
worldwide, non-cognitive symptoms are the real core symptoms
of dementia. However, difficulty in accessing care and treatment
facilities due to long travel distances makes it challenging to
implement traditional psycho-social interventions. In this context,
computer-based cognitive interventions and telemedicine could
offer a promising solution.

Demographic background

Argentina has a total area of 3,745,997 km² and a total population of 40,117,096
inhabitants, resulting in an average density of 10.7 inhabitants per km². The
population is mostly concentrated in the provinces near the centre of the
country [1].

Ageing of the Argentinian population has progressed steadily over the decades. This was reflected in the 2010 census which revealed that elderly people

represented 10.2% of the population. Provinces that are further from the country's metropolitan centre are more acutely affected by this population ageing due to migration of the younger population. Meanwhile, the centre of the country is also impacted by this problem due to low birth rates. The predominance of women among older adults [1] is clearly observed.

In 2009, the United Nations placed Argentina among the countries with the oldest populations in Latin America. Projections for 2030 are worrying, given that the population of those aged over 65 years will double and the population of those aged over 80 years is expected to triple. Since dementia is more prevalent among older adults, regions that could be most affected by this disease are those with a projected increase in their elderly population such as Argentina [2].

Epidemiological studies

In their 2004 Argentinian study, Larraya *et al.* [3] reported cognitive impairment in 23% of subjects aged over 60 years. Moreover, in a pilot study conducted in Cañuelas (Buenos Aires) on a sample of 1453 individuals, Arizaga *et al.* [4] reported a prevalence of cognitive impairment of 16.9%, 23.3%, and 42.5% in subjects aged 60–69 years, 70–79 years, and 80 years or over, respectively. Cognitive impairment was also found to be significantly correlated with age, functional illiteracy, cranial trauma, high blood pressure, inactivity, and depression. Of note, Larraya *et al.*'s study included only institutionalized subjects, while the study by Arizaga *et al.* was only the pilot phase of an overall project. There are no comprehensive epidemiological studies conducted in Argentina that provide all the information necessary to develop public health strategies.

Therefore, Latin America, including Argentina, faces the same challenges in dealing with dementia as rich countries do, but with limited availability of epidemiological data and a much lower level of preparedness, as well as relatively little awareness of the disease [5]. For example, Gleichgerrcht *et al.* [6] reported that, even among neurologists, a substantial number of practising physicians who diagnose dementia will do so without providing a specific diagnosis of the type of dementia.

The diagnostic process

In Argentina, the diagnostic process in dementia and subsequent care and support for dementia patients necessitate costly services and infrastructure (e.g. cognitive disorder clinics, multidisciplinary teamwork), which are often available only in select affluent urban areas. Another huge challenge is related to diagnosing dementia in people with a low level of education and limited literacy skills. A total of 3.7% of the population of those aged over 15 years in Argentina do not have any level of education, while 30.7% have incomplete primary education, and 43.1% have complete primary, but incomplete secondary, education [1]. To cope with this situation, existing cognitive and functional tests must be adapted and relevant norms developed [5].

Of the types of dementia diagnosed, AD is the most prevalent type. In 2011, findings from the first Central Registry of Cognitive Pathologies [7] were published by the Argentinian government. This study showed that, in a sample of 292 subjects, MCI was diagnosed in 17.4% and dementia in 83.6%. Of those diagnosed with dementia, 50.2% received a diagnosis of a purely neurodegenerative process, 13.7% dementia of a purely vascular origin, 33.6% dementia with a degenerative aetiology with a vascular component, and 2.5% dementia of an apparently secondary origin from another systemic or traumatic pathology. In addition, among all dementia types, AD, in any of its forms, was the commonest type and diagnosed in 70.5% of subjects. The other next commonest dementia types were mixed vascular dementia (cortico-subcortical) (6.6%) and dementia with Lewy bodies (5.4%). This same study also showed that the time interval between the onset of symptoms and diagnosis was approximately 12 months and that the commonest comorbidity in patients with dementia in Argentina was hypertension [7].

Treatments

Regarding pharmacological treatment, the most commonly used antidementia drugs are donepezil and memantine, either alone or in combination. Antidepressants and antipsychotics are used in a third of dementia patients, of which the most commonly used are sertraline and paroxetine, followed by risperidone and quetiapine. Anxiolytics and hypnotics are prescribed in less than half of dementia patients. These figures show the enormous importance given to the specific treatment of behavioural and psychological symptoms of dementia. Polypharmacy is currently not a common problem in patients with cognitive disorders treated by specialists in Argentina [7].

Concerning MCI cases, Serrano *et al.* [8] carried out a survey among professionals from the Dementias Group of the Neurological Society of Argentina and from the Psychogeriatric Group of the Argentinian Association of Psychiatrists. A total of 24 (16 neurologists and eight psychiatrists) experts from Argentina and Brazil and 30 GPs agreed to answer a questionnaire on MCI (adapted from the Dubois inventory). The results indicated that 92% of these experts considered MCI to be an ambiguous entity, and not necessarily a 'pre-dementia' stage; 63% felt MCI was likely to worsen over time, and 83% would initiate treatment for MCI cases with cholinesterase inhibitors, memantine, and vitamin E. Most physicians consider MCI to be syndromic, and not limited to

AD, although they would still initiate treatment in MCI cases as they would for AD patients. This ambiguity underscores the need to standardize definitions and reconceptualize AD in its pre-dementia stage.

Non-pharmacological treatment in Argentina is usually based on interventions directed to patients, as well as to families. Thus, patients are widely recommended to take part in cognitive stimulation programmes, improve their diets, and participate in physical activity. However, difficulty in accessing care and treatment facilities due to long travel distances makes it challenging to implement traditional psycho-social interventions, and hence regular attendance to cognitive stimulation programmes is not always feasible for the majority of people with dementia. In this context, computer-based cognitive interventions and telemedicine could offer a promising solution. The development of research studies to evaluate the effectiveness of psycho-social intervention strategies, with and without the use of technologies, would help to meet the needs of the increasing ageing population in this country.

Caregivers

When caring for a family member with dementia, culture and ethnicity play a significant role in the caregiver's stress burden and coping mechanism [9]. Latino cultures, in particular, place great emphasis on the family underpinned by the cultural value of *familismo*, which encourages reliance on family members for support, a strong sense of obligation to care for family members in need, and reliance on relatives to provide guidance in life [10]. It is estimated that a primary caregiver for a patient with moderate AD devotes over 70 hours a week to caregiving [11]. The culture of *familismo* influences the emotional distress experienced by the caregiver through dysfunctional thoughts generally related to depression symptoms and to poor health outcomes [12]. Furthermore, since family-centred care is highly favoured in Latin America, including Argentina [10], caregivers who consider placing a relative in nursing homes or adult day care often experience feelings of guilt and shame. In Argentina, support groups, such as Alzheimer Argentina, are available to provide advice, guidance, and support for families and caregivers. Psycho-education for family and caregivers is an effective intervention to guide them in their caregiving role, as well as educate them about key components of caregiving (e.g. financial management) and promote their well-being through protective measures (e.g. exercise, social stimulation).

Economic impact

Moreover, the economic cost of dementia is high worldwide. In an Argentinian study carried out on 104 patients with dementia (AD, $n = 44$; frontotemporal dementia, $n = 34$; vascular dementia, $n = 26$), Rojas *et al.* [13] estimated that the annual direct costs were US$4625 for AD, US$4924 for frontotemporal dementia, and US$5112 for vascular dementia ($P > 0.05$ between groups). In a post hoc analysis, vascular dementia showed higher hospitalization costs than AD ($P < 0.001$) and lower medication costs compared to frontotemporal dementia ($P < 0.001$). AD exhibited higher anti-dementia drug costs, while frontotemporal dementia had higher psychotropic costs. In a multivariate analysis, depression, activities of daily living, and caregiver burden were correlated with direct costs ($r^2 = 0.76$). Overall, costs increased in the presence of behavioural symptoms, depression, and functional impairment of activities of daily living.

Finally, in Argentina and worldwide, non-cognitive symptoms are the real core symptoms of dementia and are the primary reason for a patient and their family to seek medical attention. It is evident that effective treatment of behavioural symptoms in a patient with dementia produces not only an improvement in behavioural performance, but also enhances their intellectual potential. Behavioural symptoms in dementia patients limit their social participation and are perhaps the commonest cause of early institutionalization—which undoubtedly impacts on the future of dementia care and clearly increases the costs generated by this disease.

Conclusion

Dementia is a global problem that demands comprehensive solutions. The challenge in Argentina is to overcome the difficulty for patients and their families in accessing care and support facilities due to long travel distances and also to find new approaches to improving care and treatment for dementia, as well as preventing the disease. We need to continue to work towards helping to deliver a healthier future for people living with dementia, as well as their families.

References

1. **National Institute of Statistics and Censuses (INDEC)**. *SSD system sociodemographic statistics: older adults area.* Buenos Aires: INDEC; 2010.
2. **CEPAL-CELADE**. *Aging and the elderly: socio-demographic indicators for Latin America and the Caribbean.* New York, NY: United Nations; 2009.
3. **Larraya F, Grasso L, Mari G**. Prevalence of dementia of Alzheimer's type, vascular dementia and other DSM-IV and ICD-10 dementias in the Republic of Argentina. *Revista Neurologica Argentina.* 2004;**29**:148–53.
4. **Arizaga RL, Gogorza RE, Allegri RF**, *et al.* Cognitive impairment and risk factor prevalence in a population over 60 in Argentina. *Dementia and Neuropsychologia.* 2014;**8**:364–70.
5. **Manes F**. The huge burden of dementia in Latin America. *The Lancet Neurology.* 2016;**15**:29.

6. Gleichgerrcht E, Flichtentrei D, Manes F. How much do physicians in Latin America know about behavioral variant frontotemporal dementia? *Journal of Molecular Neuroscience*. 2011;**45**:609–17.

7. Melcon CM, Bartoloni L, Katz M, *et al.* [Proposal for a Centralized Registry of Cases of Cognitive Impairment in Argentina (ReDeCAr) based on the national epidemiological surveillance system]. *Neurologia Argentina*. 2010;**2**:161–6.

8. Serrano CM, Allegri RF, Caramelli P, Taragano FE, Cámera L. [Mild cognitive impairment: survey on attitudes of medical specialists and generalists]. *Medicina (Buenos Aires)*. 2007;**67**:19–25.

9. Elnasseh AG, Trujillo MA, Peralta SV, *et al.* Family dynamics and personal strengths among dementia caregivers in Argentina. *International Journal of Alzheimer's Disease*. 2016;**2016**:2386728.

10. Gelman CR. Familismo and its impact on the family caregiving of Latinos with Alzheimer's disease: a complex narrative. *Research on Aging*. 2014;**36**:40–71.

11. Losada A, Marquez-Gonzalez M, Knight BG, Yanguas J, Sayegh P, Romero-Moreno R. Psychosocial factors and caregivers' distress: effects of familism and dysfunctional thoughts. *Aging and Mental Health*. 2010;**14**:193–202.

12. Karlawish J, Barg FK, Augsburger D, Beaver J, Ferguson A, Nunez J. What Latino Puerto Ricans and non-Latinos say when they talk about Alzheimer's disease. *Alzheimers and Dementia*. 2011;**7**:161–70.

13. Rojas G, Bartoloni L, Dillon C, Serrano CM, Iturry M, Allegri RF. Clinical and economic characteristics associated with direct costs of Alzheimer's, frontotemporal and vascular dementia in Argentina. *International Psychogeriatrics*. 2011;**23**:554–61.

Chapter 43

Brazil

Paulo R Canineu, Marta LGF Pereira, Florindo Stella, and Orestes V Forlenza

Summary

In Brazil, since 2002, through the National Health System, patients with mild/moderate Alzheimer's disease have access to cholinesterase inhibitors free of charge. Yet, the country has no comprehensive nationwide dementia programme, and new public health policies are needed to organize health services so to improve the quality of dementia care. There are many important initiatives at local or regional levels, supported by academic, public health, governmental, and private organizations. Although fragmented, these initiatives have yielded a wide range of services in relevant areas of dementia care, particularly early diagnosis, treatment, and rehabilitation, as well as educational programmes. General knowledge about dementia, as well as treatment protocols and available support programmes, is highly variable across the country, particularly in primary care settings. The main challenges in dementia care in Brazil are to increase awareness of the disease and develop professional skills, to promote a multidisciplinary approach to treatment and support in all stages of the disease, and to design a national plan aimed at reducing the risk for dementia.

Availability of a National Dementia Strategy

Brazil does not have a national programme dedicated to the study and management of dementia-related problems in a wide-reaching way [1]. Most available epidemiological and clinical data on dementia have been generated by independent efforts of scientific researchers from distinct parts of Brazil, and communication between academic experts and policymakers is still very limited. Although extensive scientific research data are available in specific areas of dementia, these have not translated into a comprehensive appraisal of the problem in the country. Likewise, optimal services may be restricted to academic and specialty facilities that, with a few exceptions, are usually offered in tertiary medical care. This renders the quality of psycho-geriatric assistance in Brazil very heterogeneous, such that a substantial part of the population may not have access to the best services. Of course, the geographic differences and social, and economic disparities in the country and the relative concentration of referral services in Southern and more developed regions also contribute to this heterogeneity in service quality. Therefore, rather than having a nationwide picture of the problem, we have distinct regional portraits and fragmented assistance programmes. University-based services usually work independently or in academic collaboration with other institutions, generally with the purpose of conducting scientific research dedicated to specific themes in dementia, in addition to offering medical treatment and multidisciplinary care for dementia patients at the highest possible standard, albeit with limited accessibility. Thus, there is need for a closer interaction between the scientific community/clinical experts and policymakers.

The Brazilian Alzheimer's Association (ABRAz) [2], affiliated to ADI, has been working since 1992 on many important programmes at a national level. These initiatives are largely dedicated to promoting awareness of the disease, providing social and psycho-educational support to patients, families, and caregivers, and sensitizing governmental agencies to critical needs. The ABRAz has regional/local offices throughout the country, gathering professional mentoring from both medical and non-medical specialists, including physicians, nurses, social workers, physiotherapists, psychologists, and caregivers, among others [2, 3]. Despite its active efforts and determination in the pursuit of its goals, the ABRAz has not received consistent support from governmental authorities or from academic faculties. Nevertheless, a number of fruitful initiatives with tangible benefits to the clients have been accomplished. For instance, the ABRAz established a partnership with the Federal University of the State of Acre (which is located in a remote area of the country to the southwest of the Amazon rainforest) to enhance the provision of specialty neurology and geriatric services by the university for diagnosis and pharmacological treatment of dementia, home care services, and general support to the public. Short courses on dementia were promoted, including thematic lectures dedicated to GPs and specialists, in addition to open lectures and publications to the lay public. The outcome of this partnership has shown that, through synergistic efforts with the Brazilian academic community, the ABRAz has been able to facilitate the provision of specialized care for patients with dementia and their caregivers in remote areas of Brazil. Therefore, it is crucial to sensitize governmental agencies and policymakers to the need for implementing new and more widespread support programmes to deal with dementia-related problems, as these programmes are essential to organizing and administering health services, and ultimately to improving the quality of care provided to dementia patients in Brazil.

Positive aspects of dementia care in Brazil

Several important initiatives deserve to be highlighted, despite the lack of a unified National Strategy to establish a global and comprehensive approach to the diagnosis, treatment, and prevention of dementia in Brazil. There are a growing number of specialized centres that conduct relevant research in several sub-themes of dementia and provide clinical assistance to patients and care-givers, either within or in joint effort with local universities. In addition, older adults with cognitive problems have access to outpatient facilities for screening and diagnosis. More recently, several of these specialized centres have joined efforts to define common procedures and assessment protocols that will en-able multi-centred data analyses. The majority of these centres provide treat-ment for different stages of dementia, including appropriate pharmacological and non-pharmacological interventions, usually by trained specialists in neur-ology, psychiatry, and geriatric medicine, as well as by multidisciplinary, non-medical staff. These centres are generally university-based and located mostly in the main state capitals and major cities of Brazil, and have been considered to be national references for health professionals working in other regions of the country. Promising attempts have been made to establish mutual cooper-ation agreements among these centres, despite a lack of an effective integration among the centres.

Also, there are numerous private initiatives in many parts of Brazil, with specialized professionals working in the field of dementia on highly complex projects. In recent years, well-structured clinical research laboratories have fo-cused their work on the neuropsychological and biological aspects of dementia. Many of these groups have contributed to the validation of relevant cognitive tests and neuropsychological assessment protocols, in order to establish local normative data and enable international cooperation. In many cities, collab-orations have been established between health professionals and local ABRAz committees, or other similar groups, to provide training courses for caregivers of elderly people and dementia patients.

As it happens worldwide, the high economic costs of dementia are a major limitation to the development of large-scale programmes dedicated to the management of dementia [4–8]. In this regard, the Brazilian government's ini-tiative to provide medications for the treatment of AD is noteworthy. Thus, through the National Health System, patients with a well-established diagnosis of mild and moderate AD have access to treatment with cholinesterase inhibitors, which are prescribed by their doctors—galantamine, rivastigmine, and donepezil. These anti-dementia drugs may be dispensed free of charge through a special distribution system—the so-called 'high-cost pharmacy', which also includes expensive medications required for the treatment of other complex diseases that would otherwise be unaccessible to the majority of the population. This programme was launched in 2002 by the Brazilian National Health System [Sistema Único de Saúde (SUS)], although patients can have access to this benefit, irrespective of whether they receive treatment within or outside the public health system; in other words, the programme also accepts prescriptions issued by physicians from the private health system. Applicants for free prescriptions are required to undergo a simple diagnostic protocol, which includes documentation of the cognitive/functional status, as assessed by the MMSE and the Clinical Dementia Rating (CDR) Scale, as well as additional investigations (laboratory testing and neuroimaging) to confirm the clinical picture is compatible with a diagnosis of AD [9, 10]. These diagnostic procedures, in the recent past, have been performed predominantly by neurologists, geriatric psychiatrists, and geriatricians at specialized facilities, but have been recently extended to GPs and other medical specialists, thus reinforcing the distribution of the programme to remote areas of the country.

Current challenges in dementia care

Wide-reaching, comprehensive, and homogeneous neuropsychiatric and psychosocial care is possibly the most relevant challenge in dementia care in Brazil. As stated previously, Brazil has several academically oriented expert groups that are technically qualified in medical and biological research, as well as well-trained health professionals able to provide first-class clinical assistance to patients with dementia, despite the social, political, and economical restraints of a developing country such as Brazil. However, the care service capacity of these clinics is too low to meet the massive demand, given the current estimate of 1.5 million patients with AD in Brazil and the fact that care needs will continue to grow steadily as the population ages [2, 3]. In addition, not every clinical centre is fully prepared to perform the necessary diagnostic procedures for an early detection of dementia, or to apply complex diagnostic technologies in difficult cases. In remote areas, health professionals often face difficulties in establishing an actual diagnosis of probable AD, especially in the earlier stages of cognitive impairment, and sometimes fail to provide the necessary guidance to families about the clinical course of the disease and the required healthcare interventions.

Second, there is an urgent need for a central database to gather epidemiological, clinical, and prognostic data on the management of dementia and related disorders. This would support the development of large-scale policies related to, for example, the evaluation of actual needs, assessment of clinical benefits of existing programmes, pharmacoeconomic modelling, etc. Another challenge refers to the need of a national plan to increase awareness of dementia and its underlying mechanisms to healthcare professionals and the general public. Given the vast size of the country, such initiatives would benefit from telemedicine technologies and well-planned strategies to facilitate the provision of long-distance education and regular meetings, as well as the dissemination of videos and texts, with a view to updating health professionals on scientific and technological advances in dementia. When designing any such training and education programmes, it is also fundamental to overcome the social, educational, and cultural differences across distinct regions of the country, particularly due to illiteracy, limited access to information, and regional beliefs.

Moreover, regarding the high direct and indirect financial costs of dementia [5–8, 11], one must recognize that pharmacological treatment represents only part of the investment. Although much has been achieved through the universalization of access to anti-dementia drugs through the National Health System, non-pharmacological interventions and caregiver support, which may substantially inflate treatment costs, currently rely on individual/family resources in Brazil.

Approaches to present challenges and measures of success

Brazil has many highly qualified health professionals and scientists, as well as experts from different clinical specialties, who contribute to improving the level of care in dementia and related disorders. However, this does not diminish the importance of conveying to the authorities the reality regarding the growing number of cases of AD and other dementia types, which, in the very near future, will require more substantial public investments than the current level of investment in the country[12].

This challenge demands a reciprocal collaboration between the different hierarchical levels of the government and academia. The objectives of such integration include the development of strategies that would allow a rational use of financial resources and the creation of primary healthcare centres with trained staff, as well as the implementation of training programmes for health professionals and caregivers, especially in areas with difficult or limited access to diagnostic and treatment facilities. Therefore, public authorities need to focus on the burden of dementia and recognize it as a major public health problem. Leading scientists and clinical experts need to work jointly with policymakers to build a national plan.

Future perspectives in dementia care, treatment, and prevention

As it has been recognized in several countries, an accurate diagnosis, combined with the implementation of therapeutic interventions (both pharmacological and non-pharmacological), ideally in the early stages of the disease, is necessary to preserve the patient's functionality and quality of life and to attenuate the burden of the disease on families and caregivers. It is expected that health authorities in Brazil, supported by patient associations and the community, will make an effort to create specialized services in strategic regions to offer technically appropriate and humanized therapies and support. Also, healthcare professionals' training must encompass both technical abilities and a humanistic approach. In addition, identification and control of risk factors of dementia (hypertension, diabetes, dyslipidaemia, sedentary lifestyle, obesity, poor diet, psychiatric disorders such as depression, alcohol abuse, and smoking) should be prioritized [13]. In parallel, protective factors (such as education, physical activity, engaging in social activities, improving eating habits, cognitive stimulation, and treating psychiatric disorders) should be systematically reinforced [14].

References

1. **Cieto BB, Valera GG, Soares GB, Cintra RHS, Vale FAC.** Dementia care in public health in Brazil and the world. *Dementia e Neuropsychologia*. 2014;**8**:40–6.
2. **Associação Brasileira de Alzheimer.** Available from: http://www.abraz.org.br [accessed 13 August 2018].
3. **Caovilla VP, Canineu PR.** *Voce não está sozinho. Nós continuamos com você.* São Paulo: Novo Seculo Editora; 2013.
4. **Ballard C, Gauthier S, Corbett A, Brayne C, Aarsland D, Jones E.** Alzheimer's disease. *The Lancet.* 2011;**377**:1019–31.
5. **World Health Organization**. *Dementia: a public health priority.* Geneva: World Health Organization; 2012. Available from: http://www.who.int/mental_health/publications/dementia_report_2012/en/ [accessed 13 August 2018].
6. **Wimo A, Prince M.** *World Alzheimer Report 2010: the global economic impact of dementia.* London: Alzheimer's Disease International; 2010. Available from: https://www.alz.co.uk/research/files/WorldAlzheimerReport2010.pdf [accessed 13 August 2018].

7. **Wimo A, Winblad B, Jonsson L.** The worldwide societal costs of dementia: estimates for 2009. *Alzheimer's and Dementia.* 2010;**6**:98–103.

8. **Castro DM, Dillon C, Machnicki G, Allegri RF.** The economic cost of Alzheimer's disease: family or public-health burden? *Dementia e Neuropsychologia.* 2010;**4**:262–7.

9. **Carias CM, Vieira FS, Giordano CV, Zucchi P.** Medicamentos de dispensação excepcional: histórico e gastos do Ministério da Saúde do Brasil. *Revista de Saúde Pública.* 2011;**45**:233–40.

10. **Camacho ACLF, Coelho MJ.** Políticas públicas para a saúde do idoso: revisão sistemática. *Revista Brasileira de Enfermagem.* 2010;**63**:279–84.

11. **Rosow K, Holzapfel A, Karlawish JH, Baumgart M, Bain LJ, Khachaturian AS.** Countrywide strategic plans on Alzheimer's disease: developing the framework for the international battle against Alzheimer's disease. *Alzheimer's and Dementia.* 2011;**7**:615–21.

12. **Scazufca M, Menezes PR, Vallada HP,** *et al.* High prevalence of dementia among older adults from poor socioeconomic backgrounds in São Paulo, Brazil. *International Psychogeriatrics.* 2008;**20**:394–405.

13. **Prince MJ.** The 10/66 dementia research group: 10 years on. *Indian Journal of Psychiatry.* 2009;**51**(Suppl 1):S8–15.

14. **Shinohara M, Sato N, Shimamura M,** *et al.* Possible modification of Alzheimer's disease by statins in midlife: interactions with genetic and non-genetic risk factors. *Frontiers in Aging Neuroscience.* 2014;**6**:71.

Chapter 44

Chile

Andrea Slachevsky and Jean Gajardo

Summary

Currently, it is estimated there are about 200,000 people living with dementia in Chile, and this number is projected to triple by 2020. Dementia has increasingly become an important condition for society, health, and social policy. Dementia care falls mostly under the family responsibility, with limited involvement from the health sector which is usually in terms of diagnosis in secondary healthcare. Chile is currently implementing its first National Plan for Dementia. Civil society and academic efforts over the last few years have helped to create a favourable setting that has paved the way for several milestones in dementia care in the country: a national awareness campaign, enhanced research, increased public funding for day care centres, and the development of a National Dementia Plan with a multisectoral approach to address the complex needs of people with dementia and their caregivers.

Facts on dementia in Chile

It is estimated that more than 200,000 people (1% of the total population) live with dementia in Chile, according to 2018 figures, with a projected increase to 600,000 people (3% of the population) by 2050 (see Fig. 44.1). There are no Chilean epidemiological studies on the prevalence and incidence of dementia. Therefore, data on dementia have mainly emerged from two national surveys that were not particularly designed to generate data on cognitive disorders: the National Survey of Dependency in the Elderly (NSDE) [1] and the National Survey of Health (NSH) [2].

The NSDE is a cross-sectional study conducted in 2008 and 2009, with a probabilistic sample of 4860 community-dwelling subjects aged 60 years and above. This study assessed dementia using a version of the MMSE and the Functional Activities Questionnaire (FAQ) validated for the Chilean population. The crude

prevalence of dementia in people aged 60 years and above was estimated to be
7.0% (women 7.7%, men 5.9%; $P = 0.15$). In both men and women, there was a
significant increase in prevalence with age ($P < 0.0001$), rising to 13% in those
aged 75–79 years and 36.2% in those aged 85 years and above. The prevalence of
dementia was also higher in rural contexts and in people with low educational
levels, reaching up to 25.2% in high illiteracy groups. The adjusted model for
dementia suggested no association with gender, but an independent positive
association with rural residence and age, as well as a negative association with
attained educational level [3] (see Fig. 44.2).

The NSH, which was conducted in 2009–2010, used the same criteria for dementia and reported a prevalence of 10.4% in people aged 60 years and above

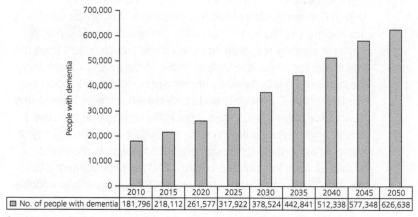

	2010	2015	2020	2025	2030	2035	2040	2045	2050
No. of people with dementia	181,796	218,112	261,577	317,922	378,524	442,841	512,338	577,348	626,638

Fig. 44.1 Predicted number of people with dementia for the next decades.

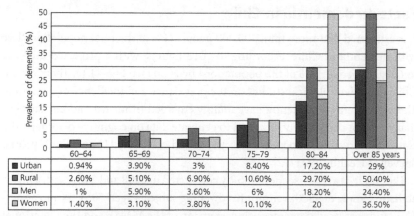

	60–64	65–69	70–74	75–79	80–84	Over 85 years
Urban	0.94%	3.90%	3%	8.40%	17.20%	29%
Rural	2.60%	5.10%	6.90%	10.60%	29.70%	50.40%
Men	1%	5.90%	3.60%	6%	18.20%	24.40%
Women	1.40%	3.10%	3.80%	10.10%	20	36.50%

Fig. 44.2 Prevalence of dementia by age group and gender in urban and rural areas.
Source data from the National Survey of Dependency in the Elderly.

(10.1% for men, 10.6% for women). The prevalence of dementia increased across age groups: 7.2% in those aged 60–69 years, 12.8% in those aged 70–79 years, and 20.9% in those aged 80 years and above. The prevalence of cognitive impairment was 5.6 times higher among adults with low educational levels (17.2%), compared to those with high educational levels (3%). This difference was statistically significant after adjusting for age and gender [1].

Dementia is also one of the most important determinants of disability in older people in Chile. From 1990 to 2010, the number of years lost due to disability as a result of dementia has increased by over 200% [4]. The number of deaths attributed to dementia has increased by 526%, making dementia as the cause of death with the highest increase in frequency during the last decade [5].

In Chile, care is mostly provided by families and relatives. In 2013, the CUIDEME study, which involved 292 family caregivers who lived in Santiago, the capital city of Chile, reported important findings regarding the negative impact of caregiving when a country lacks adequate support for caregivers. Among its findings, the study showed that 80% of family caregivers were women (spouses and daughters), of whom 63% experienced severe care burden and 47% reported psychiatric symptoms related to burden [6]. The average monthly cost of care per patient was US$943. Direct medical costs accounted for 21%, direct social costs 5%, and indirect costs 74% of the total cost. The average monthly cost was found to be inversely related to the socio-economic status (SES). The monthly cost of care was US$690 and US$1023 in high and low SES groups, respectively [7]. The high proportion of informal care reflected in the total cost of dementia is consistent with a lack of universal coverage of dementia, along with a lack of a unified public health response [8].

Moreover, it has been reported that the main unmet needs of people with dementia in Chile are related to a lack of information and education about the disease, inadequate counselling and support, and a lack of activities specifically designed for people with dementia. Thus, provision of support to people with dementia and caregivers is one of the most important interventions to address the needs of dementia patients who live at home [9].

Current actions to tackle the problem of dementia

Chile has a dual health system consisting of public and private insurance and service provision. The public component covers around 60% of the population. In 2005, Chile underwent an important health reform, called 'Explicit Guarantees System' [*Garantías Explícitas en Salud (GES)*]. The GES defines legally enforceable rights to explicit healthcare benefits for prioritized health conditions, which incrementally covered 56 conditions, representing 75% of the disease burden between 2005 and 2009. At present, 80 health conditions are included, but not dementia of any type [8].

The primary care health system in public settings has recognized the relevance of cognitive impairment and implemented a programme for the screening of cognitive and functional status. The 'Preventative Medicine Examination for the Elderly' [*Examen Anual de Medicina Preventiva del Adulto Mayor* (EMPAM)] seeks to identify people at risk of dependency for subsequent referral to various facilities for the promotion of physical and cognitive functioning. This programme is currently not covering more than 40% of the older population. A nurse or nurse assistant usually performs the examination. No information is available on the process of referral when dementia is suspected [3]. There is a scarcity of memory clinics in public hospitals where people can have access to a more comprehensive diagnostic process, including neuropsychological evaluation. Moreover, there are also important barriers to accessing evaluation at the secondary level such as waiting lists for evaluation by specialist consultations and assessments, mainly neuroimaging (brain CT and MRI scanning) and neuropsychological evaluation.

In the private healthcare system, there is no standardized assessment protocol. There have been specific efforts to standardize medical practices through the development of best practice or evidence-based guidelines for diagnosis and treatment, but these have not necessarily become a standard procedure for physicians nor a requirement for inclusion in undergraduate medical programmes [10, 11].

Therefore, without a particular dementia strategy, Chile has addressed the disease mainly at the healthcare level, focusing on diagnosis (usually performed in secondary healthcare centres) and interventions provided in facilities that indirectly support people with dementia and their caregivers (e.g. the National Programme for Depression in adults, Home Visits Programme for advanced dependency) [12]. The main resources derive from specific facilities in secondary healthcare centres that focus mainly on diagnosis but do not include non-pharmacological interventions that have proven to be a key element for positive outcomes in dementia treatment. Care is also influenced by the limited support given to people with dementia and their caregivers.

Similar to the global picture, a high proportion of people with dementia remain undiagnosed, and therefore without access to opportunities for support. NGOs have played a relevant role in trying to fill this gap in terms of lack of support, by providing psycho-social support (financed through private funding or by the users themselves).

The road so far: achievements and barriers

AD and other dementia types have progressively become a public health issue since the nineties. Efforts from different organizations have helped to raise awareness of dementia as a relevant health condition among the public. Among these, the NGO Professional Corporation of Alzheimer's and other dementias [*Corporación Profesional de Alzheimer y otras demencias* (COPRAD)], together with Alzheimer Corporation Chile (*Corporación Alzheimer Chile*) and other professional organizations, have conducted a public campaign to raise awareness of dementia, called '*No te olvido*' (I don't forget about you). This public campaign sought to gain the attention of different sectors, including relevant stakeholders, politicians, and the media. Scientific organizations, such as the Chilean Society of Neurology, Psychiatry, and Neurosurgery (SONEPSYN) and the Chilean Society of Geriatrics and Gerontology, have also played an important role, by promoting dementia as a subject of interest in academia, research, and public policymaking.

Parallel to these actions, in 2013, on the initiative of a multidisciplinary team of professionals, the National Service for the Elderly [*Servicio Nacional del Adulto Mayor* (SENAMA)] funded a project to design, implement, and evaluate the first adult day care centre to support people with dementia and their caregivers. This project, called 'Kintun', became part of a health policy in 2015, and currently new day care centres are being established across the country. Kintun[1] has become a national reference for evidence-based practice in dementia care in primary care settings, promoting the support of families and people with dementia through respite, education and training, home visits, and environment adaptation, as well as promoting awareness and dementia education in the community.

It is important to underline that the former President of Chile Michelle Bachelet's government incorporated two goals related to dementia in their programme for 2014–2018: (1) to formulate a National Dementia Plan and (2) to create support centres for people with dementia and their caregivers. In line with previous goals, in March 2015, the Chilean Government signed the agreement for Global Action against Dementia at the first World Health Organization Ministerial Conference on Dementia held in Geneva, Switzerland. This represented a milestone in Chile's campaign for dementia advocacy.

---

[1] Kintun is a concept from Mapuche (the native Chilean population) that translates into English roughly as 'to look at' or 'to search for', and represents the philosophy of a project that seeks to promote the participation and connection of people with dementia through person-centred and activity-based strategies.

In 2015, the Ministry of Health set up a panel of experts and various social agents, with the aim to build the foundations for a National Plan of Dementias (*Plan Nacional de Demencias*) [13]. The plan has been subject to public consultation, and was launched and its implementation started in 2017. This health policy was developed further to recommendations from the WHO, the Pan American Health Organization, and NGOs such as ADI. Moreover, the Ministry of Health has launched a new programme at the primary care level to promote healthy ageing, which intersects with dementia prevention in several components of the programme.

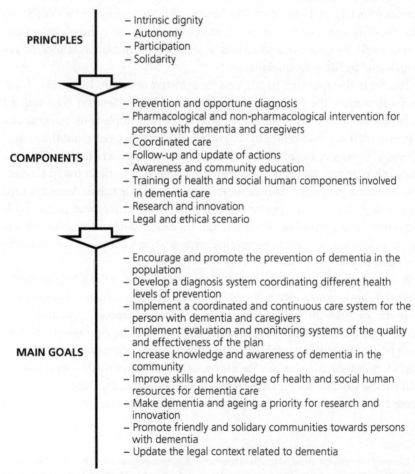

PRINCIPLES
- Intrinsic dignity
- Autonomy
- Participation
- Solidarity

COMPONENTS
- Prevention and opportune diagnosis
- Pharmacological and non-pharmacological intervention for persons with dementia and caregivers
- Coordinated care
- Follow-up and update of actions
- Awareness and community education
- Training of health and social human components involved in dementia care
- Research and innovation
- Legal and ethical scenario

MAIN GOALS
- Encourage and promote the prevention of dementia in the population
- Develop a diagnosis system coordinating different health levels of prevention
- Implement a coordinated and continuous care system for the person with dementia and caregivers
- Implement evaluation and monitoring systems of the quality and effectiveness of the plan
- Increase knowledge and awareness of dementia in the community
- Improve skills and knowledge of health and social human resources for dementia care
- Make dementia and ageing a priority for research and innovation
- Promote friendly and solidary communities towards persons with dementia
- Update the legal context related to dementia

Fig. 44.3 Principles, components, and main goals of the first version of the National Plan of Dementia for Chile.
Adapted from Ministry of Health, 2015.

Achievements and challenges

The implementation of a National Plan for Dementia, as a coordinated and multisectoral set of actions, is a key opportunity to address the challenges of AD and related cognitive disorders in Chile (see Fig. 44.3). The main components of the Plan include the development of facilities at different levels of complexity within the healthcare network, including memory clinics in secondary healthcare, a dementia programme in primary healthcare, community centers for dementia care, and a social support system [14]. The Plan also highlights the importance of prevention and training and education in dementia care for health and social professionals, as well as of promoting research, and the value of solidarity among generations. It also addresses the need for an updated jurisprudence that protects the legal rights of people with dementia as citizens. Implementation of the Plan, however, faces several challenges, such as the context of an outdated health system that has not met the needs of people with dementia and their caregivers in terms of complex and multidisciplinary actions [8]. In addition, budget constraints in the context of a global economic crisis, inadequate dementia training of health and social support teams [15], and stigma and false beliefs associated with age-related cognitive decline, leading to low rates of medical consultation, represent potential barriers to the success of a National Dementia Plan.

Against this background, Chile is an example of how civil society can succeed in raising awareness of dementia, while urgently calling for the development of a National Plan for Dementia. The next step would include advocacy of the inclusion of dementia in the Explicit Health Guarantees System (GES), so the diagnosis and treatment of dementia, as well as support for people with dementia and caregivers, are granted as health rights.

References

1. Gonzalez F, Massad C, Lavanderos F, *et al.* (2009). *Encuesta nacional de dependencia de las personas mayores 2009*. Retrieved from Santiago: http://www.senama.gob.cl/storage/docs/Dependencia-Personas-Mayores-2009.pdf [accessed 09 September 2018].
2. Ministerio de Salud. *Encuesta Nacional de Salud 2009–2010*. Santiago: Ministerio de Salud; 2010. Available from:http://www.minsal.cl/portal/url/item/bcb03d7bc28b64dfe040010165012d23.pdf [accessed 13 August 2018].
3. Custodio N, Wheelock A, Thumala D, Slachevsky A. Dementia in Latin America: epidemiological evidence and implications for public policy. *Front Aging Neurosci* 2017; **9**: 221.
4. Murray C.J, Vos T, Lozano R, *et al.* (2012). Disability-adjusted life years (DALYs) for 291 diseases and injuries in 21 regions, 1990-2010: a systematic analysis for the Global Burden of Disease Study 2010. *The Lancet*. 2012;**380**:2197–223.
5. Lozano R, Naghavi M, Foreman K, *et al.* (2012). Global and regional mortality from 235 causes of death for 20 age groups in 1990 and 2010: a systematic analysis for the Global Burden of Disease Study 2010. *The Lancet*. 2012;**380**:2095–128.

6. Slachevsky A, Budinich M, Miranda-Castillo C, *et al.* (2013). The CUIDEME Study: determinants of burden in chilean primary caregivers of patients with dementia. *Journal of Alzheimer's Disease.* 2013;**35**:297–306.

7. Hojman DA, Duarte F, Ruiz-Tagle J, Budnich M, Delgado C, Slachevsky A. The cost of dementia in an unequal country: The case of Chile. *PLoS One* 2017; **12**(3): e0172204.

8. Bossert TJ, Leisewitz T. Innovation and change in the Chilean health system. *New England Journal of Medicine.* 2016;**374**:1–5.

9. Tapia Muñoz T., Slachevsky A., León-Campos, M.O., Madrid Orrego M., Caqueo-Urízar A., Rohde G.C. & Miranda-Castillo C. (In press) Predictors of unmet needs in Chilean older people with dementia: a cross-sectional study. BMC Geriatrics.

10. Behrens M. *Guías clínicas de diagnóstico y tratamiento de las demencias.* Santiago: Ediciones Sociedad de Neurología, Neurocirugía y Psiquiatría; 2007.

11. Fuentes P, Donoso A, Slachevsky A. (2006). *Guías Clínicas de Trastornos Cognitivos y Demencias en el Adulto Mayor.* Ministerio de Salud, Gobierno de Chile, Santiago, Chile.

12. Slachevsky A, Arriagada P, Maturana J, Rojas R. *Enfermedad de Alzheimer y otras Demencias en Chile: propuesta de un Plan Nacional de Alzheimer y otras demencias.* 2012. Available from: http://www.coprad.cl/wp-content/uploads/2018/01/pasos_coprad_alzheimer_chile.pdf [accessed 09 September 2018].

13. *Plan Nacional de Demencias.* (2017). Retrieved from Santiago: http://www.minsal.cl/wp-content/uploads/2017/11/PLAN-DE-DEMENCIA.pdf [accessed 09 September 2018].

14. Gajardo, J., Aravena, J.M., Budinich, M., Larraín, A., Fuentes., P., y Gitlin, L. (2017). The Kintun program: From novel experiment to national policy (Innovative practice). *Dementia.* https://doi.org/10.1177/1471301217721863

15. Olavarría L, Mardones C, Delgado C, ., Slachevsky A. Chilean Health Professionals Perception of Knowledge about Dementia. *Rev Med Chil* 2016; **144**(10): 1365–8.

Chapter 45

Colombia

Jacqueline Arabia Buraye and María Cristina
Quijano Martínez

Summary
Dementia is among those diseases with an increased incidence in
older people, which, according to population projections, will have
an increasing impact in the coming years. Currently, it is estimated
that worldwide, 7% of people aged above 65 years, and 20–30%
of those aged above 80 years, present with cognitive impairment.
Colombia is not spared this reality. This chapter reviews the
prevalence of the disease, the current situation in the country, and
the challenges, as well as proposed management alternatives for
families, caregivers, and the community and clinical trial research
in families at genetic risk of developing hereditary early-onset
Alzheimer's disease.

Introduction

Since the second half of the last century, technological development and scientific progress have contributed to an increasing ageing population worldwide.
Data presented at the Second World Assembly on Ageing held in Madrid in
2002 were very significant in this regard—in the last 50 years, the average life
expectancy at birth has increased by 20 years, and it is anticipated that by 2050,
it will increase ten times more. In 2000, there were about 600 million people
aged over 60 years worldwide, and it is estimated that this population group will
increase to nearly 2 billion in the next 50 years [1].

In Colombia, the issue of ageing is so serious that the report *The Challenge
of Global Aging* has projected that, between 2010 and 2036, the proportion of
people aged over 65 years will increase from 6% to 15% of the total Colombian
population, a figure that took 69 and 115 years for the United States and France,
respectively, to reach. The impact of ageing is palpable. In 2013, according

to a Colombian statistical survey conducted by the National Administrative Department of Statistics [*Departamento Administrativo Nacional de Estadística* (DANE)] [2], there were 4,964,793 people aged above 60 years, representing 10.5% of the population, of which 650,000 were aged above 80 years.

The most recent study on this topic was conducted in Bogotá by the Administrative Department of Science, Technology, and Innovation (Colciencias)—the government agency that supports basic and applied research in Colombia—and Universidad Javeriana. The study authors [2] found that the main causes of death among people aged above 60 years were concentrated into five groups of diseases, which are, in increasing order of frequency: cardiac diseases, cerebrovascular diseases, respiratory tract diseases, hypertension, and diabetes mellitus (adult onset). These diseases are now considered as risk factors for developing dementia.

Now is the right time to say that most of the causes of dementia are preventable or modifiable in their outcome. For example, 72.9% of people aged above 75 years suffer from hypertension, which, to a large extent, has never been controlled. 'The main concern is that there is no difference in the causes of death related to dementia whether at a younger or more advanced age' [3].

Population ageing is already a reality in Colombia, and it is associated with social, economic, and health problems, for which the country is not prepared. 'Facing them—they insist—requires re-engineering all public policies in this regard' [3]. It is a huge social and political challenge that our country will have to address, in order to achieve a better quality of life for the population. It is a challenge that requires us to investigate the problems related to an ageing population, with a view to making changes in different areas—organization of the economic system, a more efficient health system, improving social health services, and training of qualified human resources, among others.

Regarding health problems of the elderly, one of the priorities concerns mental health. As it was formulated in 2002 by the United Nations in its *International Plan of Action on Aging*, in the section on the needs related to the mental health of the elderly, 'throughout the world, mental health issues are among the leading causes of disability and reduced quality of life' [1].

Dementia is among those diseases with an increased prevelance in older people, which, according to population projections, will have an increasing impact in the coming years. Currently, it is estimated that worldwide, 7% of people aged above 65 years, and 20–30% of those aged above 80 years, present with cognitive impairment [1].

The report submitted by ADI at the Summit Meeting in London (11 December 2013) showed the overall impact of dementia from 2013 to 2050, with an astonishing 17% increase in the number of people living with dementia, compared with the previous estimate given in ADI's *World Alzheimer Report 2009*. The 2013 report revealed that the number of people who suffered from dementia worldwide in 2013 was estimated to be 44 million and that it could reach 76 million by 2030 and 135 million by 2050. The report also predicted a change in the distribution of the global burden of dementia where, by 2050, 71% of people with dementia will come from low- and middle-income countries [1].

Latin America, Asia, and the Caribbean, which are affected by the greatest degree of economic inequality, will be particularly affected. The vast majority of countries in these regions struggle to implement a National Dementia Plan, while a few of those countries that do have a National Plan, such as Mexico and Peru, have not been able to develop their plans due to a lack of resources. Other Latin American countries, such as Colombia and Ecuador, do not know the national prevalence of dementia nor do they have epidemiological data or know the economic impact of Alzheimer's disease, the commonest type of dementia. These data need to be put in the context of the socio-economic burden that AD will have on these countries/continents [4].

In ADI's *World Alzheimer Report 2012*, it was estimated that the number of people with dementia totalled 40,000 in Bolivia, 256,000 in Colombia, 147,000 in Peru, and 1.33 million in Brazil. In Uruguay, the prevalence of dementia syndromes was reported to be 5 per thousand people among those aged over 40 years, 18 per thousand among those aged 70–79 years, and increasing to 87 per thousand in those aged over 80 years [5].

Now, what is dementia? Etymologically, the word 'dementia' comes from Latin, meaning 'deprived of intelligence' [6, 7]. Some authors have pointed out how, throughout history, this term has been used in medicine in different ways but has always been linked to the loss of reasoning. In general terms, it can argued that, for the biological/medical paradigm, dementia is 'a syndrome due to a brain disease, usually chronic or progressive in nature, in which there is a deficit of multiple higher cortical functions, including memory, thinking, comprehension, calculation, learning capacity, language, and judgment' [8].

Taking into account this definition, there are serious challenges for the Andean countries in terms of loss of functionality and autonomy, because there is a need not only for medical care, but also for long-term care, which includes support and advice for the family representing a high cost of care for dementia, and the need for a multidisciplinary and multi-sectorial approach to providing comprehensive care to affected patients and their families, which goes beyond the realm of health services, requiring a high level of coordination among all components of the society. In some countries of the region, reports have revealed a lack of knowledge about, as well as a lack of sensitivity to, the issue of dementia, with no existing clear answers from the various institutions involved in dementia.

Current situation of dementia in Colombia

Even though mental health problems represent 22% of the epidemiological burden, the area of mental health is allocated only 2% of public spending on health, which is generally intended for psychiatric hospitals. A review of mental health plans confirms that the policies and programmes do not include dementia beyond its mention. In addition, while the need for actions for detection of, and care for, dementia has become evident, low budget allocations and poor implementation of practice confirm the lack of prioritization of mental healthcare in almost all countries in the region. Consequently, it is estimated that mental health services are accessible to less than 1% of the population, with less than 10% of existing dementia cases detected and treated.

The problems in health systems related to dementia include:

1. A lack of models or guidelines for dementia care.
2. A lack of specialists in the field of dementia, which is a barrier to accessibility of specialist services to people with low income, the elderly, indigenous people living in rural areas, and those with mobility restrictions due to their disability.
3. High turnover of professionals and health workers in hospitals and healthcare centres in some municipalities, which hinders timely and appropriate patient monitoring.
4. A lack of institutions specialized in elderly care such as day care centres and homes for the elderly with cognitive impairment.
5. A scarcity of prevention programmes promoting active and healthy ageing for the elderly with disabilities.
6. Poor service continuity among the different levels of care, which hinders any proposed intervention.
7. A lack of knowledge and interest by the authorities and local leaders to support programmes for the elderly with cognitive impairment.

Alternatives for the management of dementia in Colombia

The Alzheimer Foundation is a non-profit organization founded in 1998 in Cali, Colombia. In 2015, this organization developed a multi-therapeutic care model for people with dementia [9], based on the framework of a holistic approach, including individualized, humane, dignified, and specialized care, which, from a gender perspective, succeeds in recognizing the specific needs of the population it serves. This model (see Fig. 45.1) shifts emphasis from traditionally focusing on the person with dementia to adopting a comprehensive interventional approach that takes into account the patient's emotional well-being, as well as their environment, including their family and surrounding community, thus helping to positively restructure the patient's quality of life .

The model intervenes in three key attention areas: (1) the person affected by dementia, (2) the family and/or caregivers, and (3) institutions involved in health education and the community, which have been encouraged to establish a network that allows more comprehensive disease management, not only for patients, but also benefiting their surrounding environment. Thus, the Alzheimer Foundation has achieved positive results—increased awareness of dementia among families, improved patient care, and enhanced detection and prevention of dementia in the community through education.

Care is provided to patients in both individual and group formats through cognitive, physical, and psycho-social therapies, tailored according to the severity of cognitive improvement. Some of the most important patient outcomes achieved include: the revival and maintenance of cognitive skills; greater connection with the environment; increased autonomy; maintenance of the recreational and social components to retain motivation; peer interaction; a heightened sense of belonging and participative attitude towards life; increased expression of feelings; emotional control; the ability to overcome feelings of

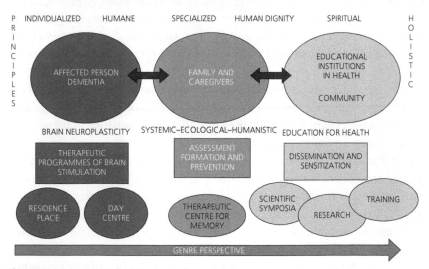

Fig. 45.1 Multi-therapeutic intervention model.

worthlessness, isolation, loneliness, and abandonment; and increased resilience to negative experiences to help them retain their sense of dignity and be recognized as human beings, regardless of their cognitive decline. Important outcomes achieved for families and caregivers include: acknowledgement of their caregiving status, network building for intra-family and social support, and redefining life projects. For the community, key achievements include: comprehensive training on the management of people with dementia, sensitization, and scientific updates on progress and advances in dementia.

Looking to the future of dementia care in Colombia, several initiatives are under way in dementia prevention. Thus, under Dr Francisco Lopera's lead, a clinical trial will be conducted on a family of 300 members, the largest group of individuals harbouring a rare genetic mutation that causes premature and hereditary AD, in which symptoms begin to appear at around the age of 45 years, i.e. much earlier than normal. The study, coordinated by the National Institutes of Health (NIH) in the United States, with the joint collaboration of the Banner Alzheimer's Institute in Arizona, the Genentech research centre (part of the pharmaceutical company Roche) in California, and the University of Antioquia in Colombia, will include the first test of a preventive drug for dementia in humans; it will study the effects of crenezumab in those 300 family members known to have a genetic risk of developing the disease but who have not yet shown symptoms. The mechanism of action of crenezumab involves the 'cleaning up' of beta-amyloid plaques that are formed in the brain of patients, which are believed to cause the progression of AD. In this 5-year study, 'sophisticated' tests will be carried out on the participants to evaluate if the drug could delay memory impairment, cognitive decline, or irreversible changes in the brain that occur during the course of the disease. As stated by Dr Lopera from the University of Antioquia: 'This trial represents a great hope for these people.'

In addition, studies in adult populations [10] are also in progress, aiming at developing scales adapted to the Colombian population, to be utilized as part of neuropsychological assessments for the detection of early-onset cognitive changes in the elderly. This would therefore allow early initiation of therapeutic interventions for cognitive impairment.

Other initiatives are aimed at increasing awareness of dementia and at dementia prevention, with the development of national sensitization and awareness campaigns to disseminate knowledge and education to the population. The Alzheimer Foundation annually runs community activities seeking to mobilize the relevant government authorities. Along with these initiatives, it is also planned for a national network of caregivers to be set up in Colombia, as well as a Caregivers School to educate families and improve the care of patients within their own environment.

While the future of dementia is still not clear, Colombia has made progress in raising awareness of the disease, and is making alliances to enable the nation to advance in dementia care.

References

1. **World Health Organization**. *Active ageing: a policy framework*. Geneva: World Health Organization; 2002.
2. **Department for National Statistics (DANE)**. *Census data 1954 to 2005 and projections 2006 to 2020*. Colombia: Department for National Statistics.
3. **Cano CA**. 'Old age: An issue for all ages', *Pesquisa Magazine*, Ageing Institute Universidad Javeriana, Bogota, 2016, https://www.javeriana.edu.co/pesquisa/tag/envejecimiento
4. **Pérez R**. *Salud. Mental health, dementia and public policy in Latin America from new and old paradigms*. Psicolibros Universitario, Montevideo, Uruguay. June 2017.
5. **Ketzoian C, Romero S, Dieguez E**, *et al*. Prevalence of demential syndromes in a population of Uruguay. Study of 'Villa del Cerro'. *Journal of Neurological Sciences*. 1997;**150**(Suppl 1):S155.
6. **Medina N**. 'The global impact of dementia', *A.L.M.A Annual Magazine*, Buenos Aires, 2014, News section, Vol 5, p. 9. www.alma-alzheimer.org.ar
7. **Manito MS, Funes HE**. Brief updates on dementia syndromic ALCLEMEON. *Argentina Journal of Clinical neuropsychiatry*. 2010;**16**:4.
8. **Kabanchik A**. Health and disease in later life, limits and psychopathological potential. and Full Member APSA XII Argentine Congress of Psychiatry Diversity and Integration. April 1996, San Miguel de Tucuminy.
9. **Gutiérez-Herrera RF**. *Alzheimer's in Iberoamerica*. Mexico: Universidad Autonoma de Nuevo Leon; 2018. pp. 227–244.
10. **Arango-Lasprilla JC, Olabarrieta Landa L, Rivera D**, *et al*. The current state of neuropsychology. In: Arango-Lasprilla JC, Rivera D (eds). *Neuropsycholology in Colombia: Regulatory data, current situation and future challenges*. Manizales, Colombia: Editorial Universidad Autónoma de Manizales; 2015. pp. 21–46.

Chapter 46

Peru

Víctor Carcelén and Waldo Cárdenas Berrocal

Summary

The Peruvian health system is highly influenced by the ageing of
the population. Public health spending as a percentage of the
gross domestic product is below the average for Latin America;
pocket spending is excessive, particularly for the purchase of drugs
and payment for diagnostic services. Infrastructure and human
resources are inadequate and unequally distributed across the
country, with significant disparities between regions. Although
Peru has a universal insurance scheme, its coverage remains low.
In addition, a high degree of institutional fragmentation persists,
which highlights the inequalities and inefficiencies that prevail
in the country. Each component of the health system operates
independently, serving different populations, with its own rules,
networks of suppliers, and therapeutic methods. Cognitive
impairment and dementia are closely linked with old age, and
their rising prevalence and increasing social impact are particularly
marked in developing countries. The prevalence of dementia
in adults aged over 65 years in Peru is 6.85%, with Alzheimer's
disease as the commonest type.

Population of Peru

If we consider that the life expectancy of a population is rising, it is necessary
to know the impact that degenerative diseases in the elderly population may
have on health systems, especially in the case of dementia as it is one of the
main public health problems. In developed countries, the crude prevalence of
dementia in people aged over 65 years is 6–9% [1, 2].

In Latin America, population-based studies are scarce; however, they have
served as a basis for establishing the prevalence of dementia, which ranges between 4.03% and 8.2% [3, 4, 5]. According to the National Institute of Statistics

and Informatics (INEI), the total population of Peru in 2015 was 31.15 million people, with almost equal gender composition, and there were 2,040,000 people aged 65 years or above, which represents 6.55% of the total population. It is estimated that by 2020, there will be about 3.7 million older adults in Peru, representing 11% of its population [6]. Peru has a high rate of migration from rural to urban areas, although this is mainly in the young population and very low among elderly people.

The prevalence of dementia in Peru is between 6.85% and 7.4%, of which AD is the commonest type. Age, female gender, and low educational level have been correlated with this high prevalence [7].

Structure of the health system of Peru

The Peruvian health system, as part of the Andean region, is highly influenced by the ageing of the population. In addition, public health spending as a percentage of the GDP is below the average for Latin America (see Fig. 46.1); pocket spending is excessive, particularly for the purchase of drugs and payment for diagnostic services.

Infrastructure and human resources in the health sector are inadequate and unequally distributed across the country, with significant disparities between regions, and access to services is also limited. Although Peru has a universal insurance scheme, its coverage remains low. In addition, a high degree of institutional fragmentation persists, which highlights the inequalities and inefficiencies that prevail in the country. In short, each component of the health

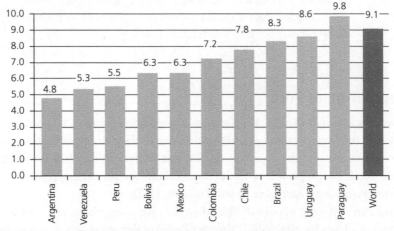

Fig. 46.1 Total expenditure on health as a percentage of the GDP (2014).
Source data from the World Bank. Available from: Gasto en salud, total (% del PIB) | Data.

system operates independently, with its own rules and provider networks, serving different populations.

The structure of the health system is highly varied and complex and still has a long way to go in the implementation of reforms to achieve the goals that are expected in the country. As shown in Fig. 46.2 [9], the health system consist of the Ministry of Public Health (MINSA) with its own directives, the Health Social Security (EsSalud), the Military Health System, and finally the private healthcare sector. Each has its own characteristics, diagnostic protocols, and therapeutic methods. There are several alternatives that have been presented to the government to address this complex health system. In addition, nearly three-quarters of the total population of Peru live in urban areas. The main challenge faced by the Peruvian health system is extension of care services to cover more than 10% of the population currently lacking access to basic healthcare [8].

It should be emphasized that, compared with other population groups, elderly people have a greater need for health services [6]. This is especially acute among those with cognitive impairment or dementia, in which case families are confronted with the need to place their loved ones in long-stay homes, which are not necessarily supervised nor do they necessarily meet legal requirements in terms of elderly care, including non-compliance with building safety

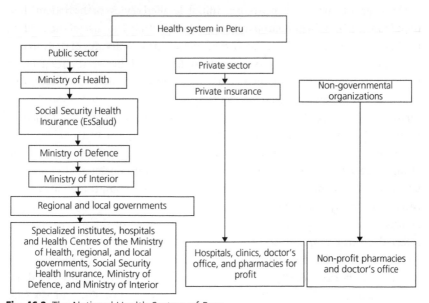

Fig. 46.2 The National Health System of Peru.

requirements (lifts, bathrooms, aisle sizes) and the availability of trained personnel for the care of the elderly.

Accurate data are lacking due to a number of long-term care homes that are not registered, but it is assumed that most older adults with dementia reside in such institutions. Also the healthcare needs of elderly people do not seem to be catered for by services provided by the health system, which often lack professional and technical personnel qualified to manage these patients.

Assessment and diagnosis

The Integrated Geriatric Assessment (IGA) is an important part of the comprehensive evaluation performed in elderly people at any healthcare level. In Peru, the MINSA has a programme called 'VACAM', which offers staff training in the use of diagnostic tools, including the MMSE [9], the clock drawing test—hands version (PDR-M) [10], and the Pfeffer Functional Activities Questionnaire (PFAQ) [11].

In EsSalud Comprehensive Geriatric Assessment (CGA), the Early Intervention Programme is used in outpatient services to identify all elderly patients. It should be mentioned that the elderly represent 8.29% of the country's population, of whom 33% are looked after by the Home Care Programme (PADOMI). Regarding health services provided by the Military Health System, the departments of geriatrics, psychiatry, and neurology are responsible for dementia diagnosis and patient monitoring.

The diagnostic process consists of an initial detailed review of the patient's history, followed by a short neuropsychological evaluation with use of the MMSE, the PDR-M test, and the PFAQ to assess functioning in activities of daily living. Thus, this will allow health professionals to distinguish between patients who suffer from some form of dementia and those going through normal ageing. Specialists in geriatric medicine, psychiatry, and neurology are responsible for further evaluating patients who have already been diagnosed with dementia, with use of blood tests and brain CT and MRI scanning, where available.

We analysed a group of patients diagnosed with dementia assigned to the Home Care Programme (PADOMI), all of whom are pensioners living in an urban area in the north of Lima. As part of their care plan, these patients received a monthly follow-up, as well as assessments conducted by various specialists as referred by their attending physician. Most of these patients were referred to hospital specialists with a diagnosis of dementia already established. As shown in Table 46.1, a total of 188 cases of dementia were identified, of which the majority (46.3%) had a diagnosis of probable AD, followed by those with a diagnosis of AD with cerebrovascular disease (14.9%) and vascular

Table 46.1 Types of dementia identified in 188 cases of dementia in a population of pensioners living in an urban area

Diagnostics	n	%
Probable Alzheimer's disease	87	46.3
Alzheimer's disease with cerebrovascular disease	28	14.9
Vascular dementia	15	8.0
Possible Alzheimer's disease	13	6.9
Dementia due to Parkinson's disease	8	4.3
Frontotemporal dementia	5	2.7
Lewy body dementia	4	2.1
Unclassified	28	14.9

dementia (8.0%)—all of which accounted for about 75% of all cases diagnosed with dementia.

References

1. **Kawas CH, Katzman R.** Epidemiology of dementia and Alzheimer's disease. In: **Terry RD, Katzman R, Bick KL, Sisodia SS** (eds). *Alzheimer's disease*, 2nd ed. Philadelphia: Lippincott Williams and Wilkins; 1999. pp. 95–116.

2. **Berr C, Wancata J, Ritchie K.** Prevalence of dementia in the elderly in Europe. *European Neuropsychopharmacology.* 2005;**15**:463–71.

3. **Ketzoian C, Rega I, Caseres R.** Estudio de prevalencia de las principales enfermedades neurológicas en una población del Uruguay. *La Prensa Médica Uruguaya.* 1997;**17**:9–26.

4. **Llibre JJ, Guerra MA, Perez-Cruz H,** *et al.* [Dementia syndrome and risk factors in adults older than 60 years old residing in Habana]. *Revista de Neurología.* 1999;**29**:908–11.

5. **Herrera E, Caramelli P, Barreiros AS, Nitrini R.** Epidemiologic survey of dementia in a community dwelling Brazilian population. *Alzheimer Disease and Associated Disorders.* 2002;**16**:103–8.

6. **Carcelén V.** [Epidemiology of aging and psycho sanitary and social implications of a mature population]. *Acta Médica Peruana.* 2005;**XXII**:118–19.

7. **Custodio N, García A, Montesinos R.** Dementia prevalence in a Lima, Peru urban community: door-to-door study. *Anales de la Facultad de Medicina.* 2008;**69**:233–8.

8. **Alcalde-Rabanal JE, Lazo-González O, Nigenda G.** [The health system of Peru]. *Salud Pública de México.* 2011;**53**(Suppl 2):s243–54.

9. **Folstein MF, Folstein SE, McHugh PR.** 'Mini-mental state': a practical method for grading the cognitive state of patients for the clinician. *Journal of Psychiatric Research.* 1975;**12**:189–98.

10. Manos P, Wu R. The ten-point clock test: a quick screen and grading method for cognitive impairment in medical and surgical patients. *International Journal of Psychiatry in Medicine*. 1994;**24**:229–44.

11. Pfeffer RI, Kurosaki TT, Harrah CH Jr, Chance JM, Filos S. Measurement of functional activities in older adults in the community. *Journal of Gerontology*. 1982;**37**:323–9.

Chapter 47

Uruguay

Robert Pérez Fernández and Rodolfo Ferrando

Summary

Uruguay has the oldest population in Latin America, with a prevalence rate of dementia similar to that in developed countries. With regard to dementia care, the key strengths of the National Health System include: equity in accessibility to diagnosis, specialized medical consultations, diagnosis made according to international standards, and the availability of anti-dementia drugs and pharmacological treatments. Its main weaknesses are delayed diagnosis, fragmented care, the use of only a curative model of care, a lack of interdisciplinary team approach, and a lack of non-pharmacological treatments, as well as a lack of communication of diagnoses to patients. In its current format, the health system does not fully guarantee the human rights of people with dementia and their families. Recent actions have been taken by the national association of relatives (AUDAS) and academic groups to address this situation through the presentation of a National Dementia Plan.

Context, prevalence, and cost of dementia in Uruguay

Uruguay, with 13.9% of its population aged 65 years or above, is the country with the oldest population in Latin America. Ageing is typical of an advanced stage of its demographic transition, similar to what occurs in developed countries [1]. Within the older population, the group of those aged 80 years and over is expected to have the highest growth rate, doubling in number by 2025. About 95% of older people live in urban areas, and almost 61% live alone or with an elderly couple [2].

This population profile leads to a higher prevalence of age-dependent diseases, compared to other countries in the region. While the country has no epidemiological studies to quantify precisely the situation, it is estimated that 54,000 people would be affected by dementia, equivalent to 11% of the population aged 65 years and over. It is also projected that this figure will increase by 107% by 2050 [3]. The cost of dementia in 2010 was estimated to be US$ 7787 per person with the disease [3]. This meant the country incurred a total cost of nearly US$421 million for the management of dementia, which represented slightly more than 1.05% of its 2010 GDP (estimated to be US$40,000 million).

Despite the impact of these figures on the country, the issue of dementia has not received the necessary attention from public policies, which, so far, have been almost non-existent and fragmented, generated from different institutions with little coordination.

The main institutions linked to dementia care

Among the main state actors linked to public policies on dementia is the Integrated National System of Health [Sistema Nacional Integrado de Salud (SNIS)], which covers medical care for the majority of older people in the country, through public and private health institutions. The SNIS is guided and supervised by the Ministry of Public Health [Ministerio de Salud Pública (MSP)]. Currently, there is a transition period due to a profound reform that seeks to change the model of care, from a curative model to one that focuses on promotion of health and disease prevention. This reform is currently under way, such that both models still coexist at present, mainly the traditional curative one.

The other relevant state institution is the Ministry of Social Development [Ministerio de Desarrolo Social (MIDES)], which has a National Institute of Older Persons [Instituto Nacional de las Personas Mayores (INMAYORES)] responsible for the management and coordination of public policies for the elderly. Since 2016, a new institutional framework has been introduced under the aegis of the MIDES—the Integrated National System of Care [Sistema Nacional Integrado de Cuidados (SNIC)], which is responsible for providing care for different vulnerable population groups, including dependent elderly people, among others. However, people with dementia have not been included in this system yet.

In the field of organized civil society, in 1991, the Uruguayan Association of Alzheimer and Similar Disorders [Asociación Uruguaya de Alzheimer y Similares (AUDAS)] was founded, which aims to promote and improve the quality of life of people with dementia, their caregivers and families, and the community. It is an active member within Alzheimer's Latin America and ADI. For several years now, AUDAS has been operating a day centre for people with dementia and also runs workshops on mental health promotion for family caregivers. In the field of academia, the current Interdisciplinary Center of Aging [*Centro Interdisciplinario de Envejecimiento* (CIEn)] at the University of the Republic, Uruguay (*Universidad de la República, Uruguay*) has, for several years, provided technical support to the work of AUDAS through teaching and internships for undergraduate and graduate students. Several interdisciplinary research projects have also been developed, including the study of psycho-social intervention strategies and their effects on the cognitive, psychological, and neurobiological domains [4], which represents a concrete attempt to promote scientific research in the area, which has so far been scarce and isolated. Also within the framework of collaboration between AUDAS and CIEn, and with the support of INMAYORES, a recent study has generated the country's first data regarding the situation of care of people with dementia [5–6].

The care of people with dementia in Uruguay

Because there is still no socio-medical approach to care in the country, the care available for people with dementia and their families focuses solely on the medical aspect of the disease, i.e. only on the patient's medical condition, thus leaving caregiving responsibilities to families, with little institutional support. This has the immediate effect of violation of human rights of those affected, who must deal with their disease from an individual perspective [6].

Regarding healthcare in Uruguay, the National Health System has some strengths, particularly in terms of its accessibility and equity, regardless of the place of residence, economic situation, or educational level (see Box 47.1).

However, the SNIS also presents some significant challenges in the provision of quality care to people with dementia and their families. In this regard, one of the

Box 47.1 Strengths of the SNIS in the care of people with dementia

♦ Equity in access to the diagnostic process, specialized medical consultations, and pharmacological treatments
♦ Diagnosis according to international standards
♦ Availability of anti-dementia drugs and psychotropic medications

main obstacles is at the theoretical and technical levels, as attention is currently focused exclusively from a biomedical perspective [6]. While the biomedical model is very important to diagnosis and pharmacological treatment, it is used in Uruguay as a sole and exclusive approach to care, overlooking other perspectives, which thus enhances the risk for iatrogenesis, because all attention is focused on the disease, and not the person, as some studies have reported [6–11].

One of the main weaknesses of the SNIS relates to the difficulties in making early diagnosis. From the first appearance of clinical symptoms to diagnosis, there is an average time interval of almost 3 years [35 ± 30.7 months, mean ± standard deviation (SD)] [6]. While these figures are similar to those of Australia [12] and the UK [13], unlike these two countries, in the case of Uruguay, the main reason for a delayed diagnosis is not due to a delay in families seeking medical help (as in developed countries), but rather due to delays between the first consultation and diagnosis within an inefficient health system (lack of protocols on dementia, difficulties and delays in finding dementia specialists, long waiting times for diagnostic tests, limited availability of diagnostic tests in some institutions, lack of information about the tests required for patients and doctors, etc.) [6]. The number of dementia specialists is limited in the country. Although there are well-trained cognitive neurologists, most clinical neurologists do not have enough training in the mental health area. This lack of training is even more critical among psychiatrists and psychologists who generally are not involved in dementia care. However, concrete work by university departments of geriatrics, psychiatry, and psychology is being done to improve this situation.

Regarding diagnostic tools, neuropsychological evaluation includes protocols validated for use in the country, which are generally available in most SNIS institutions, with a few exceptions. Structural (MRI) and functional (SPECT, PET) imaging facilities are also available in the country, although they are underutilized in general, due to problems with coverage, the tendency to medicate before reaching an accurate clinical diagnosis, and stigma associated with the disease.

In addition, another major obstacle to providing quality care is a lack of an interdisciplinary team approach for diagnosis and treatment. Care provision is highly fragmented, with each medical specialist acting individually when managing patients, with little coordination with other colleagues. This lack of team approach is clearly displayed in the diagnostic process and in the communication of the final diagnosis. Only 34% of patients are informed of their diagnosis (23% by the physician and 11% by relatives), leading to a violation of their human rights in most cases [6]. Making a diagnosis and communicating the diagnosis to the patient are the first steps in patient management and treatment. In the current situation, communicating a diagnosis takes place within the framework of a common consultation, conducted individually by health professionals who, although usually well-trained in the medical aspects of the disease, lack training on the psychological aspects, including how to communicate a diagnosis and its impact on patients, and who mostly also have a very negative view of the disease. In this context, the diagnosis focuses on the disease, and not the person, which thus introduces, in many cases, a mechanism of 'loss of personhood', as defined by Kitwood [7–8].

Another major weakness of the SNIS lies in treatment provision. Currently, the SNIS does not provide comprehensive treatments as recommended by the WHO [14]. With a lack of non-pharmacological interventions for dementia, the health system can only provide drug treatments. A negative consequence of this is that behavioural and psychological disorders can only be treated pharmacologically, because, despite their use as first-line treatment being discouraged, drugs are the only therapeutic option available in the country [6]. Moreover, acetylcholinesterase inhibitors are often prescribed indiscriminately, even when a diagnosis of AD is unclear or in other clinical situations where there is no proven benefit, leading to unnecessary costs and avoidable side effects. Prescription of psychiatric medications to control symptoms is often excessive and without proper follow-up.

Finally, a major weakness of the care system for dementia in Uruguay refers to a lack of control and influence of civil society on the quality of care. The lack of progress made by associations of families in raising awareness of care burden among family caregivers, as well as indifference from the government, means that the disease burden itself will remain as an isolated 'family' problem, rather than be considered as a public health problem.

Some challenges to improve the quality of care

Based on the strengths and weaknesses of the current care system, AUDAS has led the way in the development of a National Dementia Plan, which is expected to serve as guidance for the development of public policies to promote and protect the human rights of people with dementia and their families. The Plan was submitted to the authorities in 2016, with a view to being passed as law by the parliament. The preparation of this Plan, which took place over 20 months, involved different groups linked to dementia care, from civil society to academics.

The Plan includes actions to integrate treatments into a system of care, as well as the development of measures of prevention and destigmatization. The role of primary care and family physicians and the creation of interdisciplinary teams, for diagnosis and follow-up, are also highlighted in this Plan. Another key aspect of the Plan is the inclusion of psycho-social interventions, in addition to pharmacological treatments, into the care system that will integrate the SNIS, SNIC, and civil society, thus adopting a true socio-medical approach. At the same time, the Plan defines a series of indicators to evaluate its implementation, outcomes, and impact, while also promoting the role of research and knowledge dissemination to ensure continuous quality improvement.

Success in achieving improvement in the quality of care for people with dementia in the coming years in Uruguay will depend on the priority given to this Plan by the national authorities that so far has been postponed.

References

1. **Paredes M, Ciarniello M, Brunet M.** *Indicadores sociodemográficos de envejecimiento y vejez en Uruguay: una perspectiva comparada en el contexto de Latinoamérica.* Montevideo: Lucida Ediciones; 2010.

2. **Paredes M, Pérez R.** Personas mayores en Uruguay: configuraciones familiares, participación social y detección de dependencia. In: **Batthyány K, Berriel F, Carbajal M,** *et al.* (eds). *Las personas mayores ante el cuidado.* Montevideo: Instituto Nacional de las Personas Mayores; 2014. pp. 11–39.

3. **Alzheimer's Disease International, BUPA.** *La demencia en América: el coste y la prevalencia del Alzheimer y otros tipos de demencia.* 2013. Available from: https://www.alz.co.uk/sites/default/files/pdfs/dementia-in-the-americas-SPANISH.pdf [accessed 14 August 2018].

4. **Berriel F, Pérez R.** *Alzheimer y psicoterapia. Clínica e investigación.* Montevideo: Psicolibros; 2007.

5. **Pérez R.** Demoras, diagnósticos y tratamientos para las personas con demencia en el sistema de salud de Uruguay: un análisis de situación. In: **Batthyány K, Berriel F, Carbajal M,** *et al.* (eds). *Las personas mayores ante el cuidado.* Montevideo: Instituto Nacional de las Personas Mayores; 2014. pp. 95–130.

6. **Pérez R.** *Las dolencias de la mente. Prácticas de atención y cuidado de las personas con demencia en Uruguay.* Doctoral thesis. Remedios de Escalada: Universidad Nacional de Lanús; 2016.

7. **Kitwood T.** *Dementia reconsidered: the person comes first.* Buckinghan: Open University Press; 1997.

8. **Kitwood T.** Towards a theory of dementia care: the interpersonal process. *Ageing and Society.* 1993;**13**:51–67.

9. **Martorell-Poveda M, Paz C, Montes-Muñoz M, Jiménez-Herrera M, Burjalés-Martí M.** [Alzheimer: significance, sense and care from a transcultural perspective]. *Index de Enfermería.* 2010;**19**:106–10.

10. **Behuniak SM.** Toward a political model of dementia: power as compassionate care. *Journal of Aging Studies.* 2010;**4**:231–40.

11. **Innes A, Manthorpe J.** Developing theoretical understandings of dementia and their application to dementia care policy in the UK. *Dementia.* 2013;**12**:682–96.

12. **Speechly CM, Bridges-Webb C, Passmore E.** The pathway to dementia diagnosis. *Medical Journal of Australia.* 2008;**189**:487–9.

13. **Chrisp T, Thomas B, Goddard W, Owens A.** Dementia timeline: journeys, delays and decisions on the pathway to an early diagnosis. *Dementia.* 2011;**10**:555–70.

14. **World Health Organization, Alzheimer's Disease International.** *Dementia: a public health priority.* Geneva: World Health Organization; 2012.

Index

Note: Tables, figures, and boxes are indicated by an italic *t*, *f*, and *b* following the page number.